Modern Pharmaceutics for Cardiovascular Diseases

Modern Pharmaceutics for Cardiovascular Diseases

Editors

Ionut Tudorancea
Radu Iliescu

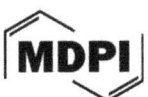

Basel • Beijing • Wuhan • Barcelona • Belgrade • Novi Sad • Cluj • Manchester

Editors

Ionut Tudorancea
Department of Physiology
Grigore T Popa University of
Medicine and Pharmacy
Iasi
Romania

Radu Iliescu
Department of Pharmacology
Grigore T Popa University of
Medicine and Pharmacy
Iasi
Romania

Editorial Office
MDPI
St. Alban-Anlage 66
4052 Basel, Switzerland

This is a reprint of articles from the Special Issue published online in the open access journal *Pharmaceutics* (ISSN 1999-4923) (available at: www.mdpi.com/journal/pharmaceutics/special_issues/mp_cardiovasculardiseases).

For citation purposes, cite each article independently as indicated on the article page online and as indicated below:

Lastname, A.A.; Lastname, B.B. Article Title. *Journal Name* **Year**, *Volume Number*, Page Range.

ISBN 978-3-0365-9980-9 (Hbk)
ISBN 978-3-0365-9979-3 (PDF)
doi.org/10.3390/books978-3-0365-9979-3

© 2024 by the authors. Articles in this book are Open Access and distributed under the Creative Commons Attribution (CC BY) license. The book as a whole is distributed by MDPI under the terms and conditions of the Creative Commons Attribution-NonCommercial-NoDerivs (CC BY-NC-ND) license.

Contents

About the Editors vii

Preface ix

Irene Paula Popa, Mihai Ștefan Cristian Haba, Minela Aida Mărănducă, Daniela Maria Tănase, Dragomir N. Șerban and Lăcrămioara Ionela Șerban et al.
Modern Approaches for the Treatment of Heart Failure: Recent Advances and Future Perspectives
Reprinted from: *Pharmaceutics* **2022**, *14*, 1964, doi:10.3390/pharmaceutics14091964 1

Alina Scridon and Alkora Ioana Balan
Targeting Myocardial Fibrosis—A Magic Pill in Cardiovascular Medicine?
Reprinted from: *Pharmaceutics* **2022**, *14*, 1599, doi:10.3390/pharmaceutics14081599 27

Ana Clara Aprotosoaie, Alexandru-Dan Costache and Irina-Iuliana Costache
Therapeutic Strategies and Chemoprevention of Atherosclerosis: What Do We Know and Where Do We Go?
Reprinted from: *Pharmaceutics* **2022**, *14*, 722, doi:10.3390/pharmaceutics14040722 52

Daniela Maria Tanase, Alina Georgiana Apostol, Claudia Florida Costea, Claudia Cristina Tarniceriu, Ionut Tudorancea and Minela Aida Maranduca et al.
Oxidative Stress in Arterial Hypertension (HTN): The Nuclear Factor Erythroid Factor 2-Related Factor 2 (Nrf2) Pathway, Implications and Future Perspectives
Reprinted from: *Pharmaceutics* **2022**, *14*, 534, doi:10.3390/pharmaceutics14030534 75

Lorena Pérez-Carrillo, Alana Aragón-Herrera, Isaac Giménez-Escamilla, Marta Delgado-Arija, María García-Manzanares and Laura Anido-Varela et al.
Cardiac Sodium/Hydrogen Exchanger (NHE11) as a Novel Potential Target for SGLT2i in Heart Failure: A Preliminary Study
Reprinted from: *Pharmaceutics* **2022**, *14*, 1996, doi:10.3390/pharmaceutics14101996 93

Dragan Copic, Martin Direder, Klaudia Schossleitner, Maria Laggner, Katharina Klas and Daniel Bormann et al.
Paracrine Factors of Stressed Peripheral Blood Mononuclear Cells Activate Proangiogenic and Anti-Proteolytic Processes in Whole Blood Cells and Protect the Endothelial Barrier
Reprinted from: *Pharmaceutics* **2022**, *14*, 1600, doi:10.3390/pharmaceutics14081600 103

Deborah M. Eaton, Thomas G. Martin, Michael Kasa, Natasa Djalinac, Senka Ljubojevic-Holzer and Dirk Von Lewinski et al.
HDAC Inhibition Regulates Cardiac Function by Increasing Myofilament Calcium Sensitivity and Decreasing Diastolic Tension
Reprinted from: *Pharmaceutics* **2022**, *14*, 1509, doi:10.3390/pharmaceutics14071509 123

Leticia González, Juan Francisco Bulnes, María Paz Orellana, Paula Muñoz Venturelli and Gonzalo Martínez Rodriguez
The Role of Colchicine in Atherosclerosis: From Bench to Bedside
Reprinted from: *Pharmaceutics* **2022**, *14*, 1395, doi:10.3390/pharmaceutics14071395 140

Jelena Vekic, Aleksandra Zeljkovic, Aleksandra Stefanovic, Natasa Bogavac-Stanojevic, Ioannis Ilias and José Silva-Nunes et al.
Novel Pharmaceutical and Nutraceutical-Based Approaches for Cardiovascular Diseases Prevention Targeting Atherogenic Small Dense LDL
Reprinted from: *Pharmaceutics* **2022**, *14*, 825, doi:10.3390/pharmaceutics14040825 162

Rocco Mollace, Micaela Gliozzi, Roberta Macrì, Annamaria Tavernese, Vincenzo Musolino and Cristina Carresi et al.
Efficacy and Safety of Novel Aspirin Formulations: A Randomized, Double-Blind, Placebo-Controlled Study
Reprinted from: *Pharmaceutics* **2022**, *14*, 187, doi:10.3390/pharmaceutics14010187 . . . . **179**

Minela Aida Maranduca, Daniela Maria Tanase, Cristian Tudor Cozma, Nicoleta Dima, Andreea Clim and Alin Constantin Pinzariu et al.
The Impact of Angiotensin-Converting Enzyme-2/Angiotensin 1-7 Axis in Establishing Severe COVID-19 Consequences
Reprinted from: *Pharmaceutics* **2022**, *14*, 1906, doi:10.3390/pharmaceutics14091906 . . . . **190**

About the Editors

Ionut Tudorancea

Ionut Tudorancea is the M.D. PhD Lecturer at Grigore T. Popa University of Medicine and Pharmacy, Department of Physiology.

My expertise is related but not limited to the following areas of cardiovascular systems: hypertension, blood pressure, cardiac arrhythmias, heart rate variability, heart failure, chronic heart failure;, cardiovascular physiology, electrocardiography, cardiac implantable devices, pharmacology and experimental medicine.

Radu Iliescu

Radu Iliescu MD, PhD, FAHA is a Professor at University of Medicine and Pharmacy "Gr. T. Popa" Iasi.

His experience covers: Twenty years of experience in cardiovascular and renal research; Published over 40 research papers and chapters in top peer-reviewed journals and books; Peer review for various medical journals, grant review study sections, committee member for national and international professional societies.

His goals are: develop basic and applied cardiovascular research in an integrated academic and pharmaceutical industry environment for targeted therapeutic approaches; develop novel education paradigms for the formation of basic and clinical scientists.

His interesting research fields include: integrative physiology; molecular biology and transgenic technology; mathematical modeling; medical devices; profiling therapeutic targets; and medical education.

Preface

Dear colleagues,

Observational studies have shown that cardiovascular diseases are the leading cause of mortality in the world, and it is estimated that disturbances such as ischemic heart disease and stroke account for approximately 80% of cardiovascular disease mortality. Although various non-pharmaceutical strategies addressed to the primary prevention of cardiovascular diseases such as tobacco control policies, reducing the consumption of harmful food, and increasing physical activity still represent a key strategy, they are often insufficient. Moreover, despite the availability of a plethora of pharmaceutic approaches specifically targeting mechanisms involved in cardiovascular diseases over recent years, the burden of these pathologies has only been marginally alleviated. Therefore, new pharmaceutical and non-pharmaceutical strategies are necessary for both primary and secondary prevention to reduce the burden of cardiovascular diseases.

It is well known that recent advances in pharmaceutics led to the development of new drugs for cardiovascular diseases, which are able to significantly improve the short- and long-term prognosis and to possibly prevent premature deaths. The present reprint brings together original and review articles aiming to highlight the advances in the development of modern pharmaceutics for cardiovascular diseases in recent years.

We would like to thank all the authors for their contributions and efforts that made this reprint possible.

Ionut Tudorancea and Radu Iliescu
Editors

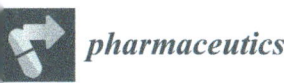

Review

Modern Approaches for the Treatment of Heart Failure: Recent Advances and Future Perspectives

Irene Paula Popa [1,†], Mihai Ștefan Cristian Haba [1,2,†], Minela Aida Mărănducă [3], Daniela Maria Tănase [2,4], Dragomir N. Șerban [3], Lăcrămioara Ionela Șerban [3], Radu Iliescu [5] and Ionuț Tudorancea [1,3,*]

1. Cardiology Clinic, "St. Spiridon" County Clinical Emergency Hospital, 700111 Iași, Romania
2. Department of Internal Medicine, "Grigore T. Popa" University of Medicine and Pharmacy, 700115 Iași, Romania
3. Department of Physiology, "Grigore T. Popa" University of Medicine and Pharmacy, 700115 Iași, Romania
4. Internal Medicine Clinic, "St. Spiridon" County Clinical Emergency Hospital, 700115 Iași, Romania
5. Department of Pharmacology, "Grigore T. Popa" University of Medicine and Pharmacy, 700115 Iași, Romania
* Correspondence: ionut.tudorancea@umfiasi.ro
† These authors contributed equally to this work.

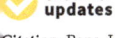

Abstract: Heart failure (HF) is a progressively deteriorating medical condition that significantly reduces both the patients' life expectancy and quality of life. Even though real progress was made in the past decades in the discovery of novel pharmacological treatments for HF, the prevention of premature deaths has only been marginally alleviated. Despite the availability of a plethora of pharmaceutical approaches, proper management of HF is still challenging. Thus, a myriad of experimental and clinical studies focusing on the discovery of new and provocative underlying mechanisms of HF physiopathology pave the way for the development of novel HF therapeutic approaches. Furthermore, recent technological advances made possible the development of various interventional techniques and device-based approaches for the treatment of HF. Since many of these modern approaches interfere with various well-known pathological mechanisms in HF, they have a real ability to complement and or increase the efficiency of existing medications and thus improve the prognosis and survival rate of HF patients. Their promising and encouraging results reported to date compel the extension of heart failure treatment beyond the classical view. The aim of this review was to summarize modern approaches, new perspectives, and future directions for the treatment of HF.

Keywords: heart failure; angiotensin receptor–neprilysin inhibitor; sodium-glucose co-transporter-2 inhibitors; soluble guanylate cyclase activator; cardiac myosin activation; autonomic modulation

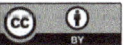

1. Introduction

Heart failure (HF) is a progressively deteriorating medical condition that is associated with a high risk of hospitalization and unscheduled hospital visits and significantly reduces the patients' life expectancy and quality of life [1]. Although epidemiological studies report that heart failure affects about 1 to 2% of the general adult population, the true prevalence of HF is likely closer to 4%, as it may be frequently undiagnosed or misdiagnosed, as in the case of heart failure with preserved ejection fraction (HFpEF). Thus, HF is a major public health issue, as well as a significant and ever-increasing socioeconomic burden [2]. The number of patients living with HF is continuously increasing due to a plethora of factors such as ageing population; improved survival following cardiac events such as myocardial infarction; and because of a rising incidence of comorbidities such as hypertension, atrial fibrillation, and type 2 diabetes [3].

Over the last 30 years, the medical management of HF has significantly progressed, thus leading to the amelioration of quality of life and outcomes, especially for patients with reduced left ventricular ejection fraction (HFrEF). The discovery of various pathological mechanisms has made this possible and it has led to a better comprehension of heart failure and thus to the development of novel and effective therapies. Despite recent advances in the pathophysiology of HF and the breakthroughs in the pharmacological and non-pharmacological management of chronic HF, the overall patients' prognosis remains poor. Thus, the research and discovery of new underlying mechanisms of HF physiopathology pave the way for the development of novel HF therapeutic approaches [4]. In this review, we aimed to summarize the current pharmacological and non-pharmacological strategies, and also we highlighted the new perspectives and future directions regarding HF treatment.

2. Pharmacological Therapies for Heart Failure

2.1. Pharmacological Therapies for HF: Angiotensin Receptor–Neprilysin Inhibitor (ARNI)

The autonomic nervous system, the renin–angiotensin–aldosterone system (RAAS), and the natriuretic peptide (NP) system play a pivotal role in the modulation of the mechanisms involved in the development and progression of HF [5]. It is well established that the RAAS overactivation in patients with HF leads to increased aldosterone levels and sympathetic tone, vasoconstriction, high levels of arterial blood pressure, and pathological cardiac remodelling [5]. NPs induce various beneficial effects such as natriuresis, vasodilation, antiproliferative properties, vascular remodeling, and a benefic modulation of RAAS. Therefore, growing evidence indicates a myriad of positive outcomes of NPs for the treatment of HF. Additionally, experimental studies have confirmed that neprilysin (a membrane-bound endopeptidase)-induced NP degradation will mitigate all the above-mentioned beneficial effects. Accordingly, the inhibition of neprilysin to increase the plasma concentration of NPs became a promising approach for the treatment of HF [6]. Unfortunately, the inhibition of the neprilysin alone resulted in elevated angiotensin II plasma levels, thus counteracting the vasodilatory effects of neprilysin [7]. To overcome this drawback, angiotensin receptor blockers were combined with neprilysin inhibitors, ushering in the notion of angiotensin receptor–neprilysin inhibitor (ARNI) [7].

Omapatrilat was the first drug developed for the inhibition of both ACE and neprilysin pathways, but the results from the OVERTURE (Omapatrilat Versus Enalapril Randomized Trial of Utility in Reducing Events) trial did not show superior benefits when compared to angiotensin-converting enzyme inhibitor (ACEi) alone in lowering heart failure hospitalization rate or mortality risk [7]. Due to an increased incidence of angioedema induced by omapatrilat reported by the OCTAVE (Omapatrilat Cardiovascular Treatment Assessment Versus Enalapril) study, further development of this medication was discontinued [8]. The PARADIGM-HF (Prospective Comparison of ARNI With ACEI to Determine Impact on Global Mortality and Morbidity in Heart Failure) trial showed promising results since the combination sacubitril–valsartan was superior to enalapril alone in decreasing the risk of death from cardiovascular causes, all-cause mortality, hospitalization for heart failure (HHF) and HF symptoms, and physical limitations [9].

At the time of enrollment, all patients in the PARADIGM-HF trial were hemodynamically stable and treated with an ACEi or angiotensin receptor blocker (ARB). The goal of the PIONEER-HF (Comparison of Sacubitril–Valsartan versus Enalapril on Effect on NT-proBNP in Patients Stabilized From an Acute Heart Failure Episode) study was to assess the safety and effectiveness of sacubitril–valsartan in comparison with enalapril in hospitalized patients with worsening HF, more than half of whom were not receiving neither an ACEi nor an ARB at the point of enrollment [10]. Surprisingly, the introduction of sacubitril–valsartan in the treatment of patients with HFrEF hospitalized for acute decompensated HF lowered N-terminal pro-B-type natriuretic peptide (NT-proBNP) levels more than enalapril alone. Moreover, the patients treated with sacubitril–valsartan showed comparable rates of worsening renal function, hyperkalemia, symptomatic hypotension, and angioedema when compared to those treated with enalapril [10]. The findings of the PIONEER-HF trial extended the indication of sacubitril–valsartan to patients hospitalized for acute decompensated HF, patients with newly diagnosed HF, and patients without previous conventional therapy with RAAS inhibitors [11]. Intriguingly, in the PARAGON-HF (Angiotensin–Neprilysin Inhibition in Heart Failure with Preserved Ejection Fraction) trial in which sacubitril–valsartan was compared to valsartan alone but in patients with HFpEF, the primary composite outcome of total HF and death from cardiovascular causes did not vary substantially between the two groups [12].

Taken together, all these data indicate that ARNI is a promising approach for the treatment of HF. Thus, in the American College of Cardiology Foundation (ACCF), American Heart Association (AHA), and Heart Failure Society of America (HFSA) guidelines, ARNI therapy became a class 1A recommendation, and it should be the primary renin–angiotensin modulator, whereas ACEi or ARB may be used if ARNI therapy is not possible [13]. Meanwhile, the latest European Society of Cardiology (ESC) guidelines give ARNI therapy a 1B recommendation class, indicating that it may be used as an alternative for ACEi in symptomatic HFrEF patients despite optimal medical therapy (OMT) to reduce the risk of HF hospitalization and death [14].

2.2. Pharmacological Therapies for HF: Sodium-Glucose Co-Transporter-2 Inhibitors (SGLT2i)

While sodium-glucose co-transporter-2 inhibitors (SGLT2i) were first developed as oral drugs to lower blood glucose by the inhibition of renal tubular sodium-glucose cotransporters, large randomized controlled studies have recently shown that SGLT2i improve cardiovascular outcomes independent of diabetes, along with reducing the risk of HF hospitalization, cardiovascular death, and all-cause mortality [15–18]. Although the mechanisms of action of SGLT2i to improve outcomes in HF are not fully understood, various hypotheses have been postulated, such as improvements in myocardial energetics and loading conditions, beneficial effects on endothelial function and inflammation, and a delay in the progression of kidney disease [19–21]. Taken together, these actions may explain the early and persistent improvements in filling pressures and ventricular remodeling, thus leading to the improvement of cardiovascular outcomes in HF patients [22–24].

In the EMPA-REG OUTCOME (Empagliflozin Cardiovascular Outcome Event Trial in Type 2 Diabetes Mellitus Patients–Removing Excess Glucose), the first trial that assessed the impact of SGLT2i on cardiovascular outcomes in patients with type 2 diabetes mellitus (T2DM), empagliflozin showed a lower rate of the primary composite outcome of cardiovascular death, and also a reduced incidence of any cause of mortality or HF hospitalization versus placebo [25]. Interestingly, the cardiovascular effects were independent of renal function and glucose levels [26]. In the CANVAS (Canagliflozin Cardiovascular Assessment Study) and CANVAS-R (Canagliflozin on Renal Endpoints in Adult Participants with Type 2 Diabetes Mellitus) trials, canagliflozin showed cardiovascular benefits since it had a lower risk of cardiovascular events and a significantly reduced exploratory endpoint of HF hospitalization [27]. In the DECLARE-TIMI 58 (Dapagliflozin Effect on Cardiovascular Events–Thrombolysis in Myocardial Infarction 58) interventional clinical trial, dapagliflozin was shown to be superior to the placebo in improving glycemic control, in reducing the relative risk of major adverse cardiac events by 16% among patients with prior myocardial infarction, and in lowering HF hospitalization and cardiovascular and all-cause mortality in patients with HFrEF [28]. The results of these three cardiovascular outcome trials (CVOT) have been confirmed by real-world studies, including CVD-REAL (Comparative Effectiveness of Cardiovascular Outcomes in New Users of SGLT-2 Inhibitors) and the ongoing EMPRISE (Empagliflozin Comparative Effectiveness and Safety Retrospective Study) [29,30].

The remarkable amount of data demonstrating the beneficial effects of SGLT2i has prompted more studies into their potential implications for cardiovascular events and mortality in broader cohorts, which are not confined to diabetes groups. On that account, an increasing number of studies, including two major randomized controlled trials, DAPA-HF (Effect of Dapagliflozin on the Incidence of Worsening Heart Failure or Cardiovascular Death in Patients with Chronic Heart Failure) and EMPEROR-Reduced (Empagliflozin Outcome Trial in Patients with Chronic Heart Failure with Reduced Ejection Fraction), examined the effects of SGLT2i in both diabetic and non-diabetic HF patients [31,32]. Almost 5000 patients with HF New York Heart Association (NYHA) class II to IV and an ejection fraction (EF) < 40% were included in the DAPA-HF trial [31]. The patients treated with SGLT2i versus the placebo group showed a significantly reduced risk of the primary composite outcome of worsening heart failure (hospitalization/urgent visit leading to intravenous therapy for HF) or death from cardiovascular causes [31]. Similar outcomes were also achieved with empagliflozin in the EMPEROR-Reduced trial [33]. Remarkably, in both of these clinical trials, SGLT2i had similar effects in patients with or without T2DM, suggesting that this class of medication has beneficial effects on HF, irrespective of its anti-diabetic actions [31–34]. Taken together, all these encouraging results from both experimental and clinical studies have led to the introduction of SGLT2i into the current clinical guidelines as a Class 1A recommendation for the treatment of HFrEF [35,36].

Approximately half of all HF patients suffer from HFpEF, and it is expected that this group of HF patients will increase due to a prolonged life expectancy and a growing prevalence of comorbidities (i.e., hypertension, diabetes, obesity) that are now recognized as direct contributors to HFpEF [37]. Unlike HFrEF, in which a plethora of drugs such as beta-blockers, RAAS inhibitors, or SGLT2i are available, in HFpEF, a lack of proven efficient therapy still exists. Thus, studies to determine if SGLT2i might be beneficial in patients with HFpEF were also conducted. The PRESERVED-HF (Dapagliflozin in PRESERVED Ejection Fraction Heart Failure) interventional clinical trial evaluated the hypothesis that dapagliflozin treatment would improve symptoms, physical limits, and exercise capacity in HFpEF patients [38]. Surprisingly, after 12 weeks of dapagliflozin treatment, a significant and consistent clinical improvement was achieved across all predefined subgroups, including patients with and without T2DM and those with EF above and below 60% [38]. The primary outcome of the DELIVER (Dapagliflozin Evaluation to Improve the Lives of Patients with Preserved Ejection Fraction Heart Failure) interventional trial was to assess whether dapagliflozin would reduce cardiovascular death, HF hospitalization, or urgent HF visits in patients with HF and a left ventricular ejection fraction (LVEF) > 40%. Moreover, in the DELIVER trial, patients with HF with improved LVEF, regardless of care setting (including during hospitalization), were also enrolled [39]. Dapagliflozin led to a statistically significant reduction in the primary composite endpoint of worsening heart failure or cardiovascular death, without a remarkable difference in benefit for patients with an LVEF of $\geq$60% or less than 60%, or in other subgroups. Furthermore, dapagliflozin resulted in a substantial decrease in the overall number of worsening heart failure events and cardiovascular mortality. The occurrence of adverse effects was comparable to that of the placebo group [39]. Since the AHA, ACCEF, and HFSA's current guidelines classified SGLT2i as class IIA, level B, for the management of HF with mildly reduced or preserved LVEF [13], the findings reported by the DELIVER study may extend clinical practice guidelines for dapagliflozin usage in HFpEF patients.

Empagliflozin is also a successful approach for HFpEF with LVEF $\leq$65% since it was able to decrease HF hospitalization and significantly improve Health-Related Quality of Life (HRQOL), as shown in the EMPEROR-Preserved (Empagliflozin Outcome Trial in Patients with Chronic Heart Failure with Preserved Ejection Fraction) trial [40–42].

In the SOLOIST-WHF (Effect of Sotagliflozin on Cardiovascular Events in Patients with Type 2 Diabetes Post Worsening Heart Failure) clinical trial, sotagliflozin, a dual SGLT1/SGLT2 antagonist, substantially reduced the incidence of fatal cardiovascular events, hospitalizations, and urgent visits for HF among diabetic patients with worsening HF compared to placebo [18]. The increased incidence of primary endpoint events at 90 days following randomization among placebo-treated patients highlighted that early treatment initiation provides a significant potential to enhance outcomes [18]. The SOLOIST-WHF trial was also designed to assess whether the advantages of SGLT2 inhibition apply to patients with HFpEF, but concise results were difficult to obtain due to the small sample size of this subgroup and early completion date [18]. In major clinical trials, including CREDENCE (Evaluation of the Effects of Canagliflozin on Renal and Cardiovascular Outcomes in Participants with Diabetic Nephropathy) and DAPA-CKD (A Study to Evaluate the Effect of Dapagliflozin on Renal Outcomes and Cardiovascular Mortality in Patients With Chronic

Kidney Disease), SGLT2i also showed significant benefits on renal and cardiovascular outcomes in patients with or without type 2 diabetes [43,44]. The ongoing trial EMPA-KIDNEY (The Study of Heart and Kidney Protection with Empagliflozin), with results expected in 2022, assesses the efficacy of empagliflozin in reducing the progression of kidney disease or cardiovascular death in patients with chronic kidney disease [45].

2.3. Pharmacological Therapies for HF: Soluble Guanylate Cyclase Activator-Vericiguat

The nitric-oxide-soluble guanylate cyclase (NO-sGC) pathway is altered in decompensated HF due to a reduced NO bioavailability and a shift in the redox state of sGC, which renders it insensitive to NO. Therefore, restoring NO-sGC-cGMP (cyclic guanosine monophosphate) signaling should have the potential to alleviate the HF burden [46,47]. Vericiguat, a new oral sGC stimulator, targets the cGMP pathway by directly activating sGC via a binding site independent of NO. Moreover, by stabilizing NO bound to its site [48], vericiguat administration results in decreased inflammation, fibrosis, and hypertrophy [49].

On the contrary, sGC activators, such as cinaciguat, operate exclusively on abnormal sGC, irrespectively of endogenous NO. In patients with HF, cinaciguat significantly decreased the pulmonary capillary wedge pressure (PCWP) at 8 h, but also increased the incidence of arterial hypotension, which determined the early withdrawal of this trial. Due to its distinctive pharmacokinetic and pharmacodynamic characteristics, vericiguat has a minor impact on arterial blood pressure values when compared with other medications of this class, reducing systolic blood pressure by almost 2 mmHg on average [50–52]. In trials comparing vericiguat to placebo, anemia and symptomatic hypotension occurred more often with vericiguat than with placebo [50]. In comparison to other sGC stimulators, such as riociguat, which failed to meet the primary endpoint in phase 2 LEPHT (Riociguat in Patients with Pulmonary Hypertension Associated with Left Ventricular Systolic Dysfunction) interventional clinical trial, modifications to the chemical composition of vericiguat have led to increased pharmacokinetic stability, superior oral bioavailability, and a prolonged half-life, allowing for once-daily oral intake [49,53].

SOCRATES-REDUCED (Phase IIb Safety and Efficacy Study of Four Dose Regimens of Vericiguat in Patients with Heart Failure with Reduced Ejection Fraction Suffering From Worsening Chronic Heart Failure) and VICTORIA (Vericiguat in Participants with Heart Failure with Reduced Ejection Fraction) are the two clinical trials that assessed the safety and effectiveness of vericiguat in HFrEF patients [50,52]. In the SOCRATES-REDUCED trial, changes in NT-proBNP levels after 12 weeks did not vary considerably between the vericiguat and placebo arms, but patients in the vericiguat group had better improvement of the LVEF [52]. The VICTORIA trial proved the effectiveness and safety of vericiguat in patients with HFrEF, with clear benefits in cardiovascular death and HF hospitalization. The patients from VICTORIA were at a higher risk than those enrolled in previous clinical HFrEF trials, as indicated by higher median NT-proBNP values (2816 pg/mL vs. 1608 pg/mL in PARADIGM-HF) as well as patients with NYHA class III or IV symptoms (40% vs. 25% in PARADIGM-HF) [9,50]. On the basis of the results of the VICTORIA study, the 2021 European Society of Cardiology (ESC) HF guidelines recommend that vericiguat may be considered in symptomatic HFrEF patients whose HF has deteriorated even with guideline-directed medical therapy (GDMT) to lower the risk of cardiovascular mortality or HF hospitalization (Class IIb; Evidence Level: B) [14].

In the VITALITY-HFpEF (Outcomes in Vericiguat-treated Patients with HFpEF) trial, the vericiguat alongside standard of care in HFpEF patients did not increase the quality of life assessed by the Kansas City Cardiomyopathy Questionnaire (KCCQ) score [54]. This may be consistent with the hypothesis that NO insufficiency is not the main condition in the development of HFpEF, as opposed to HFrEF [55].

Patients with a recent worsening HF episode and a baseline NT-proBNP value $\geq$ 8000 pg/mL appear to benefit the most from vericiguat [56]. The newly established benefit and safety of vericiguat in individuals with high-risk HF may encourage the supposition of a quintuple therapy by introducing vericiguat as a novel treatment approach for the treatment of HFrEF, alongside ACEi/ARB/ARNI, beta-blockers, MRA, and SGLTi [57]. In future medical practice, the optimal time, titrating approach, and pharmacological sequencing have yet to be determined.

2.4. Pharmacological Therapies for HF: Cardiac Myosin Activation—Omecamtiv Mecarbil

Various drugs that increase cardiovascular outcomes have been identified in patients with HFrEF, but none of them addresses the main drawback of HFrEF, which is impaired systolic function, subsequent decreased cardiac output (CO), and augmented filling pressures [58]. In addition, systolic dysfunction is frequently associated with low levels of arterial blood pressure, which makes it more difficult for patients to tolerate target dosages of GDMT [59]. To maintain optimal CO in HFrEF, present targeted therapies counteract the deleterious implications of hemodynamic and neurohormonal compensatory responses. Beta-adrenergic receptor blockers, ACEI, ARB, ARNi, MRA, hydralazine, and nitrates are evidence-based therapies that improve mortality, whereas ivabradine and digoxin provide benefits for morbidity with no significant improvements in mortality [60]. Those medications that reduce mortality also frequently enhance LVEF and decrease left ventricular end-diastolic volume (LVEDV) and left ventricular end-systolic volume (LVESV), while the majority of drugs that have no effect on mortality fail to improve LVEF [61]. Medications that improve or restore ventricular contractility by targeting underlying mechanisms of the pathophysiology of HFrEF are theoretically promising for both the acute and chronic therapy of HFrEF.

Myosin uses chemical energy to generate force for cardiac myocyte contraction, an activity which is modulated by intracellular calcium levels and regulated by several upstream signaling cascades [62]. Cardiac myosin activators are a novel class of myotropes that improve myocardial function by directly enhancing cardiac sarcomere function [63]. Although several medications have been developed to improve inotropy [64], omecamtiv mecarbil, a cardiac myosin activator, is the first one that enhances systolic function by preferentially enabling the actin–myosin interaction. Thus, omecamtiv mecarbil has the ability to increase the contractile force without any influence on cardiomyocyte calcium handling [62] and without direct impact on vascular, electrophysiological, or neurohormonal processes.

In the COSMIC-HF (Chronic Oral Study of Myosin Activation to Increase Contractility in Heart Failure) interventional clinical trial, 544 patients with HFrEF treated with omecamtiv mecarbil showed an improved left ventricular systolic function, as assessed by a rise in systolic ejection time and EF. Moreover, an improvement in the myocardial strain was also reported, while left ventricular both systolic and diastolic volumes, NT-proBNP, and heart rate (HR) decreased [65,66]. The first trial to demonstrate that selective enhancement of cardiac contractility improves cardiovascular outcomes in patients with HFrEF was GALACTIC-HF (Omecamtiv Mecarbil to Treat Chronic Heart Failure with Reduced Ejection Fraction) [58,67,68]. In this randomized, double-blind, placebo-controlled trial, patients who received omecamtiv mecarbil had a lower incidence of the composite primary outcome of an HF event or death from cardiovascular causes than those in the placebo arm [58]. Patients with an EF below the median ($\leq$28%) showed superior benefits, with a 16% reduction in the primary endpoint [59]. The premise that patients with higher systolic dysfunction would benefit the most from this therapy is plausible and supported by the mechanism of action of omecamtiv mecarbil. Interestingly, omecamtiv mecarbil showed no adverse effect on blood pressure values, heart rate, potassium homeostasis, or renal function. The slight decrease in HR was attributed to sympathetic withdrawal [59]. Although omecamtiv mecarbil treatment showed positive results on primary outcomes, this study failed to demonstrate any improvements in secondary outcomes such as the time to cardiovascular death, change in Kansas City Cardiomyopathy Questionnaire Total Symptom Score (KCCQ-TSS), time to first HF hospitalization, and time to all-cause death [58].

2.5. Pharmacological Therapies for HF: Amino Acid Orexigenic Peptide Hormone—Ghrelin

Ghrelin, first discovered in 1999, is a 28-amino acid growth hormone (GH)-releasing peptide, produced mostly by X/A-like cells of the stomach and, to a lesser degree, by the heart and other organs [69,70]. Several research and observational studies suggest that ghrelin presents a myriad of cardioprotective effects through its ability to enhance cardiac contractility; to limit ischemia/reperfusion injury, cardiac cachexia, cardiac hypertrophy, and fibrosis; to lower blood pressure by the inhibition of the sympathetic nervous system; and to ameliorate the prognosis of both myocardial infarction (MI) and HF [71–73]. By increasing NO levels and rectifying the endothelin-1/nitric oxide imbalance, ghrelin also has a pivotal role in endothelial function by inducing anti-oxidant, anti-inflammatory, and anti-apoptotic effects [74]. Although several experimental studies have documented the cardiovascular effects of ghrelin, relatively few human clinical trials have been published to date. A low dosage infusion of ghrelin for 60 min in 12 HF patients raised the mean arterial pressure and cardiac and stroke volume index without affecting the heart rate [75]. In another study including 10 patients with congestive HF, intravenous ghrelin administration for three weeks showed substantial improvement of the LVEF and a reduction in LVESV [76]. Furthermore, it improved systolic function and exercise capacity, as measured by a rise in peak workload and peak oxygen consumption during intense activity [76].

These significant and valuable cardiac effects, together with vascular protection, suggest that ghrelin is a promising candidate for the treatment of congestive heart failure and should be further investigated [74]. Synthetic ghrelin that replicates the actions of endogenous ghrelin is widely used for the treatment of metabolic conditions and obesity. However, this peptide may also function as a GH-independent mechanism in cardiomyocytes, a fact that has generally been disregarded by scientists until now [74]. Therefore, additional research is recommended to employ ghrelin as a viable heart failure treatment [77]. All the pharmacological approaches are summarized in Table 1.

Table 1. Pharmacological therapies in HF.

Drug Class		Clinical Trial/Study	Main Findings	Ongoing Trials
Dual angiotensin receptor and neprilysin inhibitors (ARNI)	Omapatrilat	OVERTURE	→not superior to an angiotensin-converting enzyme (ACE) inhibitor alone in lowering the rate of heart failure (HF) hospitalization or mortality risk [7]	1. PARAGLIDE-HF (NCT03988634) will assess the effects of sacubitril/valsartan vs. valsartan monotherapy on NT-proBNP levels, clinical outcomes, safety, and tolerability in HFpEF patients admitted for acute decompensated HF. 2. NCT04587947 will assess the effect of sacubitril/valsartan on the autonomic cardiac nerve system by monitoring HRV in HF patients. 3. TurkuPET (NCT0330042 7) will assess the effects of six weeks of sacubitril/valsartan versus valsartan on cardiac oxygen consumption and cardiac work efficiency in patients with NYHA class II and III HFrEF. 4. NCT04688294 will assess the effects of sacubitril/valsartan in the treatment of congestive HF patients, as well as the drug's adverse effects by monitoring renal function and serum electrolytes. 5. ARNICH (NCT05089539) will assess the effects of ARNI on cardiac fibrosis in HFpEF patients. 6. NCT03928158 will assess the effects of sacubitril/valsartan vs. valsartan treatments in patients with advanced LV hypertrophy and HFpEF. 7. PARABLE (NCT04687111) will assess the hypothesis that sacubitril/valsartan might improve left atrial structure and function as well as left ventricular structure and function in asymptomatic HFpEF patients. 8. ENVAD-HF (NCT04103554) will assess sacubitril/valsartan in advanced HF and left ventricular assist device recipients.
		OCTAVE	→omapatrilat group was more likely to reach blood pressure target; →increased incidence of angioedema [8]	
	Sacubitril/valsartan	PARADIGM-HF (NCT01035255)	→superior to enalapril in reducing the risks of death and heart failure hospitalization (HHF); →decreased the symptoms and physical limitations of HF; →lower incidence of renal function impairment, hyperpotassemia in sacubitril/valsartan group [9]	
		PIONEER-HF (NCT02554890)	→in acute decompensated heart failure with reduced ejection fraction (HFrEF), a greater reduction in the N-terminal pro B-type natriuretic peptide (NT-proBNP) concentration was obtained with sacubitril–valsartan than with enalapril [10]	
		PARAGON-HF (NCT01920711)	→no significant benefit in patients with HF and preserved ejection fraction (HFpEF) regarding total hospitalizations for HF and death from cardiovascular causes [12]	

Table 1. Cont.

Drug Class		Clinical Trial/Study	Main Findings	Ongoing Trials
Sodium-glucose co-transporter-2 inhibitors (SGLT2i)	Canagliflozin	CANVAS (NCT01032629 and CANVAS-R (NCT01989754)	→ in patients with type 2 diabetes (T2D) and an elevated risk of cardiovascular disease, canagliflozin treatment was associated with a lower rate of cardiovascular events; → possible benefit of canagliflozin in preventing the progression of albuminuria [16]	1. NCT05364190 will assess the efficacy and safety of the early initiation of canagliflozin treatment in hospitalized heart failure patients with volume overload (warm-wet) who require the use of an I.V loop diuretic during the hospitalization period.
		CREDENCE (NCT02065791)	→ in patients with T2D and kidney disease, canagliflozin treatment showed a lower risk of kidney failure and cardiovascular events [16]	
	Dapagliflozin	DECLARE-TIMI58 (NCT01730534)	→ in patients with T2D at risk for atherosclerotic cardiovascular disease, dapagliflozin treatment was associated with a lower rate of cardiovascular death or HHF [17]	1. DAPA-RESPONSE-AHF (NCT05406505) will assess the effect of dapagliflozin in patients with acute heart failure.
		DAPA-HF (NCT03036124)	→ in patients with HF, dapagliflozin was superior to placebo at preventing cardiovascular deaths and heart failure events, irrespective of the presence or absence of diabetes [19]	NCT05346653 will assess the effects of SGLT2i in acute decompensated heart failure.
		PRESERVED-HF (NCT03030235)	→ 12 weeks of dapagliflozin treatment significantly improved symptoms, physical limitations, and exercise function in HF with preserved ejection fraction (HFpEF) patients [38]	NCT05278962 will assess the outcomes of SGLT2i in HF patients with left ventricular assist devices.
		DELIVER (NCT03619213)	→ trial completed with results regarding the efficacy and safety of dapagliflozin in HFpEF patients available later in 2022 [39]	ICARD (NCT05420285) will assess the cardiometabolic mechanistic effects on the myocardium of dapagliflozin in HFrEF patients.
	Empagliflozin	EMPA-REG OUTCOME (NCT01131676)	→ superior to placebo in reducing cardiovascular events, including cardiovascular death, all-cause mortality, and HHF [15]	
		EMPEROR-Reduced (NCT03057977)	→ superior to placebo in improving HF outcomes (cardiovascular death or HHF) [32]	1. DRIP-AHF-1 (NCT05305495) will assess the effect of empagliflozin in acute heart failure. 2. NCT05139472 assesses the impact of empagliflozin on functional capacity in HFpEF.
		EMPEROR-Preserved (NCT03057951)	→ reduced the combined risk of cardiovascular death or HHF in HFpEF patients [40]	
		EMPA-CKD (NCT03594110)	→ ongoing trial; it assesses the effect of empagliflozin on kidney disease progression or cardiovascular death versus placebo	
	Sotagliflozin	SOLOIST-WHF (NCT03521934)	→ a significantly lower total number of deaths from cardiovascular causes and hospitalizations and urgent visits for HF than placebo [18]	
Soluble guanylate cyclase activator (sGC)	Vericiguat	SOCRATES-REDUCED (NCT01951625)	→ in patients with worsening chronic HF and reduced left ventricular ejection fraction (LVEF), no statistically significant effects on NT-proBNP levels at 12 weeks was observed in the vericiguat group [52]	1. VICTOR (NCT05093933) will assess the efficacy and safety of vericiguat in HFrEF patients, specifically those with symptomatic chronic HFrEF who have not had a recent hospitalization for heart failure or need for outpatient intravenous (IV) diuretics.
		VICTORIA (NCT02861534)	→ a lower incidence of death from cardiovascular causes or HHF in patients receiving vericiguat [50]	
		VITALITY-HFpEF (NCT03547583)	→ no improvement in the quality of life (QoL) at 24 weeks in HFpEF patients receiving vericiguat [54]	
Cardiac myosin activators	Omecamtiv mecarbil	COSMIC-HF (NCT01786512)	→ improvement of systolic ejection time, stroke volume, left ventricular end-diastolic diameter, heart rate, and NT-proBNP in the pharmacokinetic-titration group [65]	
		GALACTIC-HF (NCT02929329)	→ a lower incidence of the primary composite of an HF event or death from cardiovascular causes in the omecamtiv mecarbil group than placebo [59]	

Even though real progress has been made in the past decades in the discovery of novel pharmacological treatments for HF, the prevention of premature deaths has only been marginally alleviated. Despite the availability of a plethora of pharmaceutical approaches, proper management of HF is still challenging. Thus, further research, experimental, and clinical studies focusing on the discovery of novel drugs targeting new pathological mechanisms involved in HF are still mandatory.

Recent technological advances have made possible the development of various interventional techniques and device-based approaches for the treatment of cardiovascular diseases. In the following paragraphs, we aimed to summarize the advances made in the development of such procedures and device-based therapies for HF (other than cardiac resynchronization therapy), since these approaches complement and increase the efficiency of the classical drug-based treatments. Moreover, since many of these modern approaches interfere with various well-known described pathological mechanisms in HF, they have a real capability to increase the efficiency of existing medications and improve the prognosis and survival rate. Thus, we consider that among the classical and recently discovered drugs for the treatment of HF, non-pharmacological approaches (other than cardiac resynchronization therapy) must also be discussed.

3. Non-Pharmacological Therapies for Heart Failure

3.1. Neuromodulatory Approaches

The autonomic nervous system (ANS) plays a critical role in the regulation and homeostasis of the human body, particularly of the cardiovascular system. Since in HF ANS dysregulation has a detrimental effect on cardiac function, improving this pathological alteration by various approaches may represent a pillar in the management of HF [78]. The sympathetic and parasympathetic systems are the two major components of ANS. In the heart, the activation of the parasympathetic nervous system lowers heart rate and decreases contractility, conductance, and myocardial O_2 consumption, resulting in a reduction in cardiac output during relaxation [79]. Primarily responsible for parasympathetic innervation is the vagus nerve, encompassing all major thoracic organs [80]. Complex interactions between the sympathetic (SNS) and parasympathetic (PNS) nervous systems, as well as regional responses and feedback from the central nervous system, contribute to the modulation of cardiovascular homeostasis [81]. Briefly, excitation of the SNS causes nerve terminals to release norepinephrine (NE), whereas the adrenal glands and medulla release both norepinephrine and epinephrine. These catecholamines bind to adrenergic receptors (ARs), which are further subdivided into subtypes $\alpha 1$, $\alpha 2$, $\beta 1$, $\beta 2$, and $\beta 3$ [82]. In the human heart, β-ARs account for approximately 90% of all ARs, whereas α1-ARs account for almost 10% [83].

HF is characterized by an imbalance of the ANS, which generates a vicious cycle, meaning that the increased sympathetic activity together with reduced vagal activity promote the progression of ventricular remodeling and worsening of heart failure, and likewise, the development of HF further exacerbates the discrepancy between sympathetic and vagal activity [84]. High levels of NE over the long-term enhance myocardial stress due to chronic tachycardia increased afterload and oxygen consumption, thereby worsening ventricular remodeling. Increased catecholamines bind with their own cardiomyocyte β-receptors and stimulate G-protein-coupled receptor kinase upregulation, resulting in the downregulation and desensitization of the β1 receptors at the plasma membrane [81,85,86]. These processes are thought to be protective mechanisms by which the heart preserves itself against severe catecholaminergic toxicity, which commonly induces cyclic adenosine-monophosphate-mediated calcium overload, leading to cardiomyocyte death [81,83,86]. The modulation of the heart PNS is achieved by nicotinic and muscarinic acetylcholine receptors (nAChR and mAChR, respectively) through the neurotransmitter acetylcholine (ACh) [81,87]. Experimental and clinical HF studies have reported that an increased HR, together with a reduced HR variability, is the consequence of PNS dysfunction [88,89].

Cardiac sympathetic denervation (CSD) is a surgical antiadrenergic intervention that has significant antiarrhythmic effects, as demonstrated by both preclinical and clinical studies, being effective in severe ventricular arrhythmias [90,91]. CSD decreases automaticity and repolarization heterogeneity and prolongs repolarization. It exerts its effects by interfering with both efferent and afferent neurons [92]. Left-sided sympathetic denervation has been utilized effectively in refractory instances of long QT syndrome, catecholaminergic polymorphic ventricular tachycardia [93], and ventricular arrhythmias in patients with structural heart disease [94–96].

Renal denervation (RDNx) is a catheter-based procedure used to ablate renal nerves as a solution to ameliorate the pathophysiology of HF by lowering the activity of the sympathetic nervous system. In both HF experimental and clinical studies, RDNx is able to induce antihypertensive effects but also improve adverse cardiac remodeling [97–100]. The REACH-pilot study was the first to evaluate the value of RDNx in HF symptomatic patients. In the study, RDNx was related to improvements in both symptoms and exercise ability. There was neither a substantial fall in blood pressure nor a decline in renal function, and some patients were able to limit their usage of diuretics [101]. In the clinical studies conducted so far, RDNx seems to be safe and well tolerated in patients with HFrEF by improving HF symptoms and modestly lowering systolic and diastolic blood pressure without worsening renal function [102]. Further insights into the mechanisms by which RDNx improves the physiopathology of HF are required. In this regard, clinical trials with control arms such as RE-ADAPT-HF (A Prospective, Multicenter, Randomized, Blinded, Sham-controlled, Feasibility Study of Renal Denervation in Patients with Chronic Heart Failure) and UNLOAD-HFpEF (Renal Denervation to Treat Heart Failure with Preserved Ejection Fraction) are ongoing, with the results expected in the next years.

Vagus nerve stimulation (VNS). During an inflammatory response, the vagus nerve acts as an afferent and efferent pathway between the brain and peripheral organs, including the heart [103]. In the presence of proinflammatory cytokines in the periphery, the sensory afferents of the vagus nerve are activated and transmit the signal to the brain. This signal induces the release of acetylcholine from the vagus nerve efferents into the reticuloendothelial system, which limits inflammation by reducing the synthesis and release of proinflammatory cytokines [104]. Thus, it is comprehensible that VNS might reduce the proinflammatory state, which is already recognized as a critical pathogenic mechanism in HF, particularly in HFpEF, since it is associated with promoting cardiac remodeling [104]. Schwartz and colleagues were the first to describe the efficacy of long-term VNS in patients with heart failure. They reported an improvement in functional status, quality of life, and left ventricular volume in HFrEF after vagus nerve stimulation [105]. However, larger clinical studies of VNS in patients with HFrEF, such as NECTAR-HF (Neural Cardiac Therapy for Heart Failure Study), INOVATE-HF (Increase of Vagal Tone in Chronic Heart Failure), and ANTHEM-HF (Autonomic Neural Regulation Therapy to Enhance Myocardial Function in Heart Failure) have not reliably reproduced the advantages so far [106–108]. The inconsistency may be the result of extensive variation in stimulation settings, targets, and systems. ANTHEM HFrEF (Autonomic Regulation Therapy to Enhance Myocardial Function and Reduce Progression of Heart Failure with Reduced Ejection Fraction) is an adaptive, open-label, randomized, controlled study that is now enrolling and is expected to provide more insights regarding the efficiency of VNS on HF outcomes [109].

Tragus nerve stimulation. One of the main drawbacks of vagus stimulation is the invasive nature of this therapy, which is accompanied by surgical risks and low patient tolerance [110]. Low-level tragus stimulation (LLTS) is a non-invasive transcutaneous approach that may influence autonomic function by stimulating the auricular branch of the vagus nerve (ABVN) [111]. Currently, ideal LLTS parameters are unclear. In both preclinical and clinical research, LLTS parameters have been empirically determined. In a rat model of heart failure with HFpEF, LLTS lowered both systolic and diastolic blood pressure. Furthermore, left ventricular hypertrophy, circumferential strain, and diastolic function were improved. It has also reduced inflammatory cell infiltration and fibrosis within the ventricle and induced downregulation of pro-inflammatory and pro-fibrotic genes [112]. Human trials of LLTS in HF patients are very limited. In a prospective, randomized, double-blind, 2 × 2 cross-over trial, 1 h of LLTS improved the longitudinal mechanics of the left ventricle and the heart rate variability (HRV) in patients with HFrEF [113]. In a pilot, randomized, sham-controlled research including patients with HFrEF, 1 h of LLTS improved microcirculation as assessed by flow-mediated vasodilatation [114].

Cardiac contractility modulation (CCM) is a novel approach that employs non-excitatory electrical impulses to the interventricular septum during the absolute refractory period [115]. Implantation is similar to a conventional transvenous pacemaker device, except two right ventricular leads are used. Mechanistic research has shown an increase in left ventricular contractility and positive global effects on reverse remodeling, mostly as a result of calcium handling improvements by phosphorylation of phospholamban and upregulation of SERCA-2A [116]. Increases in functional ability and quality of life have been shown in clinical trial data, but long-term outcome data are limited [117]. After two pilot studies to validate the safety and feasibility of CCM in patients with HFrEF [118], FIX-HF-3 was the first observational trial to evaluate the clinical efficacy of CCM treatment in 25 patients [119]. At a 2-month follow-up, improvements were found in LVEF, 6 min walk distance (6MWD), NYHA functional class, and quality of life in HFrEF NYHA III patients [120]. This was accompanied by the first randomized, double-blind crossover trial (FIX-CHF-4), which included patients with severe HFrEF, defined as LVEF < 35%, NYHA class II-III, and a narrow QRS duration. Those who were medically optimized were compared to those who received additional CCM therapy, with measures taken after 12 weeks in each group. Peak VO2 as assessed by cardiopulmonary exercise testing (CPEX) improved similarly in both groups (0.4 mL/kg/min), which strongly indicated a placebo effect. After the 6-month treatment period, however, only those with CCM showed a consistent improvement linked with QoL indicators. In a recent randomized controlled study, FIX-HF-5C (Evaluation of the Safety and Effectiveness of the OPTIMIZER System in Subjects with Heart Failure), which enrolled patients with NYHA class III or IV symptoms, QRS length of 130 ms, and LVEF between 25 and 45%, patients in the CCM arm had statistically significant improvements in NYHA class, 6MWD, and quality of life, as well as a composite reduction in HFrEF hospitalization and cardiovascular mortality. Moreover, a subgroup analysis of the FIX-HF-5 study revealed more substantial treatment advantages, such as that CCM therapy may provide additional benefits in patients with a relatively moderate LVEF decline [121,122].

Baroreceptor activation therapy (BAT). The carotid body and sinus are innervated by both PNS (via the vagus and glossopharyngeal fibers) and SNS (via cervical sympathetic ganglia). Electrical stimulation of carotid sinus baroreceptors generates afferent signals to the dorsal medulla, resulting in SNS reduction and enhanced vagal tone, which reduces blood pressure and heart rate [123,124]. In HF patients, these responses associated with the baroreceptor pathway are partially blunted due to carotid body alterations, leading to baroreflex dysfunction and subsequent SNS overactivation [123]. Baroreceptor sensitivity impairments in heart failure are related to higher death rates [125]. In preclinical studies, BAT was shown to diminish sympathetic tone and increase parasympathetic signaling, thus enhancing the autonomic input to the heart [126]. The BeAT-HF (Baroreflex Activation Therapy for Heart Failure) clinical trial demonstrated that BAT is safe in HFrEF patients and significantly improves patient-centered symptomatic endpoints of the QOL score, exercise capacity, and functional status [127]. Moreover, a considerable improvement in NT-proBNP levels was achieved with BAT, despite a disproportionate rise in the number of drugs in the control group [127].

Endovascular Ablation of the Right Greater Splanchnic Nerve (GSN). Exertional dyspnea, decreased aerobic capacity, and higher mortality are all linked to elevated intracardiac filling pressures at rest and during exercise in HF patients with both reduced and preserved ejection fraction [128–130]. As a result, several cardiovascular therapies aim to lower intracardiac filling pressures in these patients to enhance exertional capacity and QOL and improve cardiovascular morbidity [131].

Reduced inotropic and chronotropic reserves, as well as impaired relaxation, all contribute to higher filling pressures at rest and during activity. The vascular system is also involved in this process by reducing pulmonary arterial compliance and increasing pulmonary arterial resistance. Excessive blood volume distribution from extrathoracic compartments into the thorax is a major factor in high filling pressures in HF patients [131,132]. Splanchnic vasoconstriction mediated by the SNS causes rapid blood shifts from the splanchnic compartment to the heart and lungs, which is a typical physiological adaptative response mechanism during exercise. These rapid blood volume shifts from the splanchnic to central vasculature, however, cause an exaggerated rise in heart filling pressures in patients with HF, increasing exercise intolerance and possibly leading to HF decompensation [133,134].

Splanchnic nerve activity modulation has thereby been developed as a possible treatment approach in HF patients to reduce volume redistribution and improve symptoms and outcomes. Recent research has explored the impact of temporarily and permanently blocking the GSN over the HF spectrum. Splanchnic nerve modulation has been proven beneficial for both acute decompensated (ADHF) and chronic heart failure (CHF), according to the Splanchnic Nerve Anesthesia in Heart Failure and Abdominal Nerve Blockade in Chronic Heart Failure trials. In 11 ADHF patients with advanced HFrEF who underwent short-term blockade of the greater splanchnic nerve via anesthetic agents, there was a significant decrease in PCWP and an increase in the cardiac index [135]. Comparable outcomes were yielded from a study including 18 CHF patients who underwent the same procedure [136]. In HFpEF patients, permanent ablation of the right greater splanchnic nerve led to a decrease in intracardiac filling pressures during exercise as soon as 24 h following the intervention [137]. The Surgical Resection of the Greater Splanchnic Nerve in Subjects Having Heart Failure with Preserved Ejection Fraction two-center study has shown a substantial decrease in PCWP at the 3-month follow-up and a considerable 12-month improvement in NYHA class and QOL [132]. To ablate the right-sided GSN, a novel, endovascular, transvenous, minimally invasive procedure (splanchnic ablation for volume management-SAVM) was designed, and it has been proven to be helpful in a small, single-center open-label pilot trial [138].

REBALANCE-HF (Endovascular Ablation of the Right Greater Splanchnic Nerve in Subjects Having HFpEF) is an ongoing, multicenter, randomized, sham-controlled trial whose objective is to assess the safety of unilateral ablation of the right greater splanchnic nerve and its effectiveness in improving hemodynamics, quality of life, and exercise tolerance in patients with HFpEF [139]. The preliminary results from this trial show that GSN ablation is efficient in reducing PCWP during exercise, with improving the symptoms, but without a significant change in exercise capacity. The decrease in PCWP is substantial and it is consistent with previous results suggesting that abnormalities in venous capacitance play a significant role in the development of hemodynamic perturbations in HFpEF during exercise [140]. These findings show for the first time that endovascular GSN ablation can be used to treat HFpEF. All neuromodulatory approaches are summarized in Table 2.

3.2. Respiratory Disorders Implicated in Heart Failure

Sleep-disordered breathing, a widespread condition affecting both the circulatory and respiratory systems, is one element now recognized as contributing to the increased morbidity and mortality in HF. Two primary sleep apnea syndromes have been described: obstructive sleep apnea syndrome (OSA) and central sleep apnea syndrome (CSA) [109].

Stimulation of Phrenic Nerve. This procedure involves inserting an electrode into a brachiocephalic or pericardiophrenic vein to detect the diaphragm's contractions throughout breathing and activate the diaphragmatic nerve during apnea, with the purpose to preserve fairly constant pO_2 and pCO_2 levels and avoid SNS and RAAS overactivation [141,142]. In the pivotal trial of the remedé system (Respicardia Inc., Minnetonka, MN, USA) involving 151 patients, the stimulation of the phrenic nerve showed a substantial decrease in the apnea–hypopnea index (AHI), central apnea index, arousal index, oxygen desaturation 4% index, percentage of sleep with rapid eye movement, and sleepiness (Epworth Sleepiness Scale (ESS)) [143]. A 5-year follow-up investigation confirmed these findings [144]. According to Costanzo et al., patients who received phrenic nerve stimulation displayed an increase in the QOL and LVEF without a substantial change in end-systolic and end-diastolic volumes [141]. Large-scale clinical studies are necessary to determine the impact of phrenic nerve stimulation on mortality in individuals with HF and CSA syndrome [145].

Synchronized Diaphragmatic Therapy. Increased intrathoracic pressure exerts persistent stress on the heart muscle and may exacerbate heart failure (HF). The respiratory muscles have a substantial effect on intrathoracic pressure, and, thus, the implantation of a device coupled to an electrode that detects the heartbeat that activates the diaphragm was developed [145]. In the Stimulation of the Diaphragm in Patients with Severe Heart Failure Following Heart Surgery randomized trial including 33 subjects, an improvement in LVEF and HF symptoms, and an elevation in maximal power and oxygen consumption during exercise testing was noticed, with no considerable improvement in the six MWT, nor the BNP levels [146]. At the 1-year follow-up of the non-randomized VisOne Heart Failure trial, improvements in LVEF, QOL, and 6MWT were reported [147]. Although both trials included a limited number of patients, because of the encouraging outcomes, it might be beneficial to conduct additional research on a larger scale.

3.3. Devices for Decongestion in HF

Although loop diuretics continue to represent the backbone of decongestive treatment in HF, the occurrence of drug resistance, particularly with prolonged usage, poses a therapeutic issue that requires the development of novel approaches [145].

TARGET-1 and TARGET-2 (A Study to Evaluate the Treatment of Patients with Acute Decompensated Heart Failure (ADHF) Using an Automated Fluid Management System) trials evaluated the safety and effectiveness of controlled decongestion using the Reprieve system, which is intended to detect urine output and administer a specific amount of substitute solution to reach the predefined fluid balance. In both trials, patients experienced an increase in urine output, a decrease in body weight, and a drop in central venous pressure (CVP), while the SBP remained constant and without renal dysfunction [148]. The first human trials of the Doraya catheter, a device designed to transiently lower renal venous pressure by generating a manageable gradient in the inferior vena cava just under the renal veins, have shown encouraging results [149]. The Doraya catheter appears to represent an innovative idea for the management of AHF patients with poor diuretic response, whereas the Reprieve device is intended for AHF patients responsive to diuretics [145].

The VENUS-HF (VENUS-Heart Failure Early Feasibility Study) regarding the preCARDIA system, a device implanted into the superior vena cava to induce transient blockage, resulting in a reduction in right ventricular preload, revealed a reduction in right atrial pressure and PCWP [150]. The WhiteSwell device, intended to produce a low-pressure zone in the outflow of the thoracic duct into the venous system, has been studied in both animal and human studies. In the animal experiment, WhiteSwell not only prevented the collection of more fluid but also stimulated its discharge [151]. The orthopnea and oedema improved when the device was applied to humans. The Aquapass system is a wearable device designed to raise the skin temperature of the lower body without affecting the body's core temperature. Increasing sweat rate in HF patients appears to be a reasonable option for decongestive treatment; nevertheless, further research is required to determine the method's particular usefulness and effectiveness [152].

Table 2. Neuromodulatory approaches in HF.

Neuromodulatory Approaches	Mechanisms of Action	Clinical Trial/Study	Main Findings	Limitations
Cardiac sympathetic denervation	surgical antiadrenergic denervation	Vaseghi et al. Schwartz et al.	→antiarrhythmic effects; →improvements in HR variability and autonomic nervous system [90–96]	→limited data exist on the benefits of sympathetic denervation in HF patients.
Renal denervation	frequency-based catheter renal nerve ablation	REACH pilot study	→improvements in both symptoms and exercise ability [101]	→the RDT-PEF (Renal Denervation in Heart Failure with Preserved Ejection Fraction) trial was prematurely disrupted due to enrollment challenges, leaving it underpowered to determine whether RDN positively affected QOL, exercise function, biomarkers, and left heart remodeling in HFpEF patients [153].
		RE-ADAPT-HF UNLOAD-HFpEF	→enrolling →enrolling	→future randomized, blinded, sham-controlled clinical studies are necessary to establish the impact of RDN on the morbidity of HFrEF and HFpEF patients.
Vagus nerve stimulation (VNS)	electrical stimulation of the vagus nerve	Schwartz et al.	→improvement in functional status, quality of life (QoL), and left ventricular volume in HFrEF [105]	
		NECTAR-HF (NCT01385176)	→favorable long-term safety profile; failed to show that VNS improved clinic outcomes versus OMT [106]	→VNS has a considerable favorable effect on the functional state of the patient, but with no effect on the prognosis [107].
		INOVATE-HF (NCT01303718)	→quality of life, NYHA class, and 6 min walking distance were favorably affected by vagus nerve stimulation; failed to show that VNS improved clinic outcomes versus OMT [107]	→the lack of a control group in the ANTHEM-HF trial is a considerable limitation; to avoid the placebo effect and validate the procedure's safety, a randomised, controlled clinical trial is required [108].
		ANTHEM-HF (NCT01823887)	→chronic open-loop left- or right-side VNS is feasible and well tolerated in HFrEF patients [108]	→no significant echocardiographic improvements nor reduction levels of NTpro BNP have been documented in any study [107].
		ANTHEM-HFrEF (NCT03425422)	→enrolling; test the impact of Vitaria system on cardiovascular mortality and HF hospitalization in patients with HF and reduced EF (HFrEF) [109]	
Tragus nerve stimulation	non-invasive transcutaneous approach to VNS that stimulates the auricular branch of the vagus nerve	Zhou et al.	→lowered both systolic and diastolic blood pressure; →left ventricular hypertrophy, circumferential strain, and diastolic function; →reduced inflammatory cell infiltration and fibrosis within the ventricle and induced downregulation of pro-inflammatory and pro-fibrotic genes [112]	→previous research has a number of limitations, including the absence of a well-controlled placebo group and longitudinal data and the limited sample populations; the optimal stimulation settings have yet to be established. →longitudinal data are required to assess the long-term impact of LLTS.
		Tran et al.	→improved the longitudinal mechanics of the left ventricle and the heart rate variability (HRV) in patients with HFrEF [113]	
		Dasari et al.	→improved microcirculation [114]	→moreover, there is no validated biomarker for measuring the efficacy of LLTS [154].

Table 2. Cont.

Neuromodulatory Approaches	Mechanisms of Action	Clinical Trial/Study	Main Findings	Limitations
Cardiac contractility modulation (CCM)	myocardial non-excitatory electrical impulses delivered during the absolute refractory period that increases left ventricular contractility as a result of calcium handling improvements by phosphorylation of phospholamban and upregulation of SERCA-2A	FIX-HF-3	→improvements in LVEF, 6 min walk distance (6MWD), NYHA functional class, and quality of life in HFrEF NYHA III patients [119,120]	→the impact of CCM on parameters such as left ventricular diastolic volumes has not been investigated systematically.
		FIX-CHF-4	→consistent improvement linked with QoL indicators at 6 months of therapy in HFrEF patients who received CCM [121]	→CCM may only be effective when administered to viable, non-necrotic myocardium; however, this has not been fully investigated in preclinical or clinical research.
		FIX-HF-5 (NCT00112125)	→subgroup analysis revealed improvements in ventilatory anaerobic threshold were observed in patients with ejection fraction ranging from 25% to 45% [121,122]	→likewise, the advantages of CCM in CRT "non-responder" patients are inadequately documented. →in the study conducted by Kuschyk et al., there was an increased number of adverse outcomes, including two fatalities.
		FIX-HF-5C (NCT01381172)	→statistically significant improvements in NYHA class, 6MWD, QoL, a composite reduction in hospitalization, and cardiovascular mortality [122]	→prospective trial results are inadequate, and it is essential that this disparity be settled prior to expanding usage in populations with medically optimal adjusted HFrEF, narrow QRS duration, and persistent symptoms [116].
Baroreceptor activation therapy (BAT)	electrical stimulation of carotid sinus baroreceptors lowers SNS activity and increases parasympathetic tone	BeAT-HF (NCT02627196)	→BAT is safe and effective; →BAT significantly improved QoL and 6MWD, and reduced NT-proBNP levels [127]	→BAT requires larger-scale studies with extended follow-up periods, a wider cohort of patients, and defined outcomes, including mortality risks, before this procedure can be included in HF clinical practice [155].
Splanchnic nerve modulation (SNM)	modulation of splanchnic nerve activity reduces cardiac filling pressures	REBALANCE-HF (NCT04592445)	→the preliminary results from this ongoing trial show that GSN ablation is efficient in reducing PCWP during exercise, with improving the symptoms but without a significant change in exercise capacity [140]	→the safety and effectiveness of SNM in the management of HF must be explored more extensively; the latest scientific studies are centered on limited patient groups with minimal follow-up; the aforementioned proof-of-concept clinical trials lacked a control group [132].

3.4. Ongoing Trials for Non-Pharmacological Therapies for HF

In the ALLEVIATE-HF-1 (NCT04583527), ALLEVIATE-HF-2 (NCT04838353), and ALLEVIATE-HFrEF (NCT05133089) studies, patients with HFpEF, HFmEF, and HFrEF will be enrolled for treatment through a no-implant interatrial shunt, using clinical, echocardiographic, and invasive hemodynamic data. The transcatheter system is designed to lower left atrial pressure by developing a therapeutic interatrial shunt, without the need for a permanent cardiac implant or open-heart surgery.

RELIEVE-HF (Reducing Lung Congestion Symptoms in Advanced Heart Failure-NCT03499236), a randomized clinical trial, is evaluating the impact of the V-Wave Ventura Interatrial Shunt System on heart failure patients, including the ability to lower hospitalizations and improve symptoms, exercise capacity, and quality of life. This small, hourglass-shaped device facilitates blood to flow from the left to the right atrium, lowering the pressure on the left side during physical activity.

It is a certainty now that the technological advances from the last years have paved the way for the development of non-pharmacological approaches that may efficiently complement classical HF therapy. Although further experimental studies are required to elucidate the underlying mechanisms through which many of these therapies act, the promising and encouraging results reported to date compel us to extend the HF treatment beyond the classical view.

4. Future Perspectives of HF Management—Artificial Intelligence

A late-breaking discovery presented at the European Society of Cardiology's (ESC) Heart Failure 2022 congress was a voice analysis software that can be used by heart failure patients at home that can detect fluid in the lungs in up to 80% of cases, three weeks prior to an unexpected hospitalization or escalation in outpatient medication therapy [156]. As cardiovascular illnesses evolve, advances in therapeutic and diagnostic approaches are required, and artificial intelligence (AI) is now being rapidly integrated into the field of cardiovascular medicine. By analyzing colossal databases more effectively than the human brain, AI has the potential to improve medical diagnosis, treatment, risk prediction, clinical care, and drug development [157]. For healthcare providers, AI has the potential to reduce the risk of adverse events, patient waiting times, and per capita expenditures while boosting accessibility, productivity, and overall patient experience [158]. AI also has the potential to reduce workloads and margin of error for physicians, as well as to improve patient–doctor interactions and therapeutic decision making [159,160]. For patients, AI can improve their health and well-being by increasing their knowledge, shared decision making, and self-efficacy in disease management [160].

For accurate quantitative and qualitative evaluation of heart failure, AI has been incorporated into different cardiac imaging techniques, such as echocardiography, cardiac magnetic resonance imaging, and cardiac computed tomography. Machine learning algorithms have been found to deliver a near-instantaneous echocardiography evaluation. Knackstedt et al. showed that the LVEF and longitudinal strain could be determined in less than 8 s [161]. This quick and precise evaluation might also have applications outside the cardiology department, such as in the emergency room, where point-of-care ultrasound scans are becoming more popular [162]. AI has been also shown to be of crucial importance in cardiac magnetic resonance imaging, especially for ventricular segmentation [163]. Laser et al. compared knowledge-based reconstruction of right ventricular volumes to the gold standard of direct cardiac MRI, finding that knowledge-based reconstruction offers outstanding accuracy for right ventricular 3D volumetry [164]. AI-assisted 3D visualization and cardiac image reconstruction can aid in the identification of a range of disorders [165,166]. Similarly, completely automated AI systems have provided a considerably more accurate calculation of left ventricular mass, papillary muscle identification, common carotid artery, and descending aorta measurements [167,168]. AI has been increasingly used for cardiac computed tomography, particularly for the assessment of coronary artery calcification scoring and risk stratification of future events [169]. Interestingly, AI uses various risk calculation scoring systems to estimate cardiovascular mortality and predictive models to predict the risk of future hospitalization so that proper monitoring and control may be carried out to avoid such harmful results [140–175].

Current HF healthcare services are insufficient to satisfy the demands of an ageing population with rising comorbidities and disease complexity, as well as the disparity in medical care distribution between rural and urban areas. As a result of these factors, an urgent need to develop alternative healthcare treatments has arisen. eHealth apps have the ability to relieve a large amount of the strain on healthcare services while also improving patient care. The PASSION-HF (Patient Self-Care using eHealth in Chronic Heart Failure) project intends to create a virtual doctor, a digital decision support system that offers options based on current clinical standards. Patient independence is enhanced by providing tailored HF management 24 h a day, 7 days a week. In addition, the program establishes processes and decision points at which medical experts must be involved [176].

Although AI has the potential to solve many of the fundamental challenges faced by the current HF pandemic, it is still a fast-growing field, and therefore some caution is advised. Transparency in data quality, population representativeness, and performance evaluation will be critical. Clinicians, patients, caregivers, and IT professionals should all be included in discussions about legal, technological, and regulatory problems, with ethics and equity being prioritized [177].

5. Conclusions

Heart failure is becoming an irrefutably significant disease entity as the population ages. Thus, various mechanisms contributing to the development and progression of HF have been discovered and targeted with novel medications and non-pharmacological approaches throughout the last three decades. This has improved the clinical outcome of millions of people worldwide with HF in terms of mortality, quality of life, and survival. Researchers are aiming to identify subgroups in which specific drugs and/or devices may be most successful, innovative methods for enhanced diagnosis and prediction of prognosis in HF patients, and novel tools for treating HF. New therapies will hopefully bring more benefits and extend these results to the treatment of HFpEF also, as well as other causes and phenotypes of HF.

Author Contributions: Conceptualization: I.P.P., M.Ș.C.H. and I.T.; methodology, resources: I.P.P.; writing—original draft preparation: I.P.P., M.Ș.C.H. and I.T.; writing—review and editing: D.M.T., M.A.M., D.N.Ș., L.I.Ș. and R.I; visualization and supervision: D.N.Ș., L.I.Ș. and R.I.; project administration: I.P.P. and I.T. All authors have read and agreed to the published version of the manuscript.

Funding: This research received no external funding.

Institutional Review Board Statement: Not applicable.

Informed Consent Statement: Not applicable.

Data Availability Statement: Not applicable.

Conflicts of Interest: The authors declare no conflict of interest.

References

1. Pellicori, P.; Khan, M.J.I.; Graham, F.J.; Cleland, J.G.F. New perspectives and future directions in the treatment of heart failure. *Heart Fail. Rev.* **2019**, *25*, 147–159. [CrossRef] [PubMed]
2. Groenewegen, A.; Rutten, F.H.; Mosterd, A.; Hoes, A.W. Epidemiology of heart failure. *Eur. J. Heart Fail.* **2020**, *22*, 1342–1356. [CrossRef] [PubMed]
3. Jones, N.R.; Roalfe, A.K.; Adoki, I.; Hobbs, F.D.R.; Taylor, C.J. Survival of patients with chronic heart failure in the community: A systematic review and meta-analysis. *Eur. J. Heart Fail.* **2019**, *21*, 1306–1325. [CrossRef] [PubMed]
4. Correale, M.; Tricarico, L.; Fortunato, M.; Mazzeo, P.; Nodari, S.; Di Biase, M.; Brunetti, N.D. New targets in heart failure drug therapy. *Front Cardiovasc Med.* **2021**, *8*, 665797. [CrossRef] [PubMed]
5. D'Elia, E.; Iacovoni, A.; Vaduganathan, M.; Lorini, F.L.; Perlini, S.; Senni, M. Neprilysin inhibition in heart failure: Mechanisms and substrates beyond modulating natriuretic peptides. *Eur. J. Heart Fail.* **2017**, *19*, 710–717. [CrossRef]

6. Ferrari, L.; Sada, S.; GrAM (Gruppo di Autoformazione Metodologica). Efficacy of angiotensin-neprilysin inhibition versus enalapril in patient with heart failure with a reduced ejection fraction. *Intern Emerg Med.* **2015**, *10*, 369–371. [CrossRef]
7. Kuchulakanti, P.K. ARNI in cardiovascular disease: Current evidence and future perspectives. *Future Cardiol.* **2020**, *16*, 505–515. [CrossRef]
8. Greenberg, B. Angiotensin Receptor-Neprilysin Inhibition (ARNI) in Heart Failure. *Int. J. Heart Fail.* **2020**, *2*, 73. [CrossRef]
9. McMurray, J.J.V.; Packer, M.; Desai, A.S.; Gong, J.; Lefkowitz, M.P.; Rizkala, A.R.; Rouleau, J.L.; Shi, V.C.; Solomon, S.D.; Swedberg, K.; et al. Angiotensin-neprilysin inhibition versus enalapril in heart failure. *N. Engl. J. Med.* **2014**, *371*, 993–1004. [CrossRef]
10. Velazquez, E.J.; Morrow, D.A.; DeVore, A.D.; Duffy, C.I.; Ambrosy, A.P.; McCague, K.; Rocha, R.; Braunwald, E. Angiotensin-Neprilysin Inhibition in Acute Decompensated Heart Failure. *N. Engl. J. Med.* **2018**, *380*, 539–548. [CrossRef]
11. Ambrosy, A.P.; Mentz, R.J.; Fiuzat, M.; Cleland, J.G.F.; Greene, S.J.; O'Connor, C.M.; Teerlink, J.R.; Zannad, F.; Solomon, S.D. The role of angiotensin receptor-neprilysin inhibitors in cardiovascular disease-existing evidence, knowledge gaps, and future directions. *Eur. J. Heart Fail.* **2018**, *20*, 963–972. [CrossRef] [PubMed]
12. Solomon, S.D.; McMurray, J.J.V.; Anand, I.S.; Ge, J.; Lam, C.S.P.; Maggioni, A.P.; Martinez, F.; Packer, M.; Pfeffer, M.A.; Pieske, B.; et al. Angiotensin-Neprilysin Inhibition in Heart Failure with Preserved Ejection Fraction. *N. Engl. J. Med.* **2019**, *381*, 1609–1620. [CrossRef]
13. Heidenreich, P.A.; Bozkurt, B.; Aguilar, D.; Allen, L.A.; Byun, J.J.; Colvin, M.M.; Deswal, A.; Drazner, M.H.; Dunlay, S.M.; Evers, L.R.; et al. 2022 AHA/ACC/HFSA guideline for the management of heart failure: A report of the american college of cardiology/american heart association joint committee on clinical practice guidelines. *Circulation* **2022**, *145*, e895–e1032. [CrossRef] [PubMed]
14. McDonagh, T.A.; Metra, M.; Adamo, M.; Gardner, R.S.; Baumbach, A.; Böhm, M.; Burri, H.; Butler, J.; Čelutkienė, J.; Chioncel, O.; et al. 2021 ESC Guidelines for the diagnosis and treatment of acute and chronic heart failure. *Eur. Heart J.* **2021**, *42*, 3599–3726. [CrossRef]
15. Fitchett, D.; Zinman, B.; Wanner, C.; Lachin, J.M.; Hantel, S.; Salsali, A.; Johansen, O.E.; Woerle, H.J.; Broedl, U.C.; Inzucchi, S.E. Heart failure outcomes with empagliflozin in patients with type 2 diabetes at high cardiovascular risk: Results of the EMPA-REG OUTCOME®trial. *Eur. Heart J.* **2016**, *37*, 1526–1534. [CrossRef] [PubMed]
16. Rådholm, K.; Figtree, G.; Perkovic, V.; Solomon, S.D.; Mahaffey, K.W.; de Zeeuw, D.; Fulcher, G.; Barrett, T.D.; Shaw, W.; Desai, M.; et al. Canagliflozin and heart failure in type 2 diabetes mellitus: Results from the CANVAS program. *Circulation* **2018**, *138*, 458–468. [CrossRef]
17. Kato, E.T.; Silverman, M.G.; Mosenzon, O.; Zelniker, T.A.; Cahn, A.; Furtado, R.H.M.; Kuder, J.; Murphy, S.A.; Bhatt, D.L.; Leiter, L.A.; et al. Effect of dapagliflozin on heart failure and mortality in type 2 diabetes mellitus. *Circulation* **2019**, *139*, 2528–2536. [CrossRef]
18. Bhatt, D.L.; Szarek, M.; Steg, P.G.; Cannon, C.P.; Leiter, L.A.; McGuire, D.K.; Lewis, J.B.; Riddle, M.C.; Voors, A.A.; Metra, M.; et al. Sotagliflozin in Patients with Diabetes and Recent Worsening Heart Failure. *N. Engl. J. Med.* **2021**, *384*, 117–128. [CrossRef] [PubMed]
19. Serenelli, M.; Böhm, M.; Inzucchi, S.E.; Køber, L.; Kosiborod, M.N.; Martinez, F.A.; Ponikowski, P.; Sabatine, M.S.; Solomon, S.D.; DeMets, D.L.; et al. Effect of dapagliflozin according to baseline systolic blood pressure in the Dapagliflozin and Prevention of Adverse Outcomes in Heart Failure trial (DAPA-HF). *Eur. Heart J.* **2020**, *41*, 3402–3418. [CrossRef]
20. Nassif, M.E.; Qintar, M.; Windsor, S.L.; Jermyn, R.; Shavelle, D.M.; Tang, F.; Lamba, S.; Bhatt, K.; Brush, J.; Civitello, A.; et al. Empagliflozin Effects on Pulmonary Artery Pressure in Patients With Heart Failure: Results From the EMBRACE-HF Trial. *Circulation* **2021**, *143*, 1673–1686. [CrossRef]
21. Neuen, B.L.; Young, T.; Heerspink, H.J.L.; Neal, B.; Perkovic, V.; Billot, L.; Mahaffey, K.W.; Charytan, D.M.; Wheeler, D.C.; Arnott, C.; et al. SGLT2 inhibitors for the prevention of kidney failure in patients with type 2 diabetes: A systematic review and meta-analysis. *Lancet Diabetes Endocrinol.* **2019**, *7*, 845–854. [CrossRef]
22. Santos-Gallego, C.G.; Vargas-Delgado, A.P.; Requena-Ibanez, J.A.; Garcia-Ropero, A.; Mancini, D.; Pinney, S.; Macaluso, F.; Sartori, S.; Roque, M.; Sabatel-Perez, F.; et al. Randomized trial of empagliflozin in nondiabetic patients with heart failure and reduced ejection fraction. *J. Am. Coll. Cardiol.* **2021**, *77*, 243–255. [CrossRef] [PubMed]
23. Lee, M.M.Y.; Brooksbank, K.J.M.; Wetherall, K.; Mangion, K.; Roditi, G.; Campbell, R.T.; Berry, C.; Chong, V.; Coyle, L.; Docherty, K.F.; et al. Effect of Empagliflozin on Left Ventricular Volumes in Patients With Type 2 Diabetes, or Prediabetes, and Heart Failure With Reduced Ejection Fraction (SUGAR-DM-HF). *Circulation* **2021**, *143*, 516–525. [CrossRef] [PubMed]
24. Omar, M.; Jensen, J.; Ali, M.; Frederiksen, P.H.; Kistorp, C.; Videbæk, L.; Poulsen, M.K.; Tuxen, C.D.; Möller, S.; Gustafsson, F.; et al. Associations of empagliflozin with left ventricular volumes, mass, and function in patients with heart failure and reduced ejection fraction: A substudy of the empire HF randomized clinical trial. *JAMA Cardiol.* **2021**, *6*, 836–840. [CrossRef] [PubMed]
25. Zinman, B.; Wanner, C.; Lachin, J.M.; Fitchett, D.; Bluhmki, E.; Hantel, S.; Mattheus, M.; Devins, T.; Johansen, O.E.; Woerle, H.J.; et al. Empagliflozin, cardiovascular outcomes, and mortality in type 2 diabetes. *N. Engl. J. Med.* **2015**, *373*, 2117–2128. [CrossRef]
26. Fitchett, D.; McKnight, J.; Lee, J.; George, J.; Mattheus, M.; Woerle, H.J.; Inzucchi, S.E. P4903Empagliflozin reduces heart failure irrespective of control of blood pressure, low density lipoprotein cholesterol and HbA1c. *Eur. Heart J.* **2017**, *38* (Suppl. S1), ehx493.P4903. [CrossRef]

27. Mahaffey, K.W.; Neal, B.; Perkovic, V.; de Zeeuw, D.; Fulcher, G.; Erondu, N.; Shaw, W.; Fabbrini, E.; Sun, T.; Li, Q.; et al. Canagliflozin for primary and secondary prevention of cardiovascular events: Results from the CANVAS program (canagliflozin cardiovascular assessment study). *Circulation* **2018**, *137*, 323–334. [CrossRef]
28. Wiviott, S.D.; Raz, I.; Bonaca, M.P.; Mosenzon, O.; Kato, E.T.; Cahn, A.; Silverman, M.G.; Zelniker, T.A.; Kuder, J.F.; Murphy, S.A.; et al. Dapagliflozin and cardiovascular outcomes in type 2 diabetes. *N. Engl. J. Med.* **2019**, *380*, 347–357. [CrossRef]
29. Kosiborod, M.; Cavender, M.A.; Fu, A.Z.; Wilding, J.P.; Khunti, K.; Holl, R.W.; Norhammar, A.; Birkeland, K.I.; Jørgensen, M.E.; Thuresson, M.; et al. Lower Risk of Heart Failure and Death in Patients Initiated on Sodium-Glucose Cotransporter-2 Inhibitors Versus Other Glucose-Lowering Drugs: The CVD-REAL Study (Comparative Effectiveness of Cardiovascular Outcomes in New Users of Sodium-Glucose Cotransporter-2 Inhibitors). *Circulation* **2017**, *136*, 249–259.
30. Patorno, E.; Pawar, A.; Franklin, J.M.; Najafzadeh, M.; Déruaz-Luyet, A.; Brodovicz, K.G.; Sambevski, S.; Bessette, L.G.; Santiago Ortiz, A.J.; Kulldorff, M.; et al. Empagliflozin and the risk of heart failure hospitalization in routine clinical care. *Circulation* **2019**, *139*, 2822–2830. [CrossRef]
31. McMurray, J.J.V.; Solomon, S.D.; Inzucchi, S.E.; Køber, L.; Kosiborod, M.N.; Martinez, F.A.; Ponikowski, P.; Sabatine, M.S.; Anand, I.S.; Bělohlávek, J.; et al. Dapagliflozin in Patients with Heart Failure and Reduced Ejection Fraction. *N. Engl. J. Med.* **2019**, *381*, 1995–2008. [CrossRef]
32. Anker, S.D.; Butler, J.; Filippatos, G.; Khan, M.S.; Marx, N.; Lam, C.S.P.; Schnaidt, S.; Ofstad, A.P.; Brueckmann, M.; Jamal, W.; et al. Effect of Empagliflozin on Cardiovascular and Renal Outcomes in Patients With Heart Failure by Baseline Diabetes Status: Results From the EMPEROR-Reduced Trial. *Circulation* **2021**, *143*, 337–349. [CrossRef] [PubMed]
33. Packer, M.; Anker, S.D.; Butler, J.; Filippatos, G.; Pocock, S.J.; Carson, P.; Januzzi, J.; Verma, S.; Tsutsui, H.; Brueckmann, M.; et al. Cardiovascular and Renal Outcomes with Empagliflozin in Heart Failure. *N. Engl. J. Med.* **2020**, *383*, 1413–1424. [CrossRef] [PubMed]
34. Petrie, M.C.; Verma, S.; Docherty, K.F.; Inzucchi, S.E.; Anand, I.; Belohlávek, J.; Böhm, M.; Chiang, C.-E.; Chopra, V.K.; de Boer, R.A.; et al. Effect of dapagliflozin on worsening heart failure and cardiovascular death in patients with heart failure with and without diabetes. *JAMA* **2020**, *323*, 1353–1368. [CrossRef]
35. Writing Committee; Maddox, T.M.; Januzzi, J.L.; Allen, L.A.; Breathett, K.; Butler, J.; Davis, L.L.; Fonarow, G.C.; Ibrahim, N.E.; Lindenfeld, J.; et al. 2021 update to the 2017 ACC expert consensus decision pathway for optimization of heart failure treatment: Answers to 10 pivotal issues about heart failure with reduced ejection fraction: A report of the american college of cardiology solution set oversight committee. *J. Am. Coll. Cardiol.* **2021**, *77*, 772–810. [PubMed]
36. Seferović, P.M.; Fragasso, G.; Petrie, M.; Mullens, W.; Ferrari, R.; Thum, T.; Bauersachs, J.; Anker, S.D.; Ray, R.; Çavuşoğlu, Y.; et al. Sodium-glucose co-transporter 2 inhibitors in heart failure: Beyond glycaemic control. A position paper of the Heart Failure Association of the European Society of Cardiology. *Eur. J. Heart Fail.* **2020**, *22*, 1495–1503. [CrossRef]
37. Gladden, J.D.; Chaanine, A.H.; Redfield, M.M. Heart Failure with Preserved Ejection Fraction. *Annu. Rev. Med.* **2018**, *69*, 65–79. [CrossRef]
38. Nassif, M.E.; Windsor, S.L.; Borlaug, B.A.; Kitzman, D.W.; Shah, S.J.; Tang, F.; Khariton, Y.; Malik, A.O.; Khumri, T.; Umpierrez, G.; et al. The SGLT2 inhibitor dapagliflozin in heart failure with preserved ejection fraction: A multicenter randomized trial. *Nat. Med.* **2021**, *27*, 1954–1960. [CrossRef]
39. Solomon, S.D.; McMurray, J.J.V.; Claggett, B.; de Boer, R.A.; DeMets, D.; Hernandez, A.F.; Inzucchi, S.E.; Kosiborod, M.N.; Lam, C.S.P.; Martinez, F.; et al. Dapagliflozin in Heart Failure with Mildly Reduced or Preserved Ejection Fraction. *N. Engl. J. Med.* **2022**, *10*, 184–197. [CrossRef]
40. Anker, S.D.; Butler, J.; Filippatos, G.; Ferreira, J.P.; Bocchi, E.; Böhm, M.; Inzucchi, S.E.; Kosiborod, M.N.; Lam, C.S.P.; Martinez, F.; et al. Empagliflozin in Heart Failure with a Preserved Ejection Fraction. *N. Engl. J. Med.* **2021**, *385*, 1451–1461. [CrossRef]
41. Butler, J.; Packer, M.; Filippatos, G.; Ferreira, J.P.; Zeller, C.; Schnee, J.; Brueckmann, M.; Pocock, S.J.; Zannad, F.; Anker, S.D. Effect of empagliflozin in patients with heart failure across the spectrum of left ventricular ejection fraction. *Eur. Heart J.* **2022**, *43*, 416–426. [CrossRef] [PubMed]
42. Butler, J.; Filippatos, G.; Jamal Siddiqi, T.; Brueckmann, M.; Böhm, M.; Chopra, V.K.; Pedro Ferreira, J.; Januzzi, J.L.; Kaul, S.; Piña, I.L.; et al. Empagliflozin, Health Status, and Quality of Life in Patients With Heart Failure and Preserved Ejection Fraction: The EMPEROR-Preserved Trial. *Circulation* **2022**, *145*, 184–193. [CrossRef]
43. Perkovic, V.; Jardine, M.J.; Neal, B.; Bompoint, S.; Heerspink, H.J.L.; Charytan, D.M.; Edwards, R.; Agarwal, R.; Bakris, G.; Bull, S.; et al. Canagliflozin and renal outcomes in type 2 diabetes and nephropathy. *N. Engl. J. Med.* **2019**, *380*, 2295–2306. [CrossRef] [PubMed]
44. Heerspink, H.J.L.; Stefánsson, B.V.; Correa-Rotter, R.; Chertow, G.M.; Greene, T.; Hou, F.-F.; Mann, J.F.E.; McMurray, J.J.V.; Lindberg, M.; Rossing, P.; et al. Dapagliflozin in Patients with Chronic Kidney Disease. *N. Engl. J. Med.* **2020**, *383*, 1436–1446. [CrossRef]
45. EMPA-KIDNEY Collaborative Group. Design, recruitment, and baseline characteristics of the EMPA-KIDNEY trial. *Nephrol. Dial. Transplant.* **2022**, *37*, 1317–1329. [CrossRef] [PubMed]
46. Gheorghiade, M.; Marti, C.N.; Sabbah, H.N.; Roessig, L.; Greene, S.J.; Böhm, M.; Burnett, J.C.; Campia, U.; Cleland, J.G.F.; Collins, S.P.; et al. Soluble guanylate cyclase: A potential therapeutic target for heart failure. *Heart Fail. Rev.* **2013**, *18*, 123–134. [CrossRef] [PubMed]

47. Emdin, M.; Aimo, A.; Castiglione, V.; Vergaro, G.; Georgiopoulos, G.; Saccaro, L.F.; Lombardi, C.M.; Passino, C.; Cerbai, E.; Metra, M.; et al. Targeting cyclic guanosine monophosphate to treat heart failure: JACC review topic of the week. *J. Am. Coll. Cardiol.* **2020**, *76*, 1795–1807. [CrossRef] [PubMed]
48. Stasch, J.-P.; Pacher, P.; Evgenov, O.V. Soluble guanylate cyclase as an emerging therapeutic target in cardiopulmonary disease. *Circulation* **2011**, *123*, 2263–2273. [CrossRef]
49. Follmann, M.; Ackerstaff, J.; Redlich, G.; Wunder, F.; Lang, D.; Kern, A.; Fey, P.; Griebenow, N.; Kroh, W.; Becker-Pelster, E.-M.; et al. Discovery of the soluble guanylate cyclase stimulator vericiguat (BAY 1021189) for the treatment of chronic heart failure. *J. Med. Chem.* **2017**, *60*, 5146–5161. [CrossRef]
50. Armstrong, P.W.; Pieske, B.; Anstrom, K.J.; Ezekowitz, J.; Hernandez, A.F.; Butler, J.; Lam, C.S.P.; Ponikowski, P.; Voors, A.A.; Jia, G.; et al. Vericiguat in Patients with Heart Failure and Reduced Ejection Fraction. *N. Engl. J. Med.* **2020**, *382*, 1883–1893. [CrossRef]
51. Erdmann, E.; Semigran, M.J.; Nieminen, M.S.; Gheorghiade, M.; Agrawal, R.; Mitrovic, V.; Mebazaa, A. Cinaciguat, a soluble guanylate cyclase activator, unloads the heart but also causes hypotension in acute decompensated heart failure. *Eur. Heart J.* **2013**, *34*, 57–67. [CrossRef] [PubMed]
52. Gheorghiade, M.; Greene, S.J.; Butler, J.; Filippatos, G.; Lam, C.S.P.; Maggioni, A.P.; Ponikowski, P.; Shah, S.J.; Solomon, S.D.; Kraigher-Krainer, E.; et al. Effect of Vericiguat, a Soluble Guanylate Cyclase Stimulator, on Natriuretic Peptide Levels in Patients With Worsening Chronic Heart Failure and Reduced Ejection Fraction: The SOCRATES-REDUCED Randomized Trial. *JAMA* **2015**, *314*, 2251–2262. [CrossRef] [PubMed]
53. Boettcher, M.; Thomas, D.; Mueck, W.; Loewen, S.; Arens, E.; Yoshikawa, K.; Becker, C. Safety, pharmacodynamic, and pharmacokinetic characterization of vericiguat: Results from six phase I studies in healthy subjects. *Eur. J. Clin. Pharmacol.* **2021**, *77*, 527–537. [CrossRef] [PubMed]
54. Armstrong, P.W.; Lam, C.S.P.; Anstrom, K.J.; Ezekowitz, J.; Hernandez, A.F.; O'Connor, C.M.; Pieske, B.; Ponikowski, P.; Shah, S.J.; Solomon, S.D.; et al. Effect of Vericiguat vs Placebo on Quality of Life in Patients With Heart Failure and Preserved Ejection Fraction: The VITALITY-HFpEF Random-ized Clinical Trial. *JAMA* **2020**, *324*, 1512–1521. [CrossRef] [PubMed]
55. Cruz, L.; Ryan, J.J. Nitric oxide signaling in heart failure with preserved ejection fraction. *JACC Basic Transl. Sci.* **2017**, *2*, 341–343. [CrossRef]
56. Kassis-George, H.; Verlinden, N.J.; Fu, S.; Kanwar, M. Vericiguat in Heart Failure with a Reduced Ejection Fraction: Patient Selection and Special Considerations. *Ther. Clin. Risk Manag.* **2022**, *18*, 315–322. [CrossRef]
57. Lombardi, C.M.; Cimino, G.; Pagnesi, M.; Dell'Aquila, A.; Tomasoni, D.; Ravera, A.; Inciardi, R.; Carubelli, V.; Vizzardi, E.; Nodari, S.; et al. Vericiguat for Heart Failure with Reduced Ejection Fraction. *Curr. Cardiol. Rep.* **2021**, *23*, 144. [CrossRef]
58. Teerlink, J.R.; Diaz, R.; Felker, G.M.; McMurray, J.J.V.; Metra, M.; Solomon, S.D.; Adams, K.F.; Anand, I.; Arias-Mendoza, A.; Biering-Sørensen, T.; et al. Cardiac Myosin Activation with Omecamtiv Mecarbil in Systolic Heart Failure. *N. Engl. J. Med.* **2021**, *384*, 105–116. [CrossRef]
59. Teerlink, J.R.; Diaz, R.; Felker, G.M.; McMurray, J.J.V.; Metra, M.; Solomon, S.D.; Biering-Sørensen, T.; Böhm, M.; Bonder-man, D.; Fang, J.C.; et al. Effect of ejection fraction on clinical outcomes in patients treated with omecamtiv mecarbil in GALACTIC-HF. *J. Am. Coll. Cardiol.* **2021**, *78*, 97–108. [CrossRef]
60. Writing Committee Members; Yancy, C.W.; Jessup, M.; Bozkurt, B.; Butler, J.; Casey, D.E.; Colvin, M.M.; Drazner, M.H.; Filippatos, G.; Fonarow, G.C.; et al. 2016 ACC/AHA/HFSA focused update on new pharmacological therapy for heart failure: An update of the 2013 ACCF/AHA guideline for the management of heart failure: A report of the american college of cardiology/american heart association task force on clinical practice guidelines and the heart failure society of America. *Circulation* **2016**, *134*, e282–e293.
61. Kramer, D.G.; Trikalinos, T.A.; Kent, D.M.; Antonopoulos, G.V.; Konstam, M.A.; Udelson, J.E. Quantitative evaluation of drug or device effects on ventricular remodeling as predictors of therapeutic effects on mortality in patients with heart failure and reduced ejection fraction: A meta-analytic approach. *J. Am. Coll. Cardiol.* **2010**, *56*, 392–406. [CrossRef] [PubMed]
62. Psotka, M.A.; Teerlink, J.R. Direct Myosin Activation by Omecamtiv Mecarbil for Heart Failure with Reduced Ejection Frac-tion. *Handb. Exp. Pharmacol.* **2017**, *243*, 465–490. [PubMed]
63. Malik, F.I.; Hartman, J.J.; Elias, K.A.; Morgan, B.P.; Rodriguez, H.; Brejc, K.; Anderson, R.L.; Sueoka, S.H.; Lee, K.H.; Finer, J.T.; et al. Cardiac myosin activation: A potential therapeutic approach for systolic heart failure. *Science* **2011**, *331*, 1439–1443. [CrossRef] [PubMed]
64. Ahmad, T.; Miller, P.E.; McCullough, M.; Desai, N.R.; Riello, R.; Psotka, M.; Böhm, M.; Allen, L.A.; Teerlink, J.R.; Rosano, G.M.C.; et al. Why has positive inotropy failed in chronic heart failure? Lessons from prior inotrope trials. *Eur. J. Heart Fail.* **2019**, *21*, 1064–1078. [CrossRef]
65. Teerlink, J.R.; Felker, G.M.; McMurray, J.J.V.; Solomon, S.D.; Adams, K.F.; Cleland, J.G.F.; Ezekowitz, J.A.; Goudev, A.; Macdonald, P.; Metra, M.; et al. Chronic Oral Study of Myosin Activation to Increase Contractility in Heart Failure (COSMIC-HF): A phase 2, pharmacokinetic, randomised, placebo-controlled trial. *Lancet* **2016**, *388*, 2895–2903. [CrossRef]
66. Biering-Sorensen, T.; Teerlink, J.; Felker, G.M.; McMurray, J.; Malik, F.; Honarpour, N.; Monsalvo, M.L.; Johnston, J.; Solomon, S.D. The cardiac myosin activator, omecamtiv mecarbil, improves left ventricular myocardial deformation in chronic heart failure (cosmic-hf). *J. Am. Coll. Cardiol.* **2017**, *69*, 858. [CrossRef]
67. Teerlink, J.R.; Diaz, R.; Felker, G.M.; McMurray, J.J.V.; Metra, M.; Solomon, S.D.; Legg, J.C.; Büchele, G.; Varin, C.; Kurtz, C.E.; et al. Omecamtiv Mecarbil in Chronic Heart Failure With Reduced Ejection Fraction: Rationale and Design of GALACTIC-HF. *JACC Heart Fail.* **2020**, *8*, 329–340. [CrossRef]

68. Teerlink, J.R.; Diaz, R.; Felker, G.M.; McMurray, J.J.V.; Metra, M.; Solomon, S.D.; Adams, K.F.; Anand, I.; Arias-Mendoza, A.; Biering-Sørensen, T.; et al. Omecamtiv mecarbil in chronic heart failure with reduced ejection fraction: GALACTIC-HF baseline characteristics and comparison with contemporary clinical trials. *Eur. J. Heart Fail.* **2020**, *22*, 2160–2171. [CrossRef]
69. Date, Y.; Kojima, M.; Hosoda, H.; Sawaguchi, A.; Mondal, M.S.; Suganuma, T.; Matsukura, S.; Kangawa, K.; Nakazato, M. Ghrelin, a novel growth hor-mone-releasing acylated peptide, is synthesized in a distinct endocrine cell type in the gastrointestinal tracts of rats and humans. *Endocrinology* **2000**, *141*, 4255–4261. [CrossRef]
70. Kojima, M.; Kangawa, K. Ghrelin: Structure and function. *Physiol. Rev.* **2005**, *85*, 495–522. [CrossRef]
71. Nagaya, N.; Uematsu, M.; Kojima, M.; Ikeda, Y.; Yoshihara, F.; Shimizu, W.; Hosoda, H.; Hirota, Y.; Ishida, H.; Mori, H.; et al. Chronic administration of ghrelin improves left ventricular dysfunction and attenuates development of cardiac cachexia in rats with heart failure. *Circulation* **2001**, *104*, 1430–1435. [CrossRef] [PubMed]
72. Chang, L.; Ren, Y.; Liu, X.; Li, W.G.; Yang, J.; Geng, B.; Weintraub, N.L.; Tang, C. Protective effects of ghrelin on ischemia/reperfusion injury in the isolated rat heart. *J. Cardiovasc. Pharmacol.* **2004**, *43*, 165–170. [CrossRef] [PubMed]
73. Ledderose, C.; Kreth, S.; Beiras-Fernandez, A. Ghrelin, a novel peptide hormone in the regulation of energy balance and cardiovascular function. *Recent. Pat. Endocr. Metab. Immune Drug Discov.* **2011**, *5*, 1–6. [CrossRef]
74. Gupta, S.; Mitra, A. Heal the heart through gut (hormone) ghrelin: A potential player to combat heart failure. *Heart Fail. Rev.* **2021**, *26*, 417–435. [CrossRef] [PubMed]
75. Nagaya, N.; Miyatake, K.; Uematsu, M.; Oya, H.; Shimizu, W.; Hosoda, H.; Kojima, M.; Nakanishi, N.; Mori, H.; Kangawa, K. Hemodynamic, renal, and hormonal effects of ghrelin infusion in patients with chronic heart failure. *J. Clin. Endocrinol. Metab.* **2001**, *86*, 5854–5859. [CrossRef]
76. Nagaya, N.; Moriya, J.; Yasumura, Y.; Uematsu, M.; Ono, F.; Shimizu, W.; Ueno, K.; Kitakaze, M.; Miyatake, K.; Kangawa, K. Effects of ghrelin administration on left ventricular function, exercise capacity, and muscle wasting in patients with chronic heart failure. *Circulation* **2004**, *110*, 3674–3679. [CrossRef]
77. Yuan, M.-J.; Li, W.; Zhong, P. Research progress of ghrelin on cardiovascular disease. *Biosci. Rep.* **2021**, *41*, BSR20203387. [CrossRef]
78. Sobowale, C.O.; Hori, Y.; Ajijola, O.A. Neuromodulation therapy in heart failure: Combined use of drugs and devices. *J. Innov. Cardiac. Rhythm Manag.* **2020**, *11*, 4151–4159. [CrossRef]
79. Elsevier Health Sciences. *Guyton and Hall Textbook of Medical Physiology E-Book*; Hall, J.E., Hall, M.E., Eds.; Elsevier Health Sciences: Amsterdam, The Netherlands, 2020.
80. Krahl, S.E.; Clark, K.B. Vagus nerve stimulation for epilepsy: A review of central mechanisms. *Surg. Neurol. Int.* **2012**, *3* (Suppl. S4), S255–S259. [CrossRef]
81. Florea, V.G.; Cohn, J.N. The autonomic nervous system and heart failure. *Circ. Res.* **2014**, *114*, 1815–1826. [CrossRef]
82. Bylund, D.B.; Eikenberg, D.C.; Hieble, J.P.; Langer, S.Z.; Lefkowitz, R.J.; Minneman, K.P.; Molinoff, P.B.; Ruffolo, R.R.; Trendelenburg, U. International Union of Pharmacology nomenclature of adrenoceptors. *Pharmacol. Rev.* **1994**, *46*, 121–136. [PubMed]
83. Port, J.D.; Bristow, M.R. Altered beta-adrenergic receptor gene regulation and signaling in chronic heart failure. *J. Mol. Cell Cardiol.* **2001**, *33*, 887–905. [CrossRef] [PubMed]
84. Patel, H.C.; Rosen, S.D.; Lindsay, A.; Hayward, C.; Lyon, A.R.; di Mario, C. Targeting the autonomic nervous system: Measuring autonomic function and novel devices for heart failure management. *Int. J. Cardiol.* **2013**, *170*, 107–117. [CrossRef] [PubMed]
85. Orso, F.; Fabbri, G.; Maggioni, A.P. Epidemiology of heart failure. *Handb. Exp. Pharmacol.* **2017**, *243*, 15–33.
86. Triposkiadis, F.; Karayannis, G.; Giamouzis, G.; Skoularigis, J.; Louridas, G.; Butler, J. The sympathetic nervous system in heart failure physiology, pathophysiology, and clinical implications. *J. Am. Coll. Cardiol.* **2009**, *54*, 1747–1762. [CrossRef]
87. Olshansky, B.; Sabbah, H.N.; Hauptman, P.J.; Colucci, W.S. Parasympathetic nervous system and heart failure: Patho-physiology and potential implications for therapy. *Circulation* **2008**, *118*, 863–871. [CrossRef]
88. Bibevski, S.; Dunlap, M.E. Evidence for impaired vagus nerve activity in heart failure. *Heart Fail. Rev.* **2011**, *16*, 129–135. [CrossRef]
89. Motte, S.; Mathieu, M.; Brimioulle, S.; Pensis, A.; Ray, L.; Ketelslegers, J.-M.; Montano, N.; Naeije, R.; van de Borne, P.; Entee, K.M. Respiratory-related heart rate variability in progressive experimental heart failure. *Am. J. Physiol. Heart Circ. Physiol.* **2005**, *289*, H1729–H1735. [CrossRef]
90. Buckley, U.; Yamakawa, K.; Takamiya, T.; Andrew Armour, J.; Shivkumar, K.; Ardell, J.L. Targeted stellate decentralization: Implications for sympathetic control of ventricular electrophysiology. *Heart Rhythm.* **2016**, *13*, 282–288. [CrossRef]
91. Witt, C.M.; Bolona, L.; Kinney, M.O.; Moir, C.; Ackerman, M.J.; Kapa, S.; Asirvatham, S.J.; McLeod, C.J. Denervation of the extrinsic cardiac sympathetic nervous system as a treatment modality for arrhythmia. *Europace* **2017**, *19*, 1075–1083. [CrossRef]
92. Vaseghi, M.; Barwad, P.; Malavassi Corrales, F.J.; Tandri, H.; Mathuria, N.; Shah, R.; Sorg, J.M.; Gima, J.; Mandal, K.; Sàenz Morales, L.C.; et al. Cardiac sympathetic denervation for refractory ventricular arrhythmias. *J. Am. Coll. Cardiol.* **2017**, *69*, 3070–3080. [CrossRef] [PubMed]
93. Schneider, H.E.; Steinmetz, M.; Krause, U.; Kriebel, T.; Ruschewski, W.; Paul, T. Left cardiac sympathetic denervation for the management of life-threatening ventricular tachyarrhythmias in young patients with catecholaminergic polymorphic ven-tricular tachycardia and long QT syndrome. *Clin. Res. Cardiol.* **2013**, *102*, 33–42. [CrossRef] [PubMed]
94. Shah, R.; Assis, F.; Alugubelli, N.; Okada, D.R.; Cardoso, R.; Shivkumar, K.; Tandri, H. Cardiac sympathetic denervation for refractory ventricular arrhythmias in patients with structural heart disease: A systematic review. *Heart Rhythm.* **2019**, *16*, 1499–1505. [CrossRef] [PubMed]

95. Hofferberth, S.C.; Cecchin, F.; Loberman, D.; Fynn-Thompson, F. Left thoracoscopic sympathectomy for cardiac denervation in patients with life-threatening ventricular arrhythmias. *J. Thorac. Cardiovasc. Surg.* 2014, *147*, 404–409. [CrossRef]
96. Schwartz, P.J. Cardiac sympathetic denervation to prevent life-threatening arrhythmias. *Nat. Rev. Cardiol.* 2014, *11*, 346–353. [CrossRef]
97. Schirmer, S.H.; Sayed, M.M.Y.A.; Reil, J.-C.; Ukena, C.; Linz, D.; Kindermann, M.; Laufs, U.; Mahfoud, F.; Böhm, M. Improvements in left ventricular hypertrophy and diastolic function following renal denervation: Effects beyond blood pressure and heart rate reduction. *J. Am. Coll. Cardiol.* 2014, *63*, 1916–1923. [CrossRef]
98. Chen, W.; Ling, Z.; Xu, Y.; Liu, Z.; Su, L.; Du, H.; Xiao, P.; Lan, X.; Shan, Q.; Yin, Y. Preliminary effects of renal denervation with saline irrigated catheter on cardiac systolic function in patients with heart failure: A Prospective, Randomized, Controlled, Pilot Study. *Catheter. Cardiovasc. Interv.* 2017, *89*, E153–E161. [CrossRef]
99. Schiller, A.M.; Haack, K.K.V.; Pellegrino, P.R.; Curry, P.L.; Zucker, I.H. Unilateral renal denervation improves autonomic balance in conscious rabbits with chronic heart failure. *Am. J. Physiol. Regul. Integr. Comp. Physiol.* 2013, *305*, R886–R892. [CrossRef]
100. Akinseye, O.A.; Ralston, W.F.; Johnson, K.C.; Ketron, L.L.; Womack, C.R.; Ibebuogu, U.N. Renal sympathetic denervation: A comprehensive review. *Curr. Probl. Cardiol.* 2021, *46*, 100598. [CrossRef]
101. Davies, J.E.; Manisty, C.H.; Petraco, R.; Barron, A.J.; Unsworth, B.; Mayet, J.; Hamady, M.; Hughes, A.D.; Sever, P.S.; Sobotka, P.A.; et al. First-in-man safety evaluation of renal denervation for chronic systolic heart failure: Primary outcome from REACH-Pilot study. *Int. J. Cardiol.* 2013, *162*, 189–192. [CrossRef]
102. Xia, Z.; Han, L.; Pellegrino, P.R.; Schiller, A.M.; Harrold, L.D.; Lobato, R.L.; Lisco, S.J.; Zucker, I.H.; Wang, H.-J. Safety and efficacy of renal denervation in patients with heart failure with reduced ejection fraction (HFrEF): A systematic review and meta-analysis. *Heliyon* 2022, *8*, e08847. [CrossRef] [PubMed]
103. Pavlov, V.A.; Tracey, K.J. The vagus nerve and the inflammatory reflex–linking immunity and metabolism. *Nat. Rev. Endo-crinol.* 2012, *8*, 743–754. [CrossRef] [PubMed]
104. Kittipibul, V.; Fudim, M. Tackling inflammation in heart failure with preserved ejection fraction: Resurrection of vagus nerve stimulation? *J. Am. Heart Assoc.* 2022, *11*, e024481. [CrossRef] [PubMed]
105. Schwartz, P.J.; De Ferrari, G.M.; Sanzo, A.; Landolina, M.; Rordorf, R.; Raineri, C.; Campana, C.; Revera, M.; Ajmone-Marsan, N.; Tavazzi, L.; et al. Long term vagal stimulation in patients with advanced heart failure: First experience in man. *Eur. J. Heart Fail.* 2008, *10*, 884–891. [CrossRef]
106. Zannad, F.; De Ferrari, G.M.; Tuinenburg, A.E.; Wright, D.; Brugada, J.; Butter, C.; Klein, H.; Stolen, C.; Meyer, S.; Stein, K.M.; et al. Chronic vagal stimulation for the treatment of low ejection fraction heart failure: Results of the NEural Cardiac TherApy foR Heart Failure (NECTAR-HF) randomized controlled trial. *Eur. Heart J.* 2015, *36*, 425–433. [CrossRef] [PubMed]
107. Gold, M.R.; Van Veldhuisen, D.J.; Hauptman, P.J.; Borggrefe, M.; Kubo, S.H.; Lieberman, R.A.; Milasinovic, G.; Berman, B.J.; Djordjevic, S.; Neelagaru, S.; et al. Vagus Nerve Stimulation for the Treatment of Heart Failure: The INOVATE-HF Trial. *J. Am. Coll. Cardiol.* 2016, *68*, 149–158. [CrossRef]
108. Premchand, R.K.; Sharma, K.; Mittal, S.; Monteiro, R.; Dixit, S.; Libbus, I.; DiCarlo, L.A.; Ardell, J.L.; Rector, T.S.; Amurthur, B.; et al. Autonomic regulation therapy via left or right cervical vagus nerve stimulation in patients with chronic heart failure: Results of the ANTHEM-HF trial. *J. Card. Fail.* 2014, *20*, 808–816. [CrossRef]
109. Fudim, M.; Abraham, W.T.; von Bardeleben, R.S.; Lindenfeld, J.; Ponikowski, P.P.; Salah, H.M.; Khan, M.S.; Sievert, H.; Stone, G.W.; Anker, S.D.; et al. Device Therapy in Chronic Heart Failure: JACC State-of-the-Art Review. *J. Am. Coll. Cardiol.* 2021, *78*, 931–956. [CrossRef]
110. Akdemir, B.; Benditt, D.G. Vagus nerve stimulation: An evolving adjunctive treatment for cardiac disease. *Anatol. J. Cardiol.* 2016, *16*, 804–810. [CrossRef]
111. Deuchars, S.A.; Lall, V.K.; Clancy, J.; Mahadi, M.; Murray, A.; Peers, L.; Deuchars, J. Mechanisms underpinning sympathetic nervous activity and its modulation using transcutaneous vagus nerve stimulation. *Exp. Physiol.* 2018, *103*, 326–331. [CrossRef]
112. Zhou, L.; Filiberti, A.; Humphrey, M.B.; Fleming, C.D.; Scherlag, B.J.; Po, S.S.; Stavrakis, S. Low-level transcutaneous vagus nerve stimulation attenuates cardiac remodelling in a rat model of heart failure with preserved ejection fraction. *Exp. Physiol.* 2019, *104*, 28–38. [CrossRef] [PubMed]
113. Tran, N.; Asad, Z.; Elkholey, K.; Scherlag, B.J.; Po, S.S.; Stavrakis, S. Autonomic neuromodulation acutely ameliorates left ventricular strain in humans. *J. Cardiovasc. Transl. Res.* 2019, *12*, 221–230. [CrossRef] [PubMed]
114. Dasari, T.W.; Gabor, F.; Csipo, T.; Palacios, F.S.; Yabluchanskiy, A.; Samannan, R.; Po, S. Non-invasive Neuromodulation of Vagus Activity Improves Endothelial Function in Patients with Heart Failure with Reduced Ejection Fraction: A Randomized Study. *J Card. Fail.* 2018, *24*, S59–S60. [CrossRef]
115. Abi-Samra, F.; Gutterman, D. Cardiac contractility modulation: A novel approach for the treatment of heart failure. *Heart Fail. Rev.* 2016, *21*, 645–660. [CrossRef] [PubMed]
116. Patel, P.A.; Nadarajah, R.; Ali, N.; Gierula, J.; Witte, K.K. Cardiac contractility modulation for the treatment of heart failure with reduced ejection fraction. *Heart Fail. Rev.* 2021, *26*, 217–226. [CrossRef] [PubMed]
117. Chinyere, I.R.; Balakrishnan, M.; Hutchinson, M.D. The emerging role of cardiac contractility modulation in heart failure treatment. *Curr. Opin. Cardiol.* 2022, *37*, 30–35. [CrossRef]
118. Pappone, C.; Augello, G.; Rosanio, S.; Vicedomini, G.; Santinelli, V.; Romano, M.; Agricola, E.; Maggi, F.; Buchmayr, G.; Moretti, G.; et al. First human chronic experience with cardiac contractility modulation by nonexcitatory electrical currents for treating

systolic heart failure: Mid-term safety and efficacy results from a multicenter study. *J. Cardiovasc. Electrophysiol.* **2004**, *15*, 418–427. [CrossRef]
119. Stix, G.; Borggrefe, M.; Wolpert, C.; Hindricks, G.; Kottkamp, H.; Böcker, D.; Wichter, T.; Mika, Y.; Ben-Haim, S.; Burkhoff, D.; et al. Chronic electrical stimulation during the absolute refractory period of the myocardium improves severe heart failure. *Eur. Heart J.* **2004**, *25*, 650–655. [CrossRef]
120. Borggrefe, M.M.; Lawo, T.; Butter, C.; Schmidinger, H.; Lunati, M.; Pieske, B.; Misier, A.R.; Curnis, A.; Böcker, D.; Remppis, A.; et al. Randomized, double blind study of non-excitatory, cardiac contractility modulation electrical impulses for symptomatic heart failure. *Eur. Heart J.* **2008**, *29*, 1019–1028. [CrossRef]
121. Kadish, A.; Nademanee, K.; Volosin, K.; Krueger, S.; Neelagaru, S.; Raval, N.; Obel, O.; Weiner, S.; Wish, M.; Carson, P.; et al. A randomized controlled trial evaluating the safety and efficacy of cardiac contractility modulation in advanced heart failure. *Am. Heart J.* **2011**, *161*, 329–337.e1. [CrossRef]
122. Abraham, W.T.; Kuck, K.-H.; Goldsmith, R.L.; Lindenfeld, J.; Reddy, V.Y.; Carson, P.E.; Mann, D.L.; Saville, B.; Parise, H.; Chan, R.; et al. A randomized controlled trial to evaluate the safety and efficacy of cardiac contractility modulation. *JACC Heart Fail.* **2018**, *6*, 874–883. [CrossRef] [PubMed]
123. Chatterjee, N.A.; Singh, J.P. Novel interventional therapies to modulate the autonomic tone in heart failure. *JACC Heart Fail.* **2015**, *3*, 786–802. [CrossRef]
124. Iliescu, R.; Tudorancea, I.; Lohmeier, T.E. Baroreflex activation: From mechanisms to therapy for cardiovascular disease. *Curr. Hypertens. Rep.* **2014**, *16*, 453. [CrossRef] [PubMed]
125. Buckley, U.; Shivkumar, K.; Ardell, J.L. Autonomic regulation therapy in heart failure. *Curr Heart Fail Rep.* **2015**, *12*, 284–293. [CrossRef] [PubMed]
126. Gronda, E.; Seravalle, G.; Brambilla, G.; Costantino, G.; Casini, A.; Alsheraei, A.; Lovett, E.G.; Mancia, G.; Grassi, G. Chronic baroreflex activation effects on sympathetic nerve traffic, baroreflex function, and cardiac haemodynamics in heart failure: A proof-of-concept study. *Eur. J. Heart Fail.* **2014**, *16*, 977–983. [CrossRef] [PubMed]
127. Zile, M.R.; Lindenfeld, J.; Weaver, F.A.; Zannad, F.; Galle, E.; Rogers, T.; Abraham, W.T. Baroreflex activation therapy in patients with heart failure with reduced ejection fraction. *J. Am. Coll. Cardiol.* **2020**, *76*, 1–13. [CrossRef] [PubMed]
128. Obokata, M.; Olson, T.P.; Reddy, Y.N.V.; Melenovsky, V.; Kane, G.C.; Borlaug, B.A. Haemodynamics, dyspnoea, and pulmonary reserve in heart failure with preserved ejection fraction. *Eur. Heart J.* **2018**, *39*, 2810–2821. [CrossRef]
129. Reddy, Y.N.V.; Olson, T.P.; Obokata, M.; Melenovsky, V.; Borlaug, B.A. Hemodynamic correlates and diagnostic role of cardiopulmonary exercise testing in heart failure with preserved ejection fraction. *JACC Heart Fail.* **2018**, *6*, 665–675. [CrossRef]
130. Dorfs, S.; Zeh, W.; Hochholzer, W.; Jander, N.; Kienzle, R.-P.; Pieske, B.; Neumann, F.J. Pulmonary capillary wedge pressure during exercise and long-term mortality in patients with suspected heart failure with preserved ejection fraction. *Eur. Heart J.* **2014**, *35*, 3103–3112. [CrossRef]
131. Fudim, M.; Khan, M.S.; Paracha, A.A.; Sunagawa, K.; Burkhoff, D. Targeting preload in heart failure: Splanchnic nerve blockade and beyond. *Circ. Heart Fail.* **2022**, *15*, e009340. [CrossRef]
132. Fudim, M.; Ponikowski, P.P.; Burkhoff, D.; Dunlap, M.E.; Sobotka, P.A.; Molinger, J.; Patel, M.R.; Felker, G.M.; Hernandez, A.F.; Litwin, S.E.; et al. Splanchnic nerve modulation in heart failure: Mechanistic overview, initial clinical experience, and safety considerations. *Eur. J. Heart Fail.* **2021**, *23*, 1076–1084. [CrossRef] [PubMed]
133. Burkhoff, D.; Tyberg, J.V. Why does pulmonary venous pressure rise after onset of LV dysfunction: A theoretical analysis. *Am. J. Physiol.* **1993**, *265 Pt 2*, H1819–H1828. [CrossRef]
134. Fudim, M.; Patel, M.R.; Boortz-Marx, R.; Borlaug, B.A.; DeVore, A.D.; Ganesh, A.; Green, C.L.; Lopes, R.D.; Mentz, R.J.; Patel, C.B.; et al. Splanchnic nerve block mediated changes in stressed blood volume in heart failure. *JACC Heart Fail.* **2021**, *9*, 293–300. [CrossRef]
135. Fudim, M.; Ganesh, A.; Green, C.; Jones, W.S.; Blazing, M.A.; Devore, A.D.; Felker, G.M.; Kiefer, T.L.; Kong, D.F.; Boortz-Marx, R.L.; et al. Splanchnic nerve block for decompensated chronic heart failure: Splanchnic-HF. *Eur. Hear. J.* **2018**, *39*, 4255–4256. [CrossRef] [PubMed]
136. Fudim, M.; Jones, W.S.; Boortz-Marx, R.L.; Ganesh, A.; Green, C.L.; Hernandez, A.F.; Patel, M.R. Splanchnic nerve block for acute heart failure. *Circulation* **2018**, *138*, 951–953. [CrossRef] [PubMed]
137. Gajewski, P.; Fudim, M.; Kittipibul, V.; Engelman, Z.J.; Biegus, J.; Zymliński, R.; Ponikowski, P. Early Hemodynamic Changes following Surgical Ablation of the Right Greater Splanchnic Nerve for the Treatment of Heart Failure with Preserved Ejection Fraction. *J. Clin. Med.* **2022**, *11*, 1063. [CrossRef] [PubMed]
138. Fudim, M.; Engelman, Z.J.; Reddy, V.Y.; Shah, S.J. Splanchnic nerve ablation for volume management in heart failure. *JACC Basic Transl. Sci.* **2022**, *7*, 319–321. [CrossRef]
139. Fudim, M.; Fail, P.S.; Litwin, S.E.; Shaburishvili, T.; Goyal, P.; Hummel, S.; Borlaug, B.A.; Mohan, R.C.; Patel, R.B.; Mitter, S.S.; et al. Endovascular Ablation of the Right Greater Splanchnic Nerve in Heart Failure with Preserved Ejection Fraction: Early Results of the REBALANCE-HF Trial Roll-in Cohort. *Eur. J. Heart Fail.* **2022**, *24*, 1410–1414. [CrossRef]
140. Sorimachi, H.; Burkhoff, D.; Verbrugge, F.H.; Omote, K.; Obokata, M.; Reddy, Y.N.V.; Takahashi, N.; Sunagawa, K.; Borlaug, B.A. Obesity, venous capacitance, and venous compliance in heart failure with preserved ejection fraction. *Eur. J. Heart Fail.* **2021**, *23*, 1648–1658. [CrossRef]

141. Costanzo, M.R.; Ponikowski, P.; Coats, A.; Javaheri, S.; Augostini, R.; Goldberg, L.R.; Holcomb, R.; Kao, A.; Khayat, R.N.; Oldenburg, O.; et al. Phrenic nerve stimulation to treat patients with central sleep apnoea and heart failure. *Eur. J. Heart Fail.* **2018**, *20*, 1746–1754. [CrossRef]
142. Fudim, M.; Mirro, M.; Goldberg, L.R. Synchronized diaphragmatic stimulation for the treatment of symptomatic heart failure: A novel implantable therapy concept. *JACC Basic Transl. Sci.* **2022**, *7*, 322–323. [CrossRef] [PubMed]
143. Costanzo, M.R.; Ponikowski, P.; Javaheri, S.; Augostini, R.; Goldberg, L.; Holcomb, R.; Kao, A.; Khayat, R.N.; Oldenburg, O.; Stellbrink, C.; et al. Transvenous neurostimulation for central sleep apnoea: A randomised controlled trial. *Lancet* **2016**, *388*, 974–982. [CrossRef]
144. Costanzo, M.R.; Javaheri, S.; Ponikowski, P.; Oldenburg, O.; Augostini, R.; Goldberg, L.R.; Stellbrink, C.; Fox, H.; Schwartz, A.R.; Gupta, S.; et al. Transvenous Phrenic Nerve Stimulation for Treatment of Central Sleep Apnea: Five-Year Safety and Efficacy Outcomes. *Nat. Sci. Sleep* **2021**, *13*, 515–526. [CrossRef] [PubMed]
145. Guzik, M.; Urban, S.; Iwanek, G.; Biegus, J.; Ponikowski, P.; Zymliński, R. Novel therapeutic devices in heart failure. *J. Clin. Med.* **2022**, *11*, 4303. [CrossRef] [PubMed]
146. Beeler, R.; Schoenenberger, A.W.; Bauer, P.; Kobza, R.; Bergner, M.; Mueller, X.; Schlaepfer, R.; Zuber, M.; Erne, S.; Erne, P. Improvement of cardiac function with device-based diaphragmatic stimulation in chronic heart failure patients: The randomized, open-label, crossover Epiphrenic II Pilot Trial. *Eur. J. Heart Fail.* **2014**, *16*, 342–349. [CrossRef]
147. Cleland, J.G.F.; Young, R.; Jorbenadze, A.; Shaburishvili, T.; Demyanchuk, V.; Buriak, R.; Todurov, B.; Rudenko, K.; Zuber, M.; Stämpfli, S.F.; et al. A First in Human Mul-ti-center, Open Label, Prospective Study to Evaluate Safety, Usability and Performance of the VisONE System for Heart Failure with a Reduced Left Ventricular Ejection Fraction. *J. Card. Fail.* **2020**, *26*, S64. [CrossRef]
148. Biegus, J.; Zymlinski, R.; Siwolowski, P.; Testani, J.; Szachniewicz, J.; Tycińska, A.; Banasiak, W.; Halpert, A.; Levin, H.; Ponikowski, P. Controlled decongestion by Reprieve therapy in acute heart failure: Results of the TARGET-1 and TARGET-2 studies. *Eur. J. Heart Fail.* **2019**, *21*, 1079–1087. [CrossRef]
149. Zymliński, R.; Dierckx, R.; Biegus, J.; Vanderheyden, M.; Bartunek, J.; Ponikowski, P. Novel IVC doraya catheter provides congestion relief in patients with acute heart failure. *JACC Basic Transl. Sci.* **2022**, *7*, 326–327. [CrossRef]
150. Kapur, N.K.; Kiernan, M.S.; Gorgoshvili, I.; Yousefzai, R.; Vorovich, E.E.; Tedford, R.J.; Sauer, A.J.; Abraham, J.; Resor, C.D.; Kimmelstiel, C.D.; et al. Intermittent Occlusion of the Superior Vena Cava to Improve Hemodynamics in Patients With Acutely Decompensated Heart Failure: The VENUS-HF Early Feasibility Study. *Circ. Heart Fail.* **2022**, *15*, e008934. [CrossRef]
151. Abraham, W.T.; Jonas, M.; Dongaonkar, R.M.; Geist, B.; Ueyama, Y.; Render, K.; Youngblood, B.; Muir, W.; Hamlin, R.; Del Rio, C.L. Direct Interstitial Decongestion in an Animal Model of Acute-on-Chronic Ischemic Heart Failure. *JACC Basic Transl. Sci.* **2021**, *6*, 872–881. [CrossRef]
152. Aronson, D.; Nitzan, Y.; Petcherski, S.; Bravo, E.; Habib, M.; Burkhoff, D.; Abraham, W.T. Enhancing sweat rate using a novel device for the treatment of congestion in heart failure. *Eur. Heart J.* **2021**, *42* (Suppl. S1), ehab724–ehab1056. [CrossRef]
153. Patel, H.C.; Rosen, S.D.; Hayward, C.; Vassiliou, V.; Smith, G.C.; Wage, R.R.; Bailey, J.; Rajani, R.; Lindsay, A.C.; Pennell, D.J.; et al. Renal denervation in heart failure with preserved ejection fraction (RDT-PEF): A randomized controlled trial. *Eur. J. Heart Fail.* **2016**, *18*, 703–712. [CrossRef] [PubMed]
154. Jiang, Y.; Po, S.S.; Amil, F.; Dasari, T.W. Non-invasive Low-level Tragus Stimulation in Cardiovascular Diseases. *Arrhythm. Electrophysiol. Rev.* **2020**, *9*, 40–46. [CrossRef] [PubMed]
155. Babar, N.; Giedrimiene, D. Updates on Baroreflex Activation Therapy and Vagus Nerve Stimulation for Treatment of Heart Failure With Reduced Ejection Fraction. *Cardiol. Res.* **2022**, *13*, 11. [CrossRef]
156. Speech Analysis App Predicts Worsening Heart Failure before Symptom Onset [Internet]. Available online: https://www.escardio.org/The-ESC/Press-Office/Press-releases/Speech-analysis-app-predicts-worsening-heart-failure-before-symptom-onset (accessed on 11 June 2022).
157. Ski, C.F.; Thompson, D.R.; Brunner-La Rocca, H.-P. Putting AI at the centre of heart failure care. *ESC Heart Fail.* **2020**, *7*, 3257–3258. [CrossRef]
158. Weber, G.M. Using artificial intelligence in an intelligent way to improve efficiency of a heart failure care team. *J. Card. Fail.* **2018**, *24*, 363–364. [CrossRef]
159. Johnson, K.W.; Torres Soto, J.; Glicksberg, B.S.; Shameer, K.; Miotto, R.; Ali, M.; Ashley, E.; Dudley, J.T. Artificial intelligence in cardiology. *J. Am. Coll. Cardiol.* **2018**, *71*, 2668–2679. [CrossRef]
160. Barrett, M.; Boyne, J.; Brandts, J.; Brunner-La Rocca, H.-P.; De Maesschalck, L.; De Wit, K.; Dixon, L.; Eurlings, C.; Fitzsimons, D.; Golubnitschaja, O.; et al. Artificial intelligence sup-ported patient self-care in chronic heart failure: A paradigm shift from reactive to predictive, preventive and personalised care. *EPMA J.* **2019**, *10*, 445–464. [CrossRef] [PubMed]
161. Knackstedt, C.; Bekkers, S.C.A.M.; Schummers, G.; Schreckenberg, M.; Muraru, D.; Badano, L.P.; Franke, A.; Bavishi, C.; Omar, A.M.S.; Sengupta, P.P. Fully Automated Versus Standard Tracking of Left Ventricular Ejection Fraction and Longitudinal Strain: The FAST-EFs Multicenter Study. *J. Am. Coll. Cardiol.* **2015**, *66*, 1456–1466. [CrossRef]
162. DeCara, J.M.; Lang, R.M.; Koch, R.; Bala, R.; Penzotti, J.; Spencer, K.T. The use of small personal ultrasound devices by internists without formal training in echocardiography. *Eur. J. Echocardiogr.* **2003**, *4*, 141–147. [CrossRef]
163. Bernard, O.; Lalande, A.; Zotti, C.; Cervenansky, F.; Yang, X.; Heng, P.-A.; Cetin, I.; Lekadir, K.; Camara, O.; Gonzalez Ballester, M.A.; et al. Deep Learning Techniques for Automatic MRI Cardiac Multi-Structures Segmentation and Diagnosis: Is the Problem Solved? *IEEE Trans. Med. Imaging* **2018**, *37*, 2514–2525. [CrossRef] [PubMed]

164. Laser, K.T.; Horst, J.-P.; Barth, P.; Kelter-Klöpping, A.; Haas, N.A.; Burchert, W.; Kececioglu, D.; Körperich, H. Knowledge-based reconstruction of right ventricular volumes using real-time three-dimensional echocardiographic as well as cardiac magnetic resonance images: Comparison with a cardiac magnetic resonance standard. *J. Am. Soc. Echocardiogr.* **2014**, *27*, 1087–1097. [CrossRef] [PubMed]
165. Luo, G.; Dong, S.; Wang, K.; Zuo, W.; Cao, S.; Zhang, H. Multi-Views Fusion CNN for Left Ventricular Volumes Estimation on Cardiac MR Images. *IEEE Trans. Biomed. Eng.* **2018**, *65*, 1924–1934. [CrossRef] [PubMed]
166. Bratt, A.; Kim, J.; Pollie, M.; Beecy, A.N.; Tehrani, N.H.; Codella, N.; Perez-Johnston, R.; Palumbo, M.C.; Alakbarli, J.; Colizza, W.; et al. Machine learning derived segmentation of phase velocity encoded cardiovascular magnetic resonance for fully automated aortic flow quantification. *J. Cardiovasc. Magn. Reson.* **2019**, *21*, 1. [CrossRef]
167. Kirschbaum, S.; Aben, J.-P.; Baks, T.; Moelker, A.; Gruszczynska, K.; Krestin, G.P.; van der Giessen, W.J.; Duncker, D.J.; de Feyter, P.J.; van Geuns, R.-J.M. Accurate automatic papillary muscle identification for quantitative left ventricle mass measurements in cardiac magnetic resonance imaging. *Acad. Radiol.* **2008**, *15*, 1227–1233. [CrossRef]
168. Gao, S.; van 't Klooster, R.; Brandts, A.; Roes, S.D.; Alizadeh Dehnavi, R.; de Roos, A.; Westenberg, J.J.M.; van der Geest, R.J. Quantification of common carotid artery and descending aorta vessel wall thickness from MR vessel wall imaging using a fully automated processing pipeline. *J. Magn. Reson. Imaging.* **2017**, *45*, 215–228. [CrossRef]
169. Zreik, M.; Lessmann, N.; van Hamersvelt, R.W.; Wolterink, J.M.; Voskuil, M.; Viergever, M.A.; Leiner, T.; Išgum, I. Deep learning analysis of the myocardium in coronary CT angiography for identification of patients with functionally significant coronary artery stenosis. *Med. Image Anal.* **2018**, *44*, 72–85. [CrossRef]
170. Zolfaghar, K.; Meadem, N.; Teredesai, A.; Roy, S.B.; Chin, S.-C.; Muckian, B. Big data solutions for predicting risk-of-readmission for congestive heart failure patients. In Proceedings of the 2013 IEEE International Conference on Big Data, Santa Clara, CA, USA, 6–9 October 2013; pp. 64–71.
171. Vedomske, M.A.; Brown, D.E.; Harrison, J.H. Random Forests on Ubiquitous Data for Heart Failure 30-Day Readmissions Prediction. In Proceedings of the 2013 12th International Conference on Machine Learning and Applications, Miami, FL, USA, 4–7 December 2013; pp. 415–421.
172. Basu Roy, S.; Teredesai, A.; Zolfaghar, K.; Liu, R.; Hazel, D.; Newman, S.; Marinez, A. Dynamic Hierarchical Classification for Patient Risk-of-Readmission. In *Proceedings of the 21th ACM SIGKDD International Conference on Knowledge Discovery and Data Mining—KDD, Sydney, Australia, 10–13 August 2015*; ACM Press: New York, NY, USA, 2015; pp. 1691–1700.
173. Koulaouzidis, G.; Iakovidis, D.K.; Clark, A.L. Telemonitoring predicts in advance heart failure admissions. *Int. J. Cardiol.* **2016**, *216*, 78–84. [CrossRef]
174. Kang, Y.; McHugh, M.D.; Chittams, J.; Bowles, K.H. Utilizing home healthcare electronic health records for telehomecare patients with heart failure: A decision tree approach to detect associations with rehospitalizations. *Comput. Inform. Nurs.* **2016**, *34*, 175–182. [CrossRef]
175. Kawai, A.; Patel, H.; Kaye, D.; Nanayakkara, S. 768 Machine Learning Prediction Tools for All-Cause Readmissions in Pa-tients Hospitalised for Heart Failure Using Routinely Collected Medical Record Data. *Heart Lung Circ.* **2020**, *29*, S382. [CrossRef]
176. Palant, A.; Zippel-Schultz, B.; Brandts, J.; Eurlings, C.; Barrett, M.; Murphy, M.; Furtado Da Luz Brzychcyk, E.; Hill, L.; Dixon, L.; Fitzsimons, D.; et al. *18 Heart Failure Patient and Caregiver Needs and Expectations Regarding Self-Management via Digital Health—The Passion-HF Project*; Oral Abstract Presentations; BMJ Publishing Group Ltd and British Cardiovascular Society: London, UK, 2020; pp. A12.2–A13.
177. Beam, A.L.; Manrai, A.K.; Ghassemi, M. Challenges to the reproducibility of machine learning models in health care. *JAMA* **2020**, *323*, 305–306. [CrossRef] [PubMed]

Review

Targeting Myocardial Fibrosis—A Magic Pill in Cardiovascular Medicine?

Alina Scridon [1,*,†] and Alkora Ioana Balan [1,2,†]

1 Physiology Department, University of Medicine, Pharmacy, Science and Technology "George Emil Palade" of Târgu Mureș, 540139 Targu Mures, Romania; alkora.balan@gmail.com
2 Emergency Institute for Cardiovascular Diseases and Transplantation of Târgu Mureș, 540136 Targu Mures, Romania
* Correspondence: alinascridon@gmail.com
† These authors contributed equally to this work.

Abstract: Fibrosis, characterized by an excessive accumulation of extracellular matrix, has long been seen as an adaptive process that contributes to tissue healing and regeneration. More recently, however, cardiac fibrosis has been shown to be a central element in many cardiovascular diseases (CVDs), contributing to the alteration of cardiac electrical and mechanical functions in a wide range of clinical settings. This paper aims to provide a comprehensive review of cardiac fibrosis, with a focus on the main pathophysiological pathways involved in its onset and progression, its role in various cardiovascular conditions, and on the potential of currently available and emerging therapeutic strategies to counteract the development and/or progression of fibrosis in CVDs. We also emphasize a number of questions that remain to be answered, and we identify hotspots for future research.

Keywords: antifibrotic strategies; cardiac fibrosis; cardiovascular diseases; fibrosis pathways; therapeutic strategies

1. Introduction

Cardiovascular diseases (CVDs) are the leading cause of death and morbidity, accounting for up to one-third of deaths worldwide. The prevalence of CVDs has seen a tremendous increase over the past decades, with a doubling of CVD cases between 1990 and 2019 [1]. In parallel, cardiovascular mortality has also gradually increased during this period, from 12.1 million in 1990 to 18.6 million in 2019 [1]. Metabolic, behavioral, environmental, and social factors have all been linked to increased cardiovascular risk. Whereas several of those factors are modifiable and their removal may lower the prevalence of CVDs, others, such as age, race, sex, or family history, continue to have a significant impact on the evolution of CVDs' prevalence [1].

Initially seen as an adaptive process designed to ensure wound healing and tissue repair following injury, myocardial fibrosis is now recognized as a major contributor to CVDs and CVD-related morbidity and mortality in many clinical settings [2]. Accumulating data show that most CVDs involve pathological myocardial remodeling characterized by cardiac fibrosis. In myocardial infarction, fibrosis develops as a repair mechanism for maintaining the integrity of the cardiac wall. However, over the long term, the lack of contractile capacity of the fibrous tissue along with the death of cardiac myocytes eventually lead to impaired cardiac function [2]. In many other CVDs (e.g., hypertensive heart disease, diabetic, dilated, and hypertrophic cardiomyopathy, heart failure, chronic ischemic heart disease, or cardiac arrhythmias), fibrosis is also recognized at present as a causative or at least as an aggravating factor [2]. In addition, the natural process of aging promotes cardiac fibrosis via countless pathophysiological pathways, even in the absence of concomitant heart disease [2]. Myocardial fibrosis has thus rose as a promising diagnostic and prognostic marker in CVD patients, and strategies aiming to prevent, halt, or even reverse fibrosis have emerged as promising means to prevent and/or treat various forms of CVD.

This paper aims to provide a comprehensive view on cardiac fibrosis, with a focus on the main pathophysiological pathways involved in its occurrence and progression, its role in various cardiovascular conditions, on the techniques available for fibrosis identification and quantification, and on the potential of currently available and emerging therapeutic strategies to counteract the development and/or progression of fibrosis in CVDs.

2. The Extracellular Matrix—From Physiology to Pathophysiology

The cardiac muscle and the conduction system, supported by a fibrous skeleton, constitute the basic framework of the heart. The cardiac wall consists of three overlapped layers: the epicardium, composed of fibro-elastic and adipose tissue, the myocardium, consisting of cardiomyocytes arranged in layers and surrounded by a complex network of proteins that form the extracellular matrix (ECM), and the endocardium, made up of endothelium and subendothelial connective tissue [3]. At the level of the myocardium, the ECM works as a scaffold for cellular components and contributes to the transmission of the contractile force [4]. Tension strength is mostly provided by thick type I collagen, which accounts for ≈85% of the cardiac collagen, whereas type III collagen, present in smaller amounts (≈11%), is responsible for maintaining the elasticity of the ECM [4]. In addition to collagen, the ECM also contains elastic fibers, fibronectin, glycoproteins, glycosaminoglycans, proteoglycans, latent growth factors, and proteases [4].

2.1. Cellular Components Involved in Cardiac Fibrosis

The main cellular component involved in cardiac fibrosis is represented by the ***cardiac fibroblasts***, which are responsible for maintaining ECM integrity by regulating collagen turnover [5]. In contrast to cardiomyocytes, fibroblasts are non-excitable cells. Fibroblasts are connected, however, via gap junctions, to the neighboring cardiomyocytes, thereby contributing to optimal electrical conduction within the heart [6]. In settings favoring cardiac fibrosis, such as ischemic, hypertensive, or valvular heart disease, fibroblasts transdifferentiate into ***myofibroblasts*** (Figure 1), hybrid fibroblast/cardiomyocyte cells that express numerous ultrastructural and phenotypic characteristics of muscle cells, but not excitability [7]. Although most myofibroblasts originate in the myocardium, studies have shown that they can also have hematopoietic or endothelial origin [7]. Myofibroblasts play critical roles in both myocardial repair and fibrosis [8] and can be identified in the damaged myocardium already from the early stages of the fibrotic response by highlighting cytoplasmic actin-derived stress fibers and later α-smooth muscle actin [9]. Smooth muscle myosin heavy chain, paxillin, and tensin can also be used as myofibroblast biomarkers [10].

Monocytes and ***macrophages*** are also critical for both the initial and the chronic phase of the fibrotic response, but they also contribute to resolution of fibrosis [11]. Their ability to exert both pro- and antifibrotic effects can be explained by the large heterogeneity of these cells, which is related to the presence of several specific cell subpopulations and to their variable response to microenvironmental factors [11]. Certain monocyte and macrophage subpopulations have the ability to differentiate into myofibroblasts and to secrete numerous profibrotic cytokines (such as interleukin (IL)-1β, tumor necrosis factor (TNF)-α, and IL-6), growth factors (e.g., transforming growth factor β (TGF-β), platelet-derived growth factors (PDGFs), and fibroblast growth factors (FGFs)), and proteases, thereby participating in ECM remodeling [11]. The removal of dead cells by macrophages via phagocytosis facilitates fibroblasts growth, further contributing to myocardial fibrotic remodeling [11]. In parallel, however, monocytes and macrophages also act to eliminate profibrotic stimuli via phagocytosis of apoptotic myofibroblasts, ECM cells, and residues [11]. Due to their remarkable functional plasticity, macrophages also regulate the secretion of cytokines and growth factors in response to changes in the microenvironment [11]. Other cells of hematopoietic origin, such as the ***mast cells***, have also been shown to play important roles in the fibrotic process related to myocardial infarction and various cardiomyopathies [12].

The role of mast cells in cardiac fibrosis seems to be primarily related to their increased content in granules rich in bioactive mediators, cytokines, and growth factors, including histamine and mast cell-specific proteases tryptase and chymase [12]. Although the role of Th2 *lymphocytes* in pulmonary fibrosis has been thoroughly reviewed [13], the involvement of lymphocytes in cardiac fibrosis is much less clear. A profibrotic effect of Th17 cells has been reported in experimental myocardial fibrosis models [14], but other subsets of T lymphocytes have been shown to act as fibrosis inhibitors [15]. *Neutrophils*, the first cells that arrive at the site of a tissue injury, have also been shown to play critical roles in myocardial inflammation and consequent fibrosis. After acute myocardial infarction, neutrophils accumulate at the border between the healthy and the necrotic tissue and release inflammatory mediators and proteolytic enzymes that degrade necrotic myocardial cells and ECM residues [16]. Neutrophil persistence at the site of the injury appears to also cause, however, additional damage to viable cardiomyocytes [16]. Neutrophil inhibition one week after myocardial infarction has been shown to cause a paradoxical increase in fibroblast activity and excessive collagen deposition [17], suggesting that the moment of such a therapeutic intervention may be critical. Meanwhile, in a myocarditis animal model, neutrophil extracellular traps strongly correlated with the amount of collagen deposited and inhibition of cytokines responsible for neutrophil recruitment attenuated collagen deposition in that model [18].

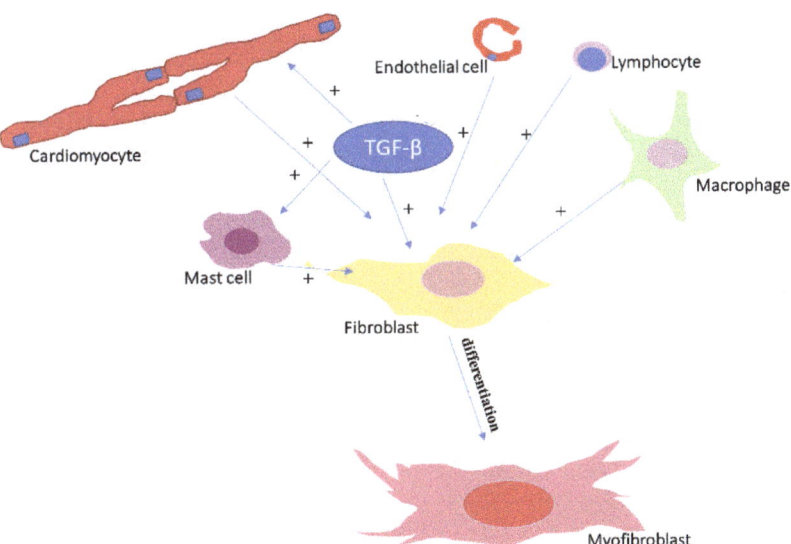

Figure 1. Interactions between different cardiac cells involved in the development of cardiac fibrosis. Cardiac cells (i.e., cardiac myocytes, macrophages, mast cells, lymphocytes, endothelial cells, and fibroblasts) regulate cardiac fibrosis in a coordinated manner. In the presence of cardiac injury, these cells release inflammatory mediators that stimulate fibroblast-to-myofibroblast differentiation, contributing to the development of fibrotic tissue. Transforming growth factor-*beta* (TGF-β) is among the most relevant of these profibrotic mediators. "+" designates a stimulatory effect.

The angiogenic response and the presence of perivascular fibrosis in settings associated with cardiac fibrosis have drawn attention toward a potential role of *endothelial cells* in cardiac remodeling and fibrosis, mainly via the secretion of endothelin, a major promotor of fibrotic matrix production, by these cells [19]. By releasing proinflammatory cytokines and chemokines, the endothelium has an important ability to recruit numerous types of fibrogenic cells [20]. In addition, endothelial cells can take, via mesenchymal transition, a mesenchymal cell phenotype, which enhances their invasiveness and migratory capacity, resistance to apoptosis, and ability to produce ECM components [7]. However, similarly to other types of cells, endothelial cells also possess antifibrotic effects via the secretion of factors such as interferon-γ-inducible protein-10/chemokine (C-X-C motif) ligand 10 and hypoxia inducible factor-1, which have been shown to protect the murine heart and the aorta from pressure overload via suppression of TGF-β signaling [21].

Cardiac myocytes can also trigger, through their death, a profibrotic inflammatory response [22]. Moreover, in certain pathological settings, even viable cardiomyocytes can promote, via pannexin-1 channels-induced ATP release, the activation of interstitial fibroblasts [23]. Deoxycorticosterone/salt-sensitive cardiomiocyte mineralocorticoid receptors have also been shown to play important roles in cardiac inflammation and fibrosis, whereas loss of these receptors has been shown to attenuate the cardiac fibrotic response [24]. Cardiomyocyte-selective TGF-β receptor II (TβRII) blockade decreased interstitial fibrosis in response to pressure overload [25], whereas cardiomyocyte-specific overexpression of angiotensin II (Ang II) type 2 receptor (AT2) was shown to exhibit antifibrotic actions mediated by the activation of the kinin–nitric oxide system [26].

2.2. Extracellular Components Involved in Cardiac Fibrosis

The accumulation of excessive amounts of fibrillar and non-fibrillar *collagen* within the myocardium represents the landmark of cardiac fibrosis [27,28]. In the remodeled heart, fibrillar collagen is represented by type I and type III collagen, the ratio between the two depending on the context that favored cardiac fibrosis development [27,28]. Cardiac myofibroblasts are the main source of cardiac collagen. Once secreted, collagen is assembled and cross-linked into a network that provides mechanical support and structural integrity to bear the increased stress and load in the presence of myocardial injury [27,28]. Non-fibrillar collagen type IV, VI, and VIII is also present in cardiac fibrosis [29]. Of these, type VI collagen has been shown to activate cardiac fibroblasts and promote myofibroblast conversion, whereas its absence has been associated with a reduction in myocardial fibrosis [29]. Other ECM components, such as amino- and proteoglycans, elastin, fibronectin, and laminin, are also present, and they play critical roles in maintaining cardiac structural integrity. Elastin provides resilience and elasticity to the cardiac wall, fibronectin fibers, organized in a fibrillar network at the cell surface, influence the structural and mechanical properties of the ECM, whereas the structural role of laminin translates into ECM cells anchoring and binding to multiple other proteins present within the matrix [4].

2.3. Types of Cardiac Fibrosis

The ability of the cardiac muscle to regenerate in response to injury is extremely low. Cardiac repair therefore occurs mainly via fibroblasts activation and differentiation into myofibroblasts, which is followed by excessive collagen deposition, fibrosis, increased ECM stiffness, and impaired cardiac contractile function [30]. Three major types of fibrotic changes have been described in the heart: replacement, interstitial, and perivascular fibrosis [30]. Replacement fibrosis is characterized by the loss and consequent fibrotic replacement of cardiac myocytes. Interstitial fibrosis includes two subtypes: reactive and infiltrative fibrosis. Reactive fibrosis occurs in response to pressure overload and is characterized by excessive ECM, without significant loss of cardiomyocytes, whereas the accumulation of insoluble proteins in the heart cells, as seen in Fabry disease, is defined as infiltrative fibrosis [30]. Finally, perivascular fibrosis involves the deposition of connective tissue around the blood vessels, as often seen in patients with hypertensive heart disease [30].

Regardless of the underlying cause, the accumulation of ECM proteins within the cardiac interstitium initially occurs as a beneficial, protective mechanism that promotes wound healing and tissue regeneration. Later, alterations in ECM composition and quality lead to fibrosis progression beyond the physiological threshold and to negative consequences on myocardial excitation–contraction coupling [31]. The distorted cardiac architecture increases ventricular stiffness and alters the contraction and relaxation of the heart, resulting in cardiac systolic and diastolic dysfunction [31]. Concomitantly, fibrosis disturbs the normal electrical activity of the heart, promoting both brady- and tachyarrhythmias [32]. Whereas conduction blocks in the sinoatrial and/or atrioventricular nodes caused by fibrosis favor bradyarrhythmias, tachyarrhythmias often occur due to the increased propensity to re-entry of the fibrotic myocardium [32].

2.4. Molecular Pathways of Myocardial Fibrosis

Extensive evidence links the activation of the *renin–angiotensin–aldosterone system* (RAAS) with the pathogenesis of cardiac fibrosis. The main effector of this system, Ang II, has a wide range of cardiac physiological and pathophysiological effects [33]. Cells present in the heart, particularly macrophages and fibroblasts, have been shown to produce both renin and the angiotensin-converting enzyme (ACE), which are required to generate Ang II. Once released, Ang II stimulates cardiac fibroblasts, directly and indirectly (via TGF-β), promoting collagen production by these cells (Figure 2) [34]. In parallel, AngII decreases the activity of matrix metalloproteinase (MMP)-1, thereby concomitantly reducing collagen degradation [33]. These profibrotic effects of Ang II occur mainly via the AT1 receptors and multiple subsequent intracellular signaling pathways [33]. Among them, the mitogen-activated protein kinase (MAPK) and the phosphoinositol-3 kinase/Akt pathways have been shown to regulate cardiac cells survival, apoptosis, and growth and to play critical roles in Ang II-induced cardiac remodeling [35,36].

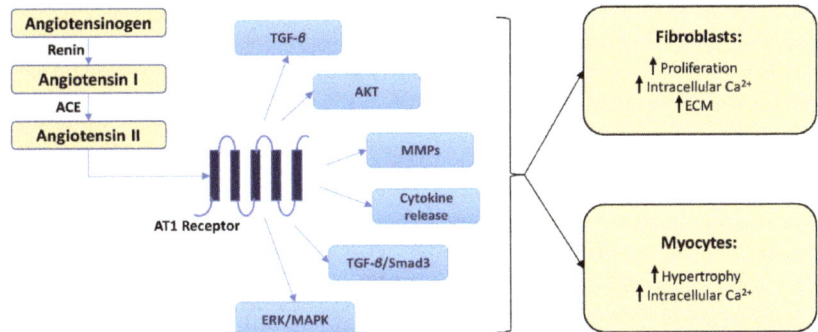

Figure 2. Pathways related to angiotensin II and their contribution to myocardial fibrosis. The figure describes the formation of angiotensin II (left part of the figure) and the consequent activation, via AT1 receptors, of numerous inflammatory and profibrotic pathways (middle part of the figure), which will eventually lead to profibrotic cardiac fibroblast and myocyte changes (right part of the figure). Myocyte hypertrophy has been shown to promote fibrosis by stimulating fibroblast activation via a complex network of downstream signal transduction pathways and by increasing the production of growth factors. "↑" designates an increase in profibrotic cardiac fibroblast and myocyte changes. ACE—angiotensin-converting enzyme; AKT—protein kinase B; AT1—angiotensin II type 1 receptor; ECM—extracellular matrix; ERK—extracellular signal-regulated kinase; MAPK—mitogen-activated protein kinase; MMPs—matrix metalloproteinases; TAK1—TGF-β-activated kinase 1; TGF-β—transforming growth factor-*beta*.

In contrast, AT2 receptor stimulation counteracts the profibrotic effects of AT1 by suppressing fibroblast proliferation and matrix synthesis [37]. Another component of the RAAS system, aldosterone, also contributes to excessive ECM accumulation by activating macrophages, cardiac myocytes and fibroblasts and increasing the expression of proinflammatory cytokines and chemokines [38].

G protein-coupled receptors (GPCRs) are cellular receptors that activate G-protein-dependent intracellular signaling pathways [39]. In parallel, several GPCR kinase- and β-arrestin2-mediated processes act as regulatory mechanisms to prevent excessive G protein activation (Figure 3) [39].

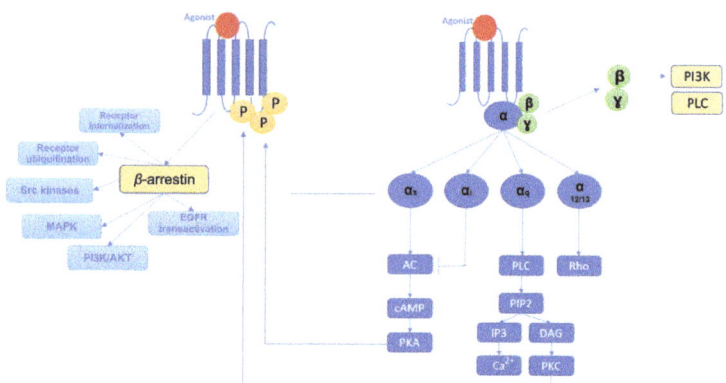

Figure 3. G protein-coupled receptors-related pathways and β-arrestin-mediated events. G-protein coupled receptors are transmembrane proteins embedded in the membrane of cardiomyocytes, fibroblasts, endothelial, and vascular smooth muscle cells that convert extracellular signals into intracellular responses. When activated by agonists (e.g., epinephrine, peptide hormones), inactive G protein heterotrimers dissociate into separate, active Gα and Gβγ subunits that differentially control downstream signal transduction. Intracellular mediators such as protein kinases A and C resulted from this process further phosphorylate the receptors and activate β-arrestin-mediated signaling, activating subsequent signaling cascades involved in cardiac fibrotic disease. AC—adenylyl cyclase; AKT—protein kinase B; cAMP—cyclic adenosine monophosphate; DAG—diacylglycerol; EGFR—epidermal growth factor receptor; IP3—inositol trisphosphate; MAPK—mitogen-activated protein kinase; PI3K—phosphoinositide 3-kinase; PIP2—phosphatidylinositol-4,5-bisphosphate; PKA—protein kinase A; PLC—phospholipase C; PKC—protein kinase C.

Several 'biased ligands' can activate signaling pathways independent of the G proteins but dependent on GPCR kinase/β-arrestin2 [39]. One such 'biased ligand' is metoprolol, which can therefore promote cardiac fibrosis and alter the cardiac diastolic function [39]. *Beta*-adrenergic receptors (βARs) are the predominant GPCR subtype expressed within the heart [40]. In physiological conditions, β1ARs represent ≈80% of the total cardiac βARs. However, in the setting of heart failure, β1ARs percentage can decrease to as low as 60%, with a concomitant increase in the proportion of β2ARs, whereas β3ARs are present in the heart in much smaller amounts [40]. Excessive β1ARs stimulation has been linked with myocyte apoptosis [40]. Meanwhile, the role of β2ARs in this setting remains controversial. Some studies suggested that β2Ars-mediated signaling could be cardioprotective [40], but in others, non-specific βARs stimulation with isoproterenol and transgenic overexpression of β2ARs were highly profibrotic [41,42], leaving this topic an open area for future research. The role of β3AR in cardiac fibrosis remains even less understood, although recent studies suggest that β3AR-mediated signaling could modulate oxidative stress-dependent paracrine signaling and consequently exhibit antifibrotic effects [43].

Endothelin-1 (ET-1), a protein synthesized by the vascular endothelium, has also been shown to play key roles in cardiac remodeling and dysfunction by promoting ECM synthesis and decreasing collagenase activity [44]. In addition, in vitro studies have shown that ET-1 increases fibroblasts' resistance to apoptosis [45], whereas ET-1 antagonization has been shown to attenuate cardiac fibrosis related to hypertension and myocardial infarction [46].

Immediately after myocardial injury, inflammatory cells, fibroblasts, and cardiomyocytes release a vast amount of cytokines and growth factors [11]. Among them, *TNF-α*, *IL-1β*, and *IL-6* levels are particularly increased in response to the inflammatory process and strongly contribute to the future development of cardiac fibrosis [47]. The role of TNF-α in cardiac fibrosis is supported by numerous experimental and clinical studies [48,49]. Meanwhile, the absence of TNF-α reduced the inflammatory response and cardiac fibrosis in mice [47], and TNF-α inhibition has been shown to improve left ventricular structure and function in patients with advanced heart failure [48]. In contrast to the vast majority of profibrotic stimuli, TNF-α does not exert its fibrotic effect by an increase but rather by a decrease in collagen synthesis, suggesting that the profibrotic effect of TNF-α is more likely to occur as a response to ECM degradation [49]. Additional mechanisms involved in TNF-α-induced fibrosis include synthesis of the matrix protein cellular communication network factor 4, favoring fibroblast proliferation, increased TGF-β1 expression, immune cell activation and proliferation, and promotion of AT1 receptors synthesis [50]. Data regarding the role of IL-1β in cardiac fibrosis are rather controversial. Some experimental studies suggested that IL-1β may promote cardiac fibroblast migration, while others reported the opposite [51]. In patients with rheumatoid arthritis, IL-1 inhibition led, however, to a significant improvement in left ventricular function [52]. In some, but not all studies, a relationship was found between low IL-6 levels and cardiac fibrosis [53,54].

The most studied fibrosis-related growth factor, **TGF-β**, has been shown to play a central role in maladaptive cardiac remodeling in both myocardial infarction and heart failure (Figure 1) [55,56]. In gain-of-function studies, cardiac overexpression of TGF-β1 increased collagen deposition and promoted cardiac fibrosis, whereas TGF-β1 deficiency has been associated with a lower degree of aging-related cardiac fibrosis [55,57]. The stimulating effect of TGF-β on cardiac fibroblasts appears to be the basis for an increased synthesis of ECM proteins [57]. Its effects on monocytes, lymphocytes, and cardiomyocytes further contribute to the profibrotic effects of TGF-β [58] as well as the reversal of the fibrosis degradation/preservation balance toward a matrix-preserving pattern via inhibition of collagenases and induction of protease inhibitors such as plasminogen activator inhibitor-1 and tissue inhibitors of metalloproteinases [57]. Meanwhile, in experimental studies, a loss of TGF-β receptors reduced cardiac fibrosis [59], further supporting the importance of TGF-β signaling cascades in cardiac fibrosis. The TGF-β signaling cascades exert their profibrotic effects through Smads, intracellular effector proteins, but also through Smad-independent pathways, both leading to fibroblast activation (Figure 4) [60].

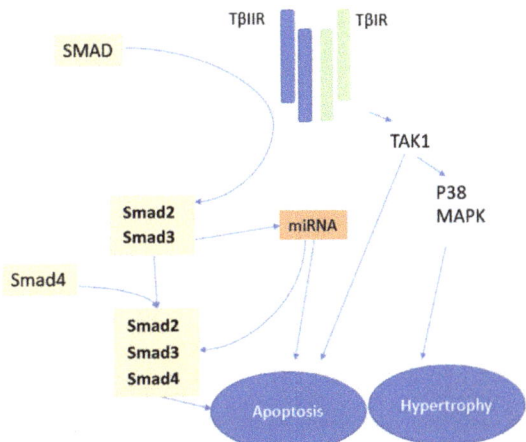

Figure 4. Transforming growth factor *beta*-related pathways and their contribution to myocardial fibrosis. Paracrine factors in fibroblasts, the most important of which is transforming growth factor-*beta*, induce profibrotic responses in cardiomyocytes. The activation of type I and II transforming growth factor-*beta* receptors regulates cell phenotypes by activating Smad- and non-Smad-related signaling pathways that eventually result in cardiomyocyte apoptosis and hypertrophy. MAPK—mitogen-activated protein kinase; TAK1—transforming growth factor-*beta*-activated kinase 1; TβIR—transforming growth factor-*beta* receptor type I; TβIIR—transforming growth factor-*beta* receptor type II.

Studies have shown Smad3 signaling to be critically involved in chronic fibrotic cardiac remodeling and to contribute to fibroblasts activation, α-smooth muscle actin expression, and synthesis of ECM [61]. In contrast, myofibroblast-specific Smad2 signaling appears to be only transiently implicated in early adverse remodeling and does not seem to play a major role in fibroblast activation [60]. Smad-independent profibrotic TGF-β-related pathways involve p38, MAPK, extracellular signal-regulated kinase, and TGF-β-activated kinase 1 (TAK1) signaling pathways activation (Figure 1) [62].

Exosomes are extracellular microvesicles that supply cells with RNA, proteins, lipids, and other biologically active signaling molecules, while acting as couriers for intercellular communication. Recent evidence indicates that in the presence of cardiac fibrosis, there is altered intercellular communication via the exosomes [63]. In addition, exosomes have been shown to alter the process of cardiac repair and to cause fibrosis via the modulation of fibroblast function [64]. During cardiac injury, exosomes promote the activation of naive fibroblasts to initiate the wound-healing process and contribute to fibroblast differentiation into myofibroblasts [64]. Injured endothelial cells have also been shown to secrete exosomes enriched with profibrotic, antiangiogenic factors, and microRNAs that will further contribute to cardiac fibrosis [65].

3. Identification and Quantification of Myocardial Fibrosis

Invasive and non-invasive methods have been developed over time in order to identify and quantify myocardial fibrosis (Table 1). Of these, myocardial biopsy is the most reliable method.

Table 1. Advantages and disadvantages of different techniques used in the evaluation and quantification of cardiac fibrosis.

Technology	Advantages	Disadvantages
Echocardiography	- favorable safety profile - non-invasive - acceptable to most patients - low cost - portable	- does not allow direct identification and quantification of fibrosis type and extent - cannot be used to measure and monitor the degree and progression of myocardial fibrosis - poor reproducibility - dependent on acoustic windows - affected by operator's skills
Cardiac magnetic resonance	- can identify macroscopic fibrosis - can identify different patterns of fibrosis - acceptable to patients - non-invasive	- potential artifacts in uncooperative patients and in the presence of tachyarrhythmias - contraindicated in patients with magnetic resonance-incompatible implants - high cost
Endomyocardial biopsy	- allows direct microscopic assessment of myocardial components and fibrotic changes	- risk of major complications - sampling error in cases of localized fibrosis - unreliable in detecting replacement fibrosis

3.1. Invasive Methods to Investigate Cardiac Fibrosis

A histological evaluation of myocardial tissue samples obtained during myomectomy, open heart surgery, or endocardial biopsy remains the gold standard for diagnosing and quantifying myocardial fibrosis [66]. Using appropriate staining methods, histological analysis of the collagen volume fraction (CVF; i.e., the ratio of the sum of connective tissue areas to the sum of all areas of connective and muscle tissue) is the most widely used method for quantitative evaluation of cardiac fibrosis [66]. No cut-off values have been defined so far; however, for CVF, the values varying considerably from one study to another. In addition, the use of this technique is strongly limited by the fact that it requires direct, invasive access to cardiac tissue samples, which carries inevitably the risk of several potentially major complications. Moreover, in settings with regional fibrosis, obtaining tissue samples does not guarantee a correct diagnosis.

3.2. Non-Invasive Methods to Evaluate Cardiac Fibrosis

Several **blood biomarkers** have been proposed to assess cellular and molecular changes that reflect the amount of fibrotic tissue of the heart. C-terminal propeptides of collagen I and N-terminal propeptides of collagen III highly correlated with total CVF, creating optimism about future clinical use [67]. However, both biomarkers have low specificity, and increased levels can also be observed in liver fibrosis [68]. High levels of galectin-3, a molecule that accelerates fibrosis by stimulating myofibroblast activation, have been associated with increased mortality and worse prognosis in heart failure. However, no associations were found between galectin-3 levels and CVF [69]. Circulating levels of miR-21, one of the regulators of fibroblast activity, have been shown to correlate with myocardial expression of type I collagen mRNA [70]. Its potential use as a blood biomarker for CVF and its cut-off values remain, however, questionable. Higher TGF-β levels have been reported in patients with heart failure compared with control [71]. However, its correlation with CVF remains to date unclear.

Cardiac magnetic resonance imaging (MRI) with T1 relaxometry can provide rapid information on cardiac edema, fibrosis, and deposition diseases, whereas replacement fibrosis can be evaluated using gadolinium MRI [72]. It should be noted, however, that this latter technique is not reliable in settings characterized by diffuse fibrosis in a homogeneous myocardium, although MRI-quantified fibrosis did correlate with cardiac function in patients with heart failure with preserved ejection fraction [73]. In the absence of edema or infiltrative disease, calculating the extracellular cardiac volume by T1 relaxometry after gadolinium injection allows evaluating even small amounts of fibrosis, and the results have been shown to correlate better with biopsy results than those obtained using other MRI-based techniques [72].

With its favorable safety profile and relative ease of use, *echocardiography* is often the first investigation used for assessing myocardial function and structure and for obtaining indirect data on cardiac fibrosis. Using speckle tracking echocardiography, one can quantify myocardial thickening, shortening, and rotation dynamics [74]. In hypertrophic cardiomyopathy, regional impairment of myocardial function assessed by speckle tracking echocardiography correlated with the presence of fibrosis detected by MRI [75]. Echocardiographic measurement of calibrated integrated backscatter is a technique developed to quantify the ultrasonic reflectivity of the myocardium in relation to the high reflectivity of the pericardium and the low reflectivity of blood [76]. In patients with dilated or hypertrophic cardiomyopathy and extensive fibrosis, the results have been shown to correlate significantly with the amount of myocardial fibrosis measured histologically [76]. The most important limitation of all echocardiographic methods remains, however, the need to obtain high-quality images.

4. Targeting Myocardial Fibrosis—A Magic Pill in Cardiovascular Medicine?

Immediately after any cardiac injury, a dynamic process of remodeling is initiated that is critical for stabilization of the cardiac wall. Expansion of non-contractile, collagen-rich tissue will lead, however, not only to scar tissue maturation but also to progressive adverse remodeling, which stands at the foundation of many CVDs. Targeting myocardial fibrosis could therefore provide tremendous benefits in many CVDs. However, because of the critical role that fibrosis plays in wound healing and tissue repair, concerns remain that fibrosis manipulation strategies may not completely innocuous. One of the major goals of novel fibrosis-oriented therapies is therefore not to withhold the process of fibrosis but rather to modify the properties of the scar tissue and to direct fibrotic pathways toward the formation of a functionally efficient fibrotic tissue.

4.1. Cardiac Antifibrotic Effects of Non-Antifibrotic Drugs

Clinical and experimental studies have shown that for numerous drugs created for various, non-antifibrotic purposes, the benefit could be at least partially linked to their antifibrotic effects (Table 2).

Table 2. Clinical and experimental studies of drugs studied for their antifibrotic effects.

Therapeutic Class	Drug	Study Type	Species	Duration	Underlying CVD	Results	References
RAAS inhibitors	Spironolactone (12.5–50.0 mg/day)	Placebo-controlled randomized trial	Human	6 months	HFrEF	Reduced PINP/PIIINP	[77]
	Lisinopril (5–20 mg/day)	Double-blind randomized trial	Human	6 months	Hypertensive heart disease	Reduced CVF and improved diastolic function	[78]
	Enalapril (5 mg/day)	Double-blind, randomized controlled clinical trial	Human	6 months	HFpEF-ESRF	Reduced PICP	[79]
	Losartan (50 mg/day)	Double-blind, randomized controlled clinical trial	Human	6 months	HFpEF-ESRF	Reduced CVF and improved diastolic function in severe fibrosis	[79]
Angiotensin receptor neprilysin inhibitor	Sacubitril-valsartan (200mg bid)	Double-blind, randomized controlled clinical trial	Human	9 months	HFpEF	No significant change in PIIINP/MMP2	[80]
Statins	Atorvastatin (40 mg/day)	Randomized open label study	Human	6 months	HFrEF	Reduction in PIIINP levels	[81]
	Rosuvastatin (40 mg/day)	Double-blind, randomized, placebo-controlled study	Human	6 months	HFrEF	No significant change in PINP/PIIINP	[82]
Pyridones	Pirfenidone	Double-blind, randomized, placebo-controlled study	Human	52 weeks	HFpEF	Ongoing	[83]
Mast cell degranulation inhibitor	Tranilast (400 mg/kg/day)	Experimental	Rat	12 weeks	2K1C renovascular hypertension	Decreased fibrotic area to total left ventricular area ratio	[84]
Endothelin receptor blocker	Bosentan (100 mg/kg/day)	Experimental	Rat	4 weeks	Myocardial hypertrophy	Decreased histological interstitial and perivascular fibrosis	[85]
Pacemaker current inhibitor	Ivabradine (5 mg bid)	Double-blind, randomized, placebo-controlled study	Human	8 months	HFrEF	Reversed LV volumes and increased LVEF	[86]
Phosphodiesterase type 5 inhibitors	Sildenafil (100 mg/day)	Double-blind, randomized, placebo-controlled study	Human	3 months	Type 2 diabetes	Improved LV contraction parameters and reduced TGF-β and MCP-1	[87]
Beta-blocker	Propranolol (40 mg/kg/day)	Preclinical	Rat	10 weeks	Left ventricular pressure overload, hypertrophy	No significant reduction in interstitial fibrosis	[88]
Calcium channel blockers	Mibefradil (10 mg/kg/day)	Preclinical	Rat	6 weeks	Myocardial infarction	Decreased infarct size and perivascular fibrosis	[89]

2K1C—two-kidney, one-clip; CVD—cardiovascular disease; CVF—collagen volume fraction; ESRF—end-stage renal disease; HFpEF—heart failure with preserved ejection fraction; HFrEF—heart failure with reduced ejection fraction; LV—left ventricle; LVEF—left ventricular ejection fraction; MCP-1—monocyte chemoattractant protein-1; MMP-2—matrix metalloproteinase-2; PICP—carboxy-terminal propeptide of procollagen type I; PINP—amino-terminal propeptide of procollagen type I; PIIINP—amino-terminal propeptide of procollagen type III; RAAS—renin-angiotensin-aldosterone system; TGF-β—transforming growth factor-beta.

Given the major role that **RAAS** plays in cardiac fibrosis pathogenesis, molecules that act at different RAAS levels have been investigated for their potential antifibrotic effects (Table 2). Aliskiren, a molecule that binds to renin and limits the initial step required for Ang II synthesis, has been shown to limit myocardial collagen deposition via Ang II-dependent and (pro)renin receptor-related pathways [90]. Already used as first-line therapy in a vast majority of CVDs, ACE inhibitors were also shown to reduce myocardial fibrosis in several animal models [33]. The decrease in myocardial collagen content induced by ACE inhibitors was related to a significant decrease in type I (but not type III) collagen as well as to an increase in gelatinase activity [91]. However, several clinical trials have failed to associate ACE inhibitors with a reduction in hospitalization and mortality in patients with various conditions characterized by extensive cardiac fibrosis, suggesting that ACE inhibition may be insufficient to effectively block the activity of multiple fibrosis pathways [92]. The blockade of Ang II AT1 receptors efficiently reduced fibrosis in both clinical and experimental settings [79,93]. Independently of their antihypertensive effects, AT1 receptor inhibitors have been associated with a more important reduction in type I collagen than ACE inhibitors [91]. Aldosterone inhibition reduced ECM, decreased fibrotic markers levels, significantly improved ventricular function in animal studies, and significantly reduced mortality in patients with heart failure and reduced ejection fraction [94]. Although in the Treatment of Preserved Cardiac Function Heart Failure With an Aldosterone Antagonist (TOPCAT) trial aldosterone inhibition failed to significantly improve the composite endpoint of cardiovascular death, aborted cardiac arrest, or hospitalization [95], a post hoc analysis of the trial indicated that this strategy may improve symptoms and hospitalization in certain patient subgroups [96].

Beta-blockers have been shown to prevent fibrosis and improve survival in animal models and to favorably affect prognosis in heart failure patients with preserved ejection fraction [97,98]. However, in humans, the antifibrotic effects of *beta*-blockers remain highly controversial (Table 2) [99]. This discordance could be at least partly related to the type of *beta*-blocker administered; there are studies suggesting that different *beta*-blockers may have opposite effects on the development of cardiac fibrosis [37]. ***Calcium channels blockers*** have also been shown to reduce cardiac fibrosis in different animal studies. The long-term administration of mibefradil, verapamil, and amlodipine reduced adverse cardiac remodeling and improved ventricular function in rats with ischemic heart failure [100]. In humans, the calcium channel blocker tetrandrine prevented myofibroblast activation and reduced cardiac fibrosis via a mechanism independent of calcium channel blockade and of the reduction in hemodynamic load [101]. Despite their anti-inflammatory effects, the ability of *statins* to alleviate cardiac fibrosis remains questionable. In rats with hypertensive heart disease, statin therapy reduced adverse cardiac remodeling, ventricular dysfunction, and progression to heart failure [102]. In patients with heart failure, statins reduced type III procollagen [81], the amount of myocardial fibrotic tissue and plasma markers of fibrosis [103]. However, in a 6-month randomized placebo-controlled study, the effect of statins on cardiac remodeling was neutral [104], whereas in another study, statin use was associated with an increase in serum collagen markers [82]. In experimental studies, *endothelin inhibitors* reduced fibrosis in multiple organs, attenuated cardiac remodeling, and significantly increased survival [105]. This did not seem to be the case, however, in patients with heart failure [106]. Adding endothelin antagonists to ACE inhibitors, *beta*-blockers, or aldosterone antagonists also does not seem to provide additional benefits in terms of cardiac remodeling in patients with heart failure [107].

4.2. Novel Targets for Cardiac Fibrosis Prevention and Therapy

Studies have identified a number of novel targets for cardiac fibrosis prevention and therapy (Table 3) [108].

Table 3. Novel targets for cardiac fibrosis prevention and therapy.

Therapeutic Target	Strategy
Cell transplantation	Direct remuscularization Stimulation of endogenous cardiovascular progenitor cells
TGF-β signaling	Suppression of TGF-β1 TGFβRII plasmid transfection ALK5 inhibition TGFβRII inhibition
Biomaterials	Hydrogel (alginate, polyester-VEGF, decellularized ECM, gelatin-HGF) Patch (alginate-neonatal rat cardiomyocytes, decellularized ECM) Glue (fibrin-fibroblast growth factor) Scaffold (fibrin–endothelial cells–smooth muscle cells)
Direct reprogramming	GMT (retrovirus/lentivirus) GMHT (retrovirus) miRNAs (miR-1, miR-133, miR-208, miR-499) Chemical/small molecule cocktails

ALK5—transforming growth factor-*beta* 1 type I receptor kinase; ECM—extracellular matrix; GMHT—Gata4/Mef2c/Hand2/Tbx5; GMT—Gata4/Mef2c/Tbx5; HGF—hepatocyte growth factor; TGF-β1—transforming growth factor-*beta* 1; TGFβRII—transforming growth factor-*beta* receptor II; VEGF—vascular endothelial growth factor.

Due to its major role in cardiac fibrosis, the *TGF-β signaling pathway* has become one of the most tempting targets in this setting. Anti-TGF-β antibodies were shown to efficiently decrease fibroblast activation and to improve diastolic function in rats with cardiac pressure overload, although they did not provide any improvement in myocyte hypertrophy or systolic function in those rats [109]. Moreover, in an experimental model of myocardial infarction, although anti-TGF-β1 antibodies reduced fibrosis, their use was associated with increased mortality and dilatation of the left ventricle [110]. Alternative approaches, such as soluble TβRII, a competitive inhibitor of TGF-β, and inhibitors of the TGFβRI kinase (ALK5) have also been investigated. Both strategies reduced collagen synthesis and cardiac fibrosis but also manifested non-negligible side effects [111,112]. GW788388, a blocker of both ALK5 and TGFβRII that has improved pharmacokinetics and minimal toxic effects, reduced left ventricular remodeling in rats with myocardial infarction [113], but the full effects of this agent remain to be established. Inhibition of TAK1 and p38-MAPK has also been investigated, and both showed promising effects on cardiac fibrosis [114,115]. Pirfenidone and tranilast, two other TGF-β inhibitors, have also shown promising results in preclinical studies [116,117]. For tranilast, clinical data on cardiac fibrosis are still lacking. Meanwhile, in a recent phase II clinical trial, pirfenidone significantly reduced myocardial fibrosis in patients with heart failure and low ejection fraction without causing serious adverse cardiac events [83]. Pirfenidone's numerous extra-cardiac, including gastrointestinal, neurological, and dermatological side effects [118], remain, however, a serious concern. In mice, both Smad3 deficiency and Smad3 inhibition efficiently reduced the amount of cardiac fibrosis and prevented the decline in left ventricular ejection fraction [119], pointing Smad3 inhibition as a promising new antifibrotic approach. Increased levels of endogline, a co-receptor of TGF-β1 and TGF-β3, have been associated with both heart failure and acute myocardial infarction [120]. Meanwhile, decreased endoglin expression reduced the amount of cardiac fibrosis and improved survival in mice with heart failure [121]. The antifibrotic effect of blocking other TGF-β-related pathways, such as the RhoA–serum response factor-myocardin-related transcription factor [122] or the transient canonical potential receptor channels pathways [123] also remains to be evaluated in future studies.

In cardiac myocytes, the *PDGF* family includes PDGF-A and -C, while PDGFRα-positive cells have been described in the cardiac interstitium. Endothelial cells express PDGF-B and -D, while pericytes and smooth muscle cells are PDGFRβ-positive [124]. All PDGFs have been shown to play a role in cardiac fibrosis. In transgenic mice, the overexpression of PDGF-C and -D has been associated with cardiac fibrosis and hypertrophy [125].

Meanwhile, PDGF blockade reduced interstitial fibrosis in rats with myocardial infarction and decreased fibroblast activation in dogs [126], and neutralizing PDGF receptor-specific antibodies suppressed cell proliferation and collagen expression in cardiac fibroblasts [127].

Elevated levels of connective tissue growth factor (*CTGF*) have been detected in myocardial infarction and heart failure and have been shown to correlate with the degree of myocardial fibrosis [128]. The profibrotic effects of CTGF appear to emerge from its ability to stimulate fibroblasts' proliferation and transformation into myofibroblasts, although its potential to intrinsically induce fibrosis seems to be rather low [129]. In some experimental studies, the overexpression of CTGF had no significant profibrotic effects [130]. Other studies indicated, however, that CTGF can exert profibrotic effects [131], and that CTGF inhibition with monoclonal antibodies enhances cardiac repair, limits fibrosis, and ensures better preservation of left ventricular systolic function post-myocardial infarction [132].

Although the exact mechanisms remain insufficiently understood, the administration of *angiotensin receptor–neprilysin inhibitors* (ARNIs), a drug complex composed of a neprilysin inhibitor precursor and a non-peptide Ang II receptor blocker, has been shown to decrease the risk of death and hospitalizations in heart failure patients [133]. Preclinical studies have shown significant improvement in ventricular remodeling following neprilysin inhibition, and clinical trials later confirmed these results in patients with heart failure treated with ARNIs [134,135]. The benefit appears to emerge from the synergistic actions of the two components of ARNIs on multiple mechanisms involved in pathological cardiac remodeling. Neprilysin inhibition increases the concentrations of vasodilator peptides, such as the atrial and brain natriuretic peptides, and bradykinin, thereby improving myocardial perfusion in the infarcted area, but also increases concomitantly the concentrations of Ang II, whose effects are efficiently counteracted by the Ang II receptor blocker [135,136]. According to preclinical data, cardiac fibrosis and adverse remodeling are counteracted by ARNIs mainly via inhibition of the Wnt/β-catenin pathway [137]. In addition, ARNIs appear to attenuate cardiomyocyte growth and to increase the capillary/cardiomyocyte ratio at the level of the border area between the infarcted and the healthy myocardium [135], and even to reduce myocardial fibrosis, as reflected by the reduction in MMP-2, MMP-9, and N-terminal propeptide of type I procollagen, leading to a reduction in left atrial size and to significant improvement in left ventricular ejection in patients with heart failure [138–140]. Disappointingly, however, ARNIs failed to reduce hospitalizations and cardiovascular death in patients with heart failure and a left ventricular ejection fraction $\geq$45% (Table 2) [141].

4.3. Targeted Blockade—Aiming to Obtain a 'Better Scar'

Although the direct manipulation of mechanisms involved in fibroblast recruitment is not currently regarded as a primary target in the management of CVDs, this strategy carries a major potential to favorably influence scar formation and tissue remodeling.

Monocyte chemoattractant protein-1 (*MCP-1*) provides key signals for the migration and infiltration of inflammatory cells and activated fibroblasts. The overexpression of MCP-1 at the cardiac level promotes fibroblast accumulation, contributing to improved cardiac function and myocardial remodeling in transgenic myocardial infarction mice [142]. Meanwhile, MCP-1 deletion significantly reduced Ang-II-induced fibrosis by reducing the uptake and differentiation of CD45+ fibroblast precursors [143]. The manipulation of MCP-1 could thus emerge as a promising strategy to influence progenitor fibroblast cells and to prevent fibrosis and adverse cardiac remodeling.

Modulation of collagen accumulation and maturation in order to obtain a myocardial collagen network adapted to the local mechanical conditions could represent another potential target in fibrosis-related CVDs. In myocardial infarction, expansion of the infarcted area is associated with poor mechanics and increased risk of rupture of the injured wall. Approaches that stimulate compaction of the infarcted area by increasing collagen cross-linking inside the scar could thus provide an option to counteract maladaptive cardiac fibrosis. Modulation of lysyl oxidases, enzymes produced by activated fibroblasts that stiffen the collagen network by boosting collagen fibers cross-linking, appears to be particularly promising in this regard [144].

Modulation of cardiomyocyte-fibroblast coupling inside the scar area, while keeping the outer area unchanged may also help to create a 'better scar'. In myocardial infarction, this would translate into increased trans-scar communication and transformation of the infarcted area into an 'electrically-transparent scar', with more homogeneous electrical activity and lower risk of re-entry [145]. This could be obtained by upregulating heterotypic connexin (Cx)-coupling with drugs such as rotigaptide, which significantly enhanced metabolic coupling in Cx43-coupled cells and attenuated gap junction closure under metabolic stress [146].

Fibroblast-derived microRNA-enriched exosomes, paracrine signaling mediators of cardiac hypertrophy and remodeling, are also regarded as highly promising. In vivo silencing of miR-21 reduced fibrosis in pressure-overload-induced disease and increased survival following myocardial infarction [70]. Other in vivo and in vitro studies suggested that miR-125b promotes profibrotic signaling in endothelial-to-mesenchymal transition and fibroblast activation [147]. miR-29 downregulation has also been associated with increased cardiac fibrosis, while miR-29 overexpression reduced collagen expression in myocardial infarction models [148]. In a mouse model of ATII-induced hypertension, mimetic miR-29 transfection also reduced the development of cardiac fibrosis via the TGF-β/Smad3 pathway [149]. More recently, miR-145, miR-30, and miR-133 have also been shown to modulate collagen deposition and to control structural ECM changes [150,151]. However, challenges in targeting microRNAs to prevent cardiac fibrosis remain, which are mainly related to their broad and non-specific effects. Nevertheless, ongoing efforts to identify the molecular targets of non-coding RNAs are promising for future clinical interventions.

Periostin targeting is also seen as a potential option in fibrosis-related CVDs. Periostin acts as a regulator of cardiac fibrosis by altering the deposition, diameter, and cross-linking of collagen fibers, by modifying the mechanical adhesion between fibroblasts and myocytes [152], and by recruiting activated fibroblasts via FAK-integrin signaling [153]. In heart failure patients, periostin distribution and expression has been associated with the amount of fibrotic tissue, suggesting that periostin may be a potential biomarker of cardiac remodeling in this setting [153]. In post-myocardial infarction mice, the genetic manipulation of periostin was shown to improve cardiac function. However, it also led to an overall increase in fibrosis [151]. Thus, the use of periostin as a potential target remains a sensitive issue.

4.4. Indirect Blockade of Fibrosis via Stimulation of Myocardial Regeneration/Repair

The targeted delivery of biomaterials composed of natural (e.g., naturally derived matrices) or synthetic (e.g., poly [N-isopropyl acrylamide]-based hydrogels) biomaterial +/− cells or growth factors has been investigated as a potential novel antifibrotic therapeutic strategy with promising results in rodent and large animal models [154]. Decellularized cardiac ECM alone can also be used as a biomaterial to control cardiac fibrosis and to provide support for the infarcted wall [154]. Transcatheter injection of processed decellularized cardiac ECM hydrogel has been shown to promote stem cells recruitment, proliferation, and differentiation into cardiac cells [155] and to be safe for administration in human patients [156]. Although the trial was not designed to assess efficacy, there was a decrease in heart failure symptoms, an increase in 6-min walk test distance, and an improvement in left ventricular remodeling in post-myocardial infarction patients [156]. Acellular patches that provide cells with tissue-specific biochemical cues important for cell migration and differentiation and tissue regeneration have also been investigated. The most used biomaterials include growth factors, ECM molecules, heparin, and thrombomodulin, which help to ensure a uniform surface coating of the polymeric cardiovascular scaffold [157]. The vascular endothelial growth factor, the insulin-like growth factor 1, the hepatocyte growth factor, the myeloid-derived growth factor, neuregulin 1, the epidermal growth factor, and the fibroblast growth factor are the most widely employed to improve the bioresponsive properties of the scaffolds [157].

Cardiac patches that use collagen as a scaffold have also been studied in combination with a variety of cell types capable of exerting paracrine effects or to directly regenerate the injured myocardium [158], whereas fibrin cardiac patches improved cell delivery in a porcine model of post-infarction left ventricular remodeling [159]. Cells that promote adipose-derived stem cell regeneration embedded into platelet-rich fibrin and patched in myocardial infarction rats significantly decreased fibrotic mediators' levels and increased the expression of antifibrotic markers [160]. The implantation of pluripotent stem cells-derived cardiomyocytes placed on collagen scaffolds into dilated mouse hearts was also shown to decrease cardiac fibrosis and to increase the expression of osteopontin, which is an acidic phosphoglycoprotein that regulates the MMPs [161]. Multiple experimental studies provided highly promising results, and there are several ongoing clinical trials that test the localized delivery of biomaterials and antifibrotic agents.

Cell-sheet implantation has been shown to attenuate remodeling, restore the damaged myocardium, and improve cardiac function in several experimental models of myocardial infarction and dilated cardiomyopathy [162]. The method was tested in patients with myocardial infarction and dilated cardiomyopathy in a phase I clinical trial [163]. Although not adequately powered, the trial indicated a decrease in pulmonary pressure and resistance, as well as in the levels of BNP, an increase in walking distances on the 6-min walk test, and an improvement in the New York Heart Association classification in the treated patients, particularly in those with ischemic heart disease [163].

4.5. Modulation of Collagen Turnover

Procollagen processing by procollagen C-proteinase(s) is critical for the maturation of soluble collagen precursors into insoluble collagen and is potentiated by procollagen C-proteinase enhancers (PCPE-1 and -2) [164]. The expression levels of these later proteins have been shown to strongly correlate with the degree of fibrosis in different animal models [164]. The effect of PCPE-1 manipulation on cardiac fibrosis has not been evaluated to date. In the mouse liver, PCPE-1 deficiency decreased, however, the amount of fibrosis [165]. Meanwhile, PCPE-2 null hearts have been associated with a decrease in CVF and with lower myocardial stiffness in mice with aortic constriction [166].

Increased collagen production via Smad7 is amidst the many mechanisms by which miR-21 promotes cardiac fibrosis [167]. Elevated miR-21 expression has been shown to negatively affect collagen cross-linking and, implicitly, CVF [168], suggesting that miR-21 silencing could inhibit collagen synthesis and could thus exhibit antifibrotic effects.

Serelaxin is a recombinant form of human relaxin-2, which is a hormone that contributes, among others, to the degradation of the ECM. The antifibrotic effect of relaxin has been reported in both the kidney and the heart [169] and appears to rely on the prevention of cardiac fibroblast-to-myofibroblast transition via TGF-β/Smad3 pathway inhibition [170]. In addition, serelaxin has been shown to be safe in patients with acute heart failure [171], making this molecule particularly appealing for future clinical research.

Alterations in the balance between MMPs and their specific tissue inhibitors (i.e., TIMPs) have been incriminated as contributors to the abnormal production of ECM [172]. Cardiac expression of TIMP-1 and -2 was shown to be significantly increased and strongly correlated with the amount of cardiac fibrosis in patients with pressure overload [172]. Meanwhile, TIMP-3 has been shown to possess an increased affinity for ECM glycosaminoglycans and to alter the fibroblast phenotype [173]. The targeted administration of TIMP-3 could thus emerge as a promising collagen-decreasing strategy. In myocardial infarction pigs, the regional delivery of exogenous TIMP-3 showed positive effects on left ventricular ejection fraction and volume as well as on the extent of the infarcted area [173].

5. Gaps in Knowledge, Ongoing and Future Research

Cardiac fibrosis is a complex syndrome that affects not only the structure but also the function of the heart, suggesting that myocardial ECM homeostasis is essential for normal cardiac functioning. Identifying widely available, inexpensive, non-invasive, and highly accurate biomarkers for in vivo quantification of not only gross but also subtle cardiac fibrosis should continue to represent a major priority, as is the case in numerous other clinical settings [174,175]. Multiple strategies have been shown to efficiently counteract fibrosis. However, incomplete knowledge regarding the complex pathogenesis of fibrosis limits advancement in this field. Understanding the activation of cardiac fibroblasts and their role in cardiac fibrosis is necessary to improve our pharmaceutical arsenal. The development of safe and effective antifibrotic strategies also depends on a detailed decipherment of the pathways involved in the antifibrotic response. The window of therapeutic opportunity also remains unknown, at present, both spatially and temporally. Cardiac fibroblasts may respond differently to different therapeutic interventions, depending on the underlying profibrotic context [176]. In reparative fibrosis that follows myocardial infarction, the blockade of fibroblasts may have discordant effects at the periphery versus the center of the scar. Therapeutic approaches designed to block cardiac fibrosis should thus focus on preventing excessive ECM deposition at the periphery of the scar and should not affect the replacement of necrotic cardiomyocytes within the scar core. The most adequate moment for blocking the different profibrotic pathways remains another pending issue at this point. Blocking mediators at the wrong time could alter cellular responses that are critical for tissue repair. In reparative fibrosis that occurs after massive acute injury (e.g., after acute myocardial infarction), the beneficial effects of fibrotic tissue clearly outweigh its harmful effects. In such settings, early antifibrotic interventions could negatively affect the healing process and promote rupture of the heart wall, whereas delayed fibrosis inhibition may be ineffective if the fibrotic process is no longer reversible.

Numerous strategies aiming to prevent, block, and even reverse cardiac fibrosis have been extremely promising in animal models. However, their evaluation in human patients delays or, if they were tested in clinical settings, the results were rather disappointing. Interspecies discordances obviously mandate caution when trying to extrapolate data from animal studies to human medicine and can contribute to the discordant results obtained with different antifibrotic agents. Other factors may play, however, even greater roles. Drug doses used in animal studies are often much higher than those suitable for clinical use, and, with very few exceptions, currently used animal models have limited ability to adequately replicate human CVDs. Whereas in humans, CVDs are most often diseases of elderly individuals, with numerous concomitant cardiac and non-cardiac conditions, treated with different medications, including with a wide variety of cardioactive drugs, and in whom treatment adherence is often questionable, most animal data arise from young, healthy animals, fully compliant to all forms of therapy and who have no concomitant diseases and no concomitant therapy [177]. Using more clinically relevant animal CVDs models would certainly increase the translational value of data obtained in animal models. Meanwhile, clinical trials on innovative strategies have either been performed on a small number of patients or the follow-up period was much too short, considering the important interspecies differences regarding the time needed for the development of fibrosis, which seems to be much longer in humans [177]. Signaling pathways, profibrotic mechanisms, and even the type of fibrosis that develops have also been shown to vary greatly depending on the underling fibrose-promoting condition, suggesting that although most cardiac diseases involve a certain degree of fibrosis, a 'one size fits all' approach is unlikely to provide the solution in cardiac antifibrotic therapy. To date, with the exception of biomaterial-based approaches, which have been largely studied in post-myocardial infarction fibrosis, antifibrotic strategies have rarely been studied targeted on a specific type of fibrosis. Thorough understanding of the pathophysiological mechanisms underlying each type of myocardial fibrosis could provide the key for safe and efficient, targeted antifibrotic therapy.

Data from clinical trials confirmed the safety of stem cells from different tissue sources, using different delivery routes, but their exact clinical benefit remains to be established. Large phase III clinical trials are in progress, and their results will be essential to determine the role of this novel, non-pharmacological approach. To fully understand the potential role of stem cell therapy in cardiac fibrosis, the mechanisms by which this therapy exerts its effects will also need to be clarified. Inhibition of the RAAS using anti-Ang II vaccines, administration of Ang (1–7), and ACE2 overexpression recently emerged as a promising new tool for myocardial fibrosis management in animal models and even in small clinical trials. Antifibrotic drugs used in different other settings would also be worth consideration. Pirfenidone, nintedanib, tranilast, bosentan, macitentan, ambrisentan, and thalidomide are drugs with excellent results in pulmonary fibrosis, and only a minority of them has been evaluated so far in CVDs. Hydralazine and ivabradine, already widely used in patients with CVDs, were shown to significantly attenuate renal fibrosis, but very few studies have assessed their cardiac antifibrotic effect (Table 2). Sildenafil was reported to exert antifibrotic effects not only in the genitals but also in the lungs and skin. A similar effect on cardiac fibrosis could thus contribute to the improvement in ventricular function associated with sildenafil usage. Bioengineering and cell transplant therapy have also demonstrated major potential in indirectly blocking fibrosis by stimulating myocardial regeneration/repair. Direct cell reprogramming and molecular targets, such as epigenetic modifiers and miRs, have also been proposed as novel promising pharmacological tools to prevent the development of cardiac scar tissue. Targeting cardiac fibrosis is still associated, however, with a number of major limitations, and the mechanisms that lead to excessive ECM formation remain incompletely understood. In the absence of myocardial regeneration, the degradation of large areas of fibrosis could result in catastrophic consequences. Future studies will need to fully elucidate the mechanisms involved in cardiac fibrosis, to identify safe and effective methods to counteract this harmful process, and to establish the most appropriate time to intervene.

6. Conclusions

Cardiac fibrosis is currently acknowledged as a central element in the vast majority of CVDs. Due to the complexity of the signaling pathways, to its dual, protective and deleterious impact, and to the numerous cell types involved in the fibrotic process, safe and effective therapies for cardiac fibrosis inhibition and/or reversal remain difficult to develop. Continuous research in this area will have to fully elucidate the mechanisms involved in cardiac fibrosis, to identify safe and effective antifibrotic methods, and to establish the most appropriate time to intervene.

Funding: This work was supported by a grant of the Romanian Ministry of Education and Research, CNCS-UEFISCDI, project number PN-III-P1-1.1-TE-2019-0370, within PNCDI III.

Institutional Review Board Statement: Not applicable.

Informed Consent Statement: Not applicable.

Data Availability Statement: Not applicable.

Conflicts of Interest: The authors declare no conflict of interest.

References

1. Roth, G.A.; Mensah, G.A.; Johnson, C.O.; Addolorato, G.; Ammirati, E.; Baddour, L.M.; Barengo, N.C.; Beaton, A.Z.; Benjamin, E.J.; Benziger, C.P.; et al. Global Burden of Cardiovascular Diseases and Risk Factors, 1990–2019: Update from the GBD 2019 Study. *J. Am. Coll. Cardiol.* **2020**, *76*, 2982–3021. [CrossRef] [PubMed]
2. Hinderer, S.; Schenke-Layland, K. Cardiac fibrosis—A short review of causes and therapeutic strategies. *Adv. Drug Deliv. Rev.* **2019**, *146*, 77–82. [CrossRef]
3. Torrent-Guasp, F.; Kocica, M.J.; Corno, A.F.; Komeda, M.; Carreras-Costa, F.; Flotats, A.; Cosin-Aguillar, J.; Wen, H. Towards new understanding of the heart structure and function. *Eur. J. Cardio-Thorac. Surg.* **2005**, *27*, 191–201. [CrossRef]
4. Burlew, B.S.; Weber, K.T. Connective Tissue and the Heart. Functional significance and regulatory mechanisms. *Cardiol. Clin.* **2000**, *18*, 435–442. [CrossRef]

5. Spinale, F.G. Myocardial Matrix Remodeling and the Matrix Metalloproteinases: Influence on Cardiac Form and Function. *Physiol. Rev.* **2007**, *87*, 1285–1342. [CrossRef] [PubMed]
6. Gaudesius, G.; Miragoli, M.; Thomas, S.P.; Rohr, S. Coupling of Cardiac Electrical Activity Over Extended Distances by Fibroblasts of Cardiac Origin. *Circ. Res.* **2003**, *93*, 421–428. [CrossRef] [PubMed]
7. Zeisberg, E.M.; Tarnavski, O.; Zeisberg, M.; Dorfman, A.L.; McMullen, J.R.; Gustafsson, E.; Chandraker, A.; Yuan, X.; Pu, W.T.; Roberts, A.B.; et al. Endothelial-to-mesenchymal transition contributes to cardiac fibrosis. *Nat. Med.* **2007**, *13*, 952–961. [CrossRef] [PubMed]
8. Willems, I.E.; Havenith, M.G.; De Mey, J.G.; Daemen, M.J. The alpha-smooth muscle actin-positive cells in healing human myocardial scars. *Am. J. Pathol.* **1994**, *145*, 868–875. [PubMed]
9. Hinz, B.; Phan, S.H.; Thannickal, V.J.; Galli, A.; Bochaton-Piallat, M.-L.; Gabbiani, G. The Myofibroblast: One Function, Multiple Origins. *Am. J. Pathol.* **2007**, *170*, 1807–1816. [CrossRef] [PubMed]
10. Santiago, J.-J.; Dangerfield, A.L.; Rattan, S.G.; Bathe, K.L.; Cunnington, R.H.; Raizman, J.E.; Bedosky, K.M.; Freed, D.H.; Kardami, E.; Dixon, I.M.C. Cardiac fibroblast to myofibroblast differentiation in vivo and in vitro: Expression of focal adhesion components in neonatal and adult rat ventricular myofibroblasts. *Dev. Dyn.* **2010**, *239*, 1573–1584. [CrossRef] [PubMed]
11. Mantovani, A.; Biswas, S.K.; Galdiero, M.R.; Sica, A.; Locati, M. Macrophage plasticity and polarization in tissue repair and remodelling. *J. Pathol.* **2012**, *229*, 176–185. [CrossRef] [PubMed]
12. Somasundaram, P.; Ren, G.; Nagar, H.; Kraemer, D.; Mendoza, L.; Michael, L.H.; Caughey, G.H.; Entman, M.L.; Frangogiannis, N.G. Mast cell tryptase may modulate endothelial cell phenotype in healing myocardial infarcts. *J. Pathol.* **2004**, *205*, 102–111. [CrossRef] [PubMed]
13. Wynn, T.A. Integrating mechanisms of pulmonary fibrosis. *J. Exp. Med.* **2011**, *208*, 1339–1350. [CrossRef] [PubMed]
14. Baldeviano, G.C.; Barin, J.G.; Talor, M.V.; Srinivasan, S.; Bedja, D.; Zheng, D.; Gabrielson, K.; Iwakura, Y.; Rose, N.R.; Cihakova, D. Interleukin-17A Is Dispensable for Myocarditis but Essential for the Progression to Dilated Cardiomyopathy. *Circ. Res.* **2010**, *106*, 1646–1655. [CrossRef]
15. Tang, T.-T.; Yuan, J.; Zhu, Z.-F.; Zhang, W.-C.; Xiao, H.; Xia, N.; Yan, X.-X.; Nie, S.-F.; Liu, J.; Zhou, S.-F.; et al. Regulatory T cells ameliorate cardiac remodeling after myocardial infarction. *Basic Res. Cardiol.* **2011**, *107*, 232. [CrossRef] [PubMed]
16. Prabhu, S.D.; Frangogiannis, N.G. The Biological Basis for Cardiac Repair After Myocardial Infarction: From inflammation to fibrosis. *Circ. Res.* **2016**, *119*, 91–112. [CrossRef] [PubMed]
17. Horckmans, M.; Ring, L.; Duchene, J.; Santovito, D.; Schloss, M.J.; Drechsler, M.; Weber, C.; Soehnlein, O.; Steffens, S. Neutrophils orchestrate post-myocardial infarction healing by polarizing macrophages towards a reparative phenotype. *Eur. Heart J.* **2017**, *38*, 187–197. [CrossRef]
18. Weckbach, L.T.; Grabmaier, U.; Uhl, A.; Gess, S.; Boehm, F.; Zehrer, A.; Pick, R.; Salvermoser, M.; Czermak, T.; Pircher, J.; et al. Midkine drives cardiac inflammation by promoting neutrophil trafficking and NETosis in myocarditis. *J. Exp. Med.* **2019**, *216*, 350–368. [CrossRef]
19. Adiarto, S.; Heiden, S.; Vignon-Zellweger, N.; Nakayama, K.; Yagi, K.; Yanagisawa, M.; Emoto, N. ET-1 from endothelial cells is required for complete angiotensin II-induced cardiac fibrosis and hypertrophy. *Life Sci.* **2012**, *91*, 651–657. [CrossRef] [PubMed]
20. Kofler, S.; Nickel, T.; Weis, M. Role of cytokines in cardiovascular diseases: A focus on endothelial responses to inflammation. *Clin. Sci.* **2005**, *108*, 205–213. [CrossRef] [PubMed]
21. Wei, H.; Bedja, D.; Koitabashi, N.; Xing, D.; Chen, J.; Fox-Talbot, K.; Rouf, R.; Chen, S.; Steenbergen, C.; Harmon, J.W.; et al. Endothelial expression of hypoxia-inducible factor 1 protects the murine heart and aorta from pressure overload by suppression of TGF-β signaling. *Proc. Natl. Acad. Sci. USA* **2012**, *109*, E841–E850. [CrossRef]
22. Piek, A.; de Boer, R.A.; Silljé, H.H.W. The fibrosis-cell death axis in heart failure. *Heart Fail. Rev.* **2016**, *21*, 199–211. [CrossRef] [PubMed]
23. Dolmatova, E.; Spagnol, G.; Boassa, D.; Baum, J.R.; Keith, K.; Ambrosi, C.; Kontaridis, M.I.; Sorgen, P.L.; Sosinsky, G.E.; Duffy, H.S. Cardiomyocyte ATP release through pannexin 1 aids in early fibroblast activation. *Am. J. Physiol. Circ. Physiol.* **2012**, *303*, H1208–H1218. [CrossRef] [PubMed]
24. Rickard, A.J.; Morgan, J.; Bienvenu, L.A.; Fletcher, E.K.; Cranston, G.A.; Shen, J.Z.; Reichelt, M.E.; Delbridge, L.M.; Young, M.J. Cardiomyocyte Mineralocorticoid Receptors Are Essential for Deoxycorticosterone/Salt-Mediated Inflammation and Cardiac Fibrosis. *Hypertension* **2012**, *60*, 1443–1450. [CrossRef] [PubMed]
25. Koitabashi, N.; Danner, T.; Zaiman, A.L.; Pinto, Y.M.; Rowell, J.; Mankowski, J.; Zhang, D.; Nakamura, T.; Takimoto, E.; Kass, D.A. Pivotal role of cardiomyocyte TGF-β signaling in the murine pathological response to sustained pressure overload. *J. Clin. Investig.* **2011**, *121*, 2301–2312. [CrossRef] [PubMed]
26. Kurisu, S.; Ozono, R.; Oshima, T.; Kambe, M.; Ishida, T.; Sugino, H.; Matsuura, H.; Chayama, K.; Teranishi, Y.; Iba, O.; et al. Cardiac Angiotensin II Type 2 Receptor Activates the Kinin/NO System and Inhibits Fibrosis. *Hypertension* **2003**, *41*, 99–107. [CrossRef] [PubMed]
27. Mukherjee, D.; Sen, S. Alteration of Cardiac Collagen Phenotypes in Hypertensive Hypertrophy: Role of Blood Pressure. *J. Mol. Cell. Cardiol.* **1993**, *25*, 185–196. [CrossRef] [PubMed]
28. Mukherjee, D.; Sen, S. Alteration of collagen phenotypes in ischemic cardiomyopathy. *J. Clin. Investig.* **1991**, *88*, 1141–1146. [CrossRef] [PubMed]

29. Naugle, J.E.; Olson, E.R.; Zhang, X.; Mase, S.E.; Pilati, C.F.; Maron, M.B.; Folkesson, H.G.; Horne, W.I.; Doane, K.J.; Meszaros, J.G. Type VI collagen induces cardiac myofibroblast differentiation: Implications for postinfarction remodeling. *Am. J. Physiol. Circ. Physiol.* **2006**, *290*, H323–H330. [CrossRef] [PubMed]
30. Graham-Brown, M.P.M.; Patel, A.S.; Stensel, D.J.; March, D.S.; Marsh, A.-M.; McAdam, J.; McCann, G.P.; Burton, J.O. Imaging of Myocardial Fibrosis in Patients with End-Stage Renal Disease: Current Limitations and Future Possibilities. *BioMed Res. Int.* **2017**, *2017*, 5453606. [CrossRef]
31. Iwanaga, Y.; Aoyama, T.; Kihara, Y.; Onozawa, Y.; Yoneda, T.; Sasayama, S. Excessive activation of matrix metalloproteinases coincides with left ventricular remodeling during transition from hypertrophy to heart failure in hypertensive rats. *J. Am. Coll. Cardiol.* **2002**, *39*, 1384–1391. [CrossRef]
32. Arisha, M.M.; Girerd, N.; Chauveau, S.; Bresson, D.; Scridon, A.; Bonnefoy, E.; Chevalier, P. In-Hospital Heart Rate Turbulence and Microvolt T-Wave Alternans Abnormalities for Prediction of Early Life-Threatening Ventricular Arrhythmia after Acute Myocardial Infarction. *Ann. Noninvasive Electrocardiol.* **2013**, *18*, 530–537. [CrossRef]
33. Brilla, C.G.; Zhou, G.; Matsubara, L.; Weber, K.T. Collagen Metabolism in Cultured Adult Rat Cardiac Fibroblasts: Response to Angiotensin II and Aldosterone. *J. Mol. Cell. Cardiol.* **1994**, *26*, 809–820. [CrossRef] [PubMed]
34. Weber, K.T.; Sun, Y.; Bhattacharya, S.K.; Ahokas, R.A.; Gerling, I.C. Myofibroblast-mediated mechanisms of pathological remodelling of the heart. *Nat. Rev. Cardiol.* **2012**, *10*, 15–26. [CrossRef] [PubMed]
35. Li, L.; Fan, D.; Wang, C.; Wang, J.-Y.; Cui, X.; Wu, D.; Zhou, Y.; Wu, L.-L. Angiotensin II increases periostin expression via Ras/p38 MAPK/CREB and ERK1/2/TGF-β1 pathways in cardiac fibroblasts. *Cardiovasc. Res.* **2011**, *91*, 80–89. [CrossRef]
36. Ock, S.; Ham, W.; Kang, C.W.; Kang, H.; Lee, W.S.; Kim, J. IGF-1 protects against angiotensin II-induced cardiac fibrosis by targeting αSMA. *Cell Death Dis.* **2021**, *12*, 688. [CrossRef] [PubMed]
37. Rompe, F.; Artuc, M.; Hallberg, A.; Alterman, M.; Ströder, K.; Thöne-Reineke, C.; Reichenbach, A.; Schacherl, J.; Dahlöf, B.; Bader, M.; et al. Direct Angiotensin II Type 2 Receptor Stimulation Acts Anti-Inflammatory Through Epoxyeicosatrienoic Acid and Inhibition of Nuclear Factor κB. *Hypertension* **2010**, *55*, 924–931. [CrossRef]
38. Sun, Y.; Zhang, J.; Lu, L.; Chen, S.S.; Quinn, M.T.; Weber, K.T. Aldosterone-Induced Inflammation in the Rat Heart: Role of oxidative stress. *Am. J. Pathol.* **2002**, *161*, 1773–1781. [CrossRef]
39. Nakaya, M.; Chikura, S.; Watari, K.; Mizuno, N.; Mochinaga, K.; Mangmool, S.; Koyanagi, S.; Ohdo, S.; Sato, Y.; Ide, T.; et al. Induction of Cardiac Fibrosis by β-Blocker in G Protein-independent and G Protein-coupled Receptor Kinase 5/β-Arrestin2-dependent Signaling Pathways. *J. Biol. Chem.* **2012**, *287*, 35669–35677. [CrossRef]
40. Communal, C.; Singh, K.; Sawyer, D.B.; Colucci, W.S. Opposing Effects of β_1- and β_2-Adrenergic Receptors on Cardiac Myocyte Apoptosis: Role of a pertussis toxin-sensitive G protein. Circulation. *Circulation* **1999**, *100*, 2210–2212. [CrossRef]
41. Benjamin, I.J.; Jalil, J.E.; Tan, L.B.; Cho, K.; Weber, K.T.; Clark, W.A. Isoproterenol-induced myocardial fibrosis in relation to myocyte necrosis. *Circ. Res.* **1989**, *65*, 657–670. [CrossRef] [PubMed]
42. Nguyen, M.-N.; Kiriazis, H.; Ruggiero, D.; Gao, X.-M.; Su, Y.; Jian, A.; Han, L.-P.; McMullen, J.R.; Du, X.-J. Spontaneous ventricular tachyarrhythmias in β2-adrenoceptor transgenic mice in relation to cardiac interstitial fibrosis. *Am. J. Physiol. Circ. Physiol.* **2015**, *309*, H946–H957. [CrossRef] [PubMed]
43. Hermida, N.; Michel, L.Y.; Esfahani, H.; Dubois-Deruy, E.; Hammond, J.; Bouzin, C.; Markl, A.; Colin, H.; Van Steenbergen, A.; De Meester, C.; et al. Cardiac myocyte β3-adrenergic receptors prevent myocardial fibrosis by modulating oxidant stress-dependent paracrine signaling. *Eur. Heart J.* **2017**, *39*, 888–898. [CrossRef] [PubMed]
44. Yamamoto, K.; Masuyama, T.; Sakata, Y.; Mano, T.; Nishikawa, N.; Kondo, H.; Akehi, N.; Kuzuya, T.; Miwa, T.; Hori, M. Roles of renin–angiotensin and endothelin systems in development of diastolic heart failure in hypertensive hearts. *Cardiovasc. Res.* **2000**, *47*, 274–283. [CrossRef]
45. Kulasekaran, P.; Scavone, C.A.; Rogers, D.S.; Arenberg, D.A.; Thannickal, V.J.; Horowitz, J.C. Endothelin-1 and Transforming Growth Factor-β1 Independently Induce Fibroblast Resistance to Apoptosis via AKT Activation. *Am. J. Respir. Cell Mol. Biol.* **2009**, *41*, 484–493. [CrossRef]
46. Wray, D.W.; Nishiyama, S.K.; Richardson, R.S. Role of α1-adrenergic vasoconstriction in the regulation of skeletal muscle blood flow with advancing age. *Am. J. Physiol. Circ. Physiol.* **2009**, *296*, H497–H504. [CrossRef]
47. Sun, M.; Chen, M.; Dawood, F.; Zurawska, U.; Li, J.Y.; Parker, T.S.; Kassiri, Z.; Kirshenbaum, L.A.; Arnold, M.; Khokha, R.; et al. Tumor Necrosis Factor-α Mediates Cardiac Remodeling and Ventricular Dysfunction After Pressure Overload State. *Circulation* **2007**, *115*, 1398–1407. [CrossRef] [PubMed]
48. Bozkurt, B.; Torre-Amione, G.; Warren, M.S.; Whitmore, J.; Soran, O.Z.; Feldman, A.M.; Mann, U.L. Results of Targeted Anti-Tumor Necrosis Factor Therapy with Etanercept (ENBREL) in Patients with Advanced Heart Failure. *Circulation* **2001**, *103*, 1044–1047. [CrossRef]
49. Okuno, T.; Andoh, A.; Bamba, S.; Araki, Y.; Fujiyama, Y.; Fujimiya, M.; Bamba, T. Interleukin-1β and Tumor Necrosis Factor-α Induce Chemokine and Matrix Metalloproteinase Gene Expression in Human Colonic Subepithelial Myofibroblasts. *Scand. J. Gastroenterol.* **2002**, *37*, 317–324. [CrossRef]
50. Zhang, W.; Chancey, A.L.; Tzeng, H.-P.; Zhou, Z.; Lavine, K.J.; Gao, F.; Sivasubramanian, N.; Barger, P.M.; Mann, D.L. The Development of Myocardial Fibrosis in Transgenic Mice with Targeted Overexpression of Tumor Necrosis Factor Requires Mast Cell–Fibroblast Interactions. *Circulation* **2011**, *124*, 2106–2116. [CrossRef]

51. Brønnum, H.; Eskildsen, T.; Andersen, D.C.; Schneider, M.; Sheikh, S.P. IL-1β suppresses TGF-β-mediated myofibroblast differentiation in cardiac fibroblasts. *Growth Factors* **2013**, *31*, 81–89. [CrossRef] [PubMed]
52. Ikonomidis, I.; Lekakis, J.P.; Nikolaou, M.; Paraskevaidis, I.; Andreadou, I.; Kaplanoglou, T.; Katsimbri, P.; Skarantavos, G.; Soucacos, P.N.; Kremastinos, D.T. Inhibition of Interleukin-1 by Anakinra Improves Vascular and Left Ventricular Function in Patients with Rheumatoid Arthritis. *Circulation* **2008**, *117*, 2662–2669. [CrossRef] [PubMed]
53. Lai, N.C.; Gao, M.H.; Tang, E.; Tang, R.; Guo, T.; Dalton, N.D.; Deng, A.; Tang, T. Pressure overload-induced cardiac remodeling and dysfunction in the absence of interleukin 6 in mice. *Lab. Investig.* **2012**, *92*, 1518–1526. [CrossRef]
54. Banerjee, I.; Fuseler, J.W.; Intwala, A.R.; Baudino, T.A. IL-6 loss causes ventricular dysfunction, fibrosis, reduced capillary density, and dramatically alters the cell populations of the developing and adult heart. *Am. J. Physiol. Circ. Physiol.* **2009**, *296*, H1694–H1704. [CrossRef]
55. Brooks, W.W.; Conrad, C.H. Myocardial Fibrosis in Transforming Growth Factor β1Heterozygous Mice. *J. Mol. Cell. Cardiol.* **2000**, *32*, 187–195. [CrossRef] [PubMed]
56. Khan, S.; Joyce, J.; Margulies, K.B.; Tsuda, T. Enhanced Bioactive Myocardial Transforming Growth Factor-β in Advanced Human Heart Failure. *Circ. J.* **2014**, *78*, 2711–2718. [CrossRef]
57. Rosenkranz, S.; Flesch, M.; Amann, K.; Haeuseler, C.; Kilter, H.; Seeland, U.; Schlüter, K.-D.; Böhm, M. Alterations of β-adrenergic signaling and cardiac hypertrophy in transgenic mice overexpressing TGF-β$_1$. *Am. J. Physiol. Circ. Physiol.* **2002**, *283*, H1253–H1262. [CrossRef] [PubMed]
58. Hanna, A.; Frangogiannis, N.G. The Role of the TGF-β Superfamily in Myocardial Infarction. *Front. Cardiovasc. Med.* **2019**, *6*, 140. [CrossRef]
59. Khalil, H.; Kanisicak, O.; Prasad, V.; Correll, R.N.; Fu, X.; Schips, T.; Vagnozzi, R.J.; Liu, R.; Huynh, T.; Lee, S.-J.; et al. Fibroblast-specific TGF-β–Smad2/3 signaling underlies cardiac fibrosis. *J. Clin. Investig.* **2017**, *127*, 3770–3783. [CrossRef]
60. Huang, S.; Chen, B.; Su, Y.; Alex, L.; Humeres, C.; Shinde, A.V.; Conway, S.J.; Frangogiannis, N.G. Distinct roles of myofibroblast-specific Smad2 and Smad3 signaling in repair and remodeling of the infarcted heart. *J. Mol. Cell. Cardiol.* **2019**, *132*, 84–97. [CrossRef]
61. Kong, P.; Shinde, A.V.; Su, Y.; Russo, I.; Chen, B.; Saxena, A.; Conway, S.J.; Graff, J.M.; Frangogiannis, N.G. Opposing Actions of Fibroblast and Cardiomyocyte Smad3 Signaling in the Infarcted Myocardium. *Circulation* **2018**, *137*, 707–724. [CrossRef] [PubMed]
62. Bageghni, S.A.; Hemmings, K.E.; Zava, N.; Denton, C.P.; Porter, K.E.; Ainscough, J.F.X.; Drinkhill, M.J.; Turner, N.A. Cardiac fibroblast-specific p38α MAP kinase promotes cardiac hypertrophy *via* a putative paracrine interleukin-6 signaling mechanism. *FASEB J.* **2018**, *32*, 4941–4954. [CrossRef] [PubMed]
63. Cosme, J.; Guo, H.; Hadipour-Lakmehsari, S.; Emili, A.; Gramolini, A.O. Hypoxia-Induced Changes in the Fibroblast Secretome, Exosome, and Whole-Cell Proteome Using Cultured, Cardiac-Derived Cells Isolated from Neonatal Mice. *J. Proteome Res.* **2017**, *16*, 2836–2847. [CrossRef] [PubMed]
64. Barile, L.; Milano, G.; Vassalli, G. Beneficial effects of exosomes secreted by cardiac-derived progenitor cells and other cell types in myocardial ischemia. *Stem Cell Investig.* **2017**, *4*, 93. [CrossRef]
65. Yue, Y.; Garikipati, V.N.S.; Verma, S.K.; Goukassian, D.A.; Kishore, R. Interleukin-10 Deficiency Impairs Reparative Properties of Bone Marrow-Derived Endothelial Progenitor Cell Exosomes. *Tissue Eng. Part A* **2017**, *23*, 1241–1250. [CrossRef]
66. Liu, T.; Song, D.; Dong, J.; Zhu, P.; Liu, J.; Liu, W.; Ma, X.; Zhao, L.; Ling, S. Current Understanding of the Pathophysiology of Myocardial Fibrosis and Its Quantitative Assessment in Heart Failure. *Front. Physiol.* **2017**, *8*, 238. [CrossRef]
67. López, B.; González, A.; Ravassa, S.; Beaumont, J.; Moreno, M.U.; José, G.S.; Querejeta, R.; Díez, J. Circulating Biomarkers of Myocardial Fibrosis: The Need for a Reappraisal. *J. Am. Coll. Cardiol.* **2015**, *65*, 2449–2456. [CrossRef] [PubMed]
68. Gudowska-Sawczuk, M.; Gruszewska, E.; Panasiuk, A.; Cylwik, B.; Swiderska, M.; Flisiak, R.; Szmitkowski, M.; Chrostek, L. High serum N-terminal propeptide of procollagen type III concentration is associated with liver diseases. *Gastroenterol. Rev.* **2017**, *12*, 203–207. [CrossRef]
69. Liu, Y.; Wu, Q.; Zhang, S.; Wang, Z.; Liu, H.; Teng, L.; Xiao, P.; Lu, Y.; Wang, X.; Dong, C.; et al. Serum Galectin-3 levels and all-cause and cardiovascular mortality in maintenance hemodialysis patients: A prospective cohort study. *BMC Nephrol.* **2022**, *23*, 5. [CrossRef]
70. Thum, T.; Gross, C.; Fiedler, J.; Fischer, T.; Kissler, S.; Bussen, M.; Galuppo, P.; Just, S.; Rottbauer, W.; Frantz, S.; et al. MicroRNA-21 contributes to myocardial disease by stimulating MAP kinase signalling in fibroblasts. *Nature* **2008**, *456*, 980–984. [CrossRef]
71. Lok, S.I.; Nous, F.M.; Van Kuik, J.; Van Der Weide, P.; Winkens, B.; Kemperman, H.; Huisman, A.; Lahpor, J.R.; De Weger, R.A.; De Jonge, N. Myocardial fibrosis and pro-fibrotic markers in end-stage heart failure patients during continuous-flow left ventricular assist device support. *Eur. J. Cardio-Thorac. Surg.* **2015**, *48*, 407–415. [CrossRef] [PubMed]
72. Everett, R.; Stirrat, C.; Semple, S.; Newby, D.; Dweck, M.; Mirsadraee, S. Assessment of myocardial fibrosis with T1 mapping MRI. *Clin. Radiol.* **2016**, *71*, 768–778. [CrossRef]
73. Flett, A.S.; Hayward, M.P.; Ashworth, M.T.; Hansen, M.; Taylor, A.M.; Elliott, P.; McGregor, C.; Moon, J. Equilibrium Contrast Cardiovascular Magnetic Resonance for the Measurement of Diffuse Myocardial Fibrosis: Preliminary Validation in Humans. Circulation. *Circulation* **2010**, *122*, 138–144. [CrossRef] [PubMed]
74. Mondillo, S.; Galderisi, M.; Mele, D.; Cameli, M.; Lomoriello, V.S.; Zacà, V.; Ballo, P.; D'Andrea, A.; Muraru, D.; Losi, M.; et al. Speckle-Tracking Echocardiography. *J. Ultrasound Med.* **2011**, *30*, 71–83. [CrossRef] [PubMed]

75. Popovic, Z.; Kwon, D.H.; Mishra, M.; Buakhamsri, A.; Greenberg, N.L.; Thamilarasan, M.; Flamm, S.D.; Thomas, J.D.; Lever, H.M.; Desai, M.Y. Association Between Regional Ventricular Function and Myocardial Fibrosis in Hypertrophic Cardiomyopathy Assessed by Speckle Tracking Echocardiography and Delayed Hyperenhancement Magnetic Resonance Imaging. *J. Am. Soc. Echocardiogr.* **2008**, *21*, 1299–1305. [CrossRef] [PubMed]
76. Mizuno, R.; Fujimoto, S.; Saito, Y.; Nakamura, S. Non-Invasive Quantitation of Myocardial Fibrosis Using Combined Tissue Harmonic Imaging and Integrated Backscatter Analysis in Dilated Cardiomyopathy. *Cardiology* **2007**, *108*, 11–17. [CrossRef]
77. Zannad, F.; Alla, F.; Dousset, B.; Perez, A.; Pitt, B. Limitation of Excessive Extracellular Matrix Turnover May Contribute to Survival Benefit of Spironolactone Therapy in Patients with Congestive Heart Failure: Insights from the randomized aldactone evaluation study (RALES). Rales Investigators. *Circulation* **2000**, *102*, 2700–2706. [CrossRef] [PubMed]
78. Brilla, C.G.; Funck, R.C.; Rupp, H. Lisinopril-Mediated Regression of Myocardial Fibrosis in Patients with Hypertensive Heart Disease. *Circulation* **2000**, *102*, 1388–1393. [CrossRef]
79. Shibasaki, Y.; Nishiue, T.; Masaki, H.; Tamura, K.; Matsumoto, N.; Mori, Y.; Nishikawa, M.; Matsubara, H.; Iwasaka, T. Impact of the Angiotensin II Receptor Antagonist, Losartan, on Myocardial Fibrosis in Patients with End-Stage Renal Disease: Assessment by Ultrasonic Integrated Backscatter and Biochemical Markers. *Hypertens. Res.* **2005**, *28*, 787–795. [CrossRef] [PubMed]
80. Zile, M.R.; Jhund, P.S.; Baicu, C.F.; Claggett, B.L.; Pieske, B.; Voors, A.A.; Prescott, M.F.; Shi, V.; Lefkowitz, M.; McMurray, J.J.; et al. Plasma Biomarkers Reflecting Profibrotic Processes in Heart Failure with a Preserved Ejection Fraction: Data from the Prospective Comparison of ARNI with ARB on Management of Heart Failure With Preserved Ejection Fraction Study. *Circ. Heart Fail.* **2016**, *9*, e002551. [CrossRef]
81. Abulhul, E.; McDonald, K.; Martos, R.; Phelan, D.; Spiers, J.P.; Hennessy, M.; Baugh, J.; Watson, C.; O'Loughlin, C.; Ledwidge, M. Long-Term Statin Therapy in Patients with Systolic Heart Failure and Normal Cholesterol: Effects on Elevated Serum Markers of Collagen Turnover, Inflammation, and B-Type Natriuretic Peptide. *Clin. Ther.* **2012**, *34*, 91–100. [CrossRef] [PubMed]
82. Ashton, E.; Windebank, E.; Skiba, M.; Reid, C.; Schneider, H.; Rosenfeldt, F.; Tonkin, A.; Krum, H. Why did high-dose rosuvastatin not improve cardiac remodeling in chronic heart failure? Mechanistic insights from the UNIVERSE study. *Int. J. Cardiol.* **2011**, *146*, 404–407. [CrossRef]
83. Lewis, G.A.; Dodd, S.; Clayton, D.; Bedson, E.; Eccleson, H.; Schelbert, E.B.; Naish, J.H.; Jimenez, B.D.; Williams, S.G.; Cunnington, C.; et al. Pirfenidone in heart failure with preserved ejection fraction: A randomized phase 2 trial. *Nat. Med.* **2021**, *27*, 1477–1482. [CrossRef] [PubMed]
84. Hocher, B.; Godes, M.; Olivier, J.; Weil, J.; Eschenhagen, T.; Slowinski, T.; Neumayer, H.-H.; Bauer, C.; Paul, M.; Pinto, Y.M. Inhibition of left ventricular fibrosis by tranilast in rats with renovascular hypertension. *J. Hypertens.* **2002**, *20*, 745–751. [CrossRef] [PubMed]
85. Visnagri, A.; Kandhare, A.D.; Ghosh, P.; Bodhankar, S.L. Endothelin receptor blocker bosentan inhibits hypertensive cardiac fibrosis in pressure overload-induced cardiac hypertrophy in rats. *Cardiovasc. Endocrinol.* **2013**, *2*, 85–97. [CrossRef]
86. Soylu, K.; Cerik, I.B.; Aksan, G.; Nar, G.; Meric, M. Evaluation of ivabradine in left ventricular dyssynchrony and reverse remodeling in patients with chronic heart failure. *J. Arrhythmia* **2020**, *36*, 762–767. [CrossRef]
87. Giannetta, E.; Isidori, A.M.; Galea, N.; Carbone, I.; Mandosi, E.; Vizza, C.D.; Naro, F.; Morano, S.; Fedele, F.; Lenzi, A. Chronic Inhibition of cGMP Phosphodiesterase 5A Improves Diabetic Cardiomyopathy: A Randomized, Controlled Clinical Trial Using Magnetic Resonance Imaging with Myocardial Tagging. *Circulation* **2012**, *125*, 2323–2333. [CrossRef] [PubMed]
88. Östman-Smith, I. Reduction by oral propranolol treatment of left ventricular hypertrophy secondary to pressure-overload in the rat. *J. Cereb. Blood Flow Metab.* **1995**, *116*, 2703–2709. [CrossRef]
89. Sandmann, S.; Bohle, R.M.; Dreyer, T.; Unger, T. The T-type calcium channel blocker mibefradil reduced interstitial and perivascular fibrosis and improved hemodynamic parameters in myocardial infarction-induced cardiac failure in rats. *Virchows Arch.* **2000**, *436*, 147–157. [CrossRef] [PubMed]
90. Zhi, H.; Luptak, I.; Alreja, G.; Shi, J.; Guan, J.; Metes-Kosik, N.; Joseph, J. Effects of Direct Renin Inhibition on Myocardial Fibrosis and Cardiac Fibroblast Function. *PLoS ONE* **2013**, *8*, e81612. [CrossRef]
91. Yamamoto, K.; Mano, T.; Yoshida, J.; Sakata, Y.; Nishikawa, N.; Nishio, M.; Ohtani, T.; Hori, M.; Miwa, T.; Masuyama, T. ACE inhibitor and angiotensin II type 1 receptor blocker differently regulate ventricular fibrosis in hypertensive diastolic heart failure. *J. Hypertens.* **2005**, *23*, 393–400. [CrossRef]
92. Cleland, J.G.; Tendera, M.; Adamus, J.; Freemantle, N.; Polonski, L.; Taylor, J. The perindopril in elderly people with chronic heart failure (PEP-CHF) study. *Eur. Heart J.* **2006**, *27*, 2338–2345. [CrossRef]
93. Lim, D.-S.; Lutucuta, S.; Bachireddy, P.; Youker, K.; Evans, A.; Entman, M.; Roberts, R.; Marian, A.J. Angiotensin II Blockade Reverses Myocardial Fibrosis in a Transgenic Mouse Model of Human Hypertrophic Cardiomyopathy. *Circulation* **2001**, *103*, 789–791. [CrossRef]
94. Pitt, B.; Zannad, F.; Remme, W.J.; Cody, R.; Castaigne, A.; Perez, A.; Palensky, J.; Wittes, J. The effect of spironolactone on morbidity and mortality in patients with severe heart failure. Randomized Aldactone Evaluation Study Investigators. *N. Engl. J. Med.* **1999**, *341*, 709–717. [CrossRef]
95. McDiarmid, A.K.; Swoboda, P.P.; Erhayiem, B.; Bounford, K.A.; Bijsterveld, P.; Tyndall, K.; Fent, G.J.; Garg, P.; Dobson, L.E.; Musa, T.A.; et al. Myocardial Effects of Aldosterone Antagonism in Heart Failure with Preserved Ejection Fraction. *J. Am. Heart Assoc.* **2020**, *9*, e011521. [CrossRef]

96. Girerd, N.; Ferreira, J.P.; Rossignol, P.; Zannad, F. A tentative interpretation of the TOPCAT trial based on randomized evidence from the brain natriuretic peptide stratum analysis. *Eur. J. Heart Fail.* **2016**, *18*, 1411–1414. [CrossRef]
97. Liu, F.; Chen, Y.; Feng, X.; Teng, Z.; Yuan, Y.; Bin, J. Effects of Beta-Blockers on Heart Failure with Preserved Ejection Fraction: A Meta-Analysis. *PLoS ONE* **2014**, *9*, e90555. [CrossRef]
98. Kobayashi, M.; Machida, N.; Mitsuishi, M.; Yamane, Y. β-blocker improves survival, left ventricular function, and myocardial remodeling in hypertensive rats with diastolic heart failure. *Am. J. Hypertens.* **2004**, *17*, 1112–1119. [CrossRef]
99. Ciulla, M.M.; Paliotti, R.; Esposito, A.; Dìiez, J.; Loópez, B.; Dahlöf, B.; Nicholls, M.G.; Smith, R.D.; Gilles, L.; Magrini, F.; et al. Different Effects of Antihypertensive Therapies Based on Losartan or Atenolol on Ultrasound and Biochemical Markers of Myocardial Fibrosis: Results of a Randomized Trial. *Circulation* **2004**, *110*, 552–557. [CrossRef] [PubMed]
100. Sandmann, S.; Claas, R.; Cleutjens, J.P.M.; Daemen, M.J.A.P.; Unger, T. Calcium Channel Blockade Limits Cardiac Remodeling and Improves Cardiac Function in Myocardial Infarction-Induced Heart Failure in Rats. *J. Cardiovasc. Pharmacol.* **2001**, *37*, 64–77. [CrossRef]
101. Teng, G.; Svystonyuk, D.; Mewhort, H.E.M.; Turnbull, J.D.; Belke, D.D.; Duff, H.J.; Fedak, P.W.M. Tetrandrine reverses human cardiac myofibroblast activation and myocardial fibrosis. *Am. J. Physiol. Circ. Physiol.* **2015**, *308*, H1564–H1574. [CrossRef] [PubMed]
102. Chang, S.-A.; Kim, Y.-J.; Lee, H.-W.; Kim, D.-H.; Kim, H.-K.; Chang, H.-J.; Sohn, D.-W.; Oh, B.-H.; Park, Y.-B. Effect of Rosuvastatin on Cardiac Remodeling, Function, and Progression to Heart Failure in Hypertensive Heart with Established Left Ventricular Hypertrophy. *Hypertension* **2009**, *54*, 591–597. [CrossRef]
103. Chang, Y.-Y.; Wu, Y.-W.; Lee, J.-K.; Lin, Y.-M.; Lin, Y.-H.; Kao, H.-L.; Hung, C.-S.; Lin, H.-J. Effects of 12 weeks of atorvastatin therapy on myocardial fibrosis and circulating fibrosis biomarkers in statin-naïve patients with hypertension with atherosclerosis. *J. Investig. Med.* **2016**, *64*, 1194–1199. [CrossRef]
104. Krum, H.; Ashton, E.; Reid, C.; Kalff, V.; Rogers, J.; Amarena, J.; Singh, B.; Tonkin, A. Double-Blind, Randomized, Placebo-Controlled Study of High-Dose HMG CoA Reductase Inhibitor Therapy on Ventricular Remodeling, Pro-Inflammatory Cytokines and Neurohormonal Parameters in Patients with Chronic Systolic Heart Failure. *J. Card. Fail.* **2007**, *13*, 1–7. [CrossRef] [PubMed]
105. Mulder, P.; Richard, V.; Derumeaux, G.; Hogie, M.; Henry, J.P.; Lallemand, F.; Compagnon, P.; Macé, B.; Comoy, E.; Letac, B.; et al. Role of Endogenous Endothelin in Chronic Heart Failure: Effect of Long-Term Treatment with an Endothelin Antagonist on Survival, Hemodynamics, and Cardiac Remodeling. *Circulation* **1997**, *96*, 1976–1982. [CrossRef]
106. Prasad, S.K.; Dargie, H.J.; Smith, G.C.; Barlow, M.M.; Grothues, F.; Groenning, B.A.; Cleland, J.G.; Pennell, D.J. Comparison of the dual receptor endothelin antagonist enrasentan with enalapril in asymptomatic left ventricular systolic dysfunction: A cardiovascular magnetic resonance study. *Heart* **2006**, *92*, 798–803. [CrossRef] [PubMed]
107. Anand, I.; McMurray, J.; Cohn, J.N.; Konstam, M.A.; Notter, T.; Quitzau, K.; Ruschitzka, F.; Lüscher, T.F. Long-term effects of darusentan on left-ventricular remodelling and clinical outcomes in the Endothelin A Receptor Antagonist Trial in Heart Failure (EARTH): Randomised, double-blind, placebo-controlled trial. *Lancet* **2004**, *364*, 347–354. [CrossRef]
108. Park, S.; Nguyen, N.B.; Pezhouman, A.; Ardehali, R. Cardiac fibrosis: Potential therapeutic targets. *Transl. Res.* **2019**, *209*, 121–137. [CrossRef]
109. Kuwahara, F.; Kai, H.; Tokuda, K.; Kai, M.; Takeshita, A.; Egashira, K.; Imaizumi, T. Transforming Growth Factor-β Function Blocking Prevents Myocardial Fibrosis and Diastolic Dysfunction in Pressure-Overloaded Rats. *Circulation* **2002**, *106*, 130–135. [CrossRef]
110. Frantz, S.; Hu, K.; Adamek, A.; Wolf, J.; Sallam, A.; Maier, S.K.; Lonning, S.; Ling, H.; Ertl, G.; Bauersachs, J. Transforming growth factor beta inhibition increases mortality and left ventricular dilatation after myocardial infarction. *Basic Res. Cardiol.* **2008**, *103*, 485–492. [CrossRef]
111. Engebretsen, K.V.; Skårdal, K.; Bjørnstad, S.; Marstein, H.S.; Skrbic, B.; Sjaastad, I.; Christensen, G.; Bjørnstad, J.L.; Tønnessen, T. Attenuated development of cardiac fibrosis in left ventricular pressure overload by SM16, an orally active inhibitor of ALK5. *J. Mol. Cell. Cardiol.* **2014**, *76*, 148–157. [CrossRef] [PubMed]
112. Okada, H.; Takemura, G.; Kosai, K.-I.; Li, Y.; Takahashi, T.; Esaki, M.; Yuge, K.; Miyata, S.; Maruyama, R.; Mikami, A.; et al. Postinfarction Gene Therapy Against Transforming Growth Factor-β Signal Modulates Infarct Tissue Dynamics and Attenuates Left Ventricular Remodeling and Heart Failure. *Circulation* **2005**, *111*, 2430–2437. [CrossRef] [PubMed]
113. Petersen, M.; Thorikay, M.; Deckers, M.; van Dinther, M.; Grygielko, E.; Gellibert, F.; de Gouville, A.; Huet, S.; Dijke, P.T.; Laping, N. Oral administration of GW788388, an inhibitor of TGF-β type I and II receptor kinases, decreases renal fibrosis. *Kidney Int.* **2008**, *73*, 705–715. [CrossRef] [PubMed]
114. Ono, K.; Ohtomo, T.; Ninomiya-Tsuji, J.; Tsuchiya, M. A dominant negative TAK1 inhibits cellular fibrotic responses induced by TGF-β. *Biochem. Biophys. Res. Commun.* **2003**, *307*, 332–337. [CrossRef]
115. See, F.; Thomas, W.; Way, K.; Tzanidis, A.; Kompa, A.; Lewis, D.; Itescu, S.; Krum, H. p38 mitogen-activated protein kinase inhibition improves cardiac function and attenuates left ventricular remodeling following myocardial infarction in the rat. *J. Am. Coll. Cardiol.* **2004**, *44*, 1679–1689. [CrossRef] [PubMed]
116. Nguyen, D.T.; Ding, C.; Wilson, E.; Marcus, G.M.; Olgin, J.E. Pirfenidone mitigates left ventricular fibrosis and dysfunction after myocardial infarction and reduces arrhythmias. *Heart Rhythm* **2010**, *7*, 1438–1445. [CrossRef] [PubMed]

117. Martin, J.; Kelly, D.J.; Mifsud, S.A.; Zhang, Y.; Cox, A.J.; See, F.; Krum, H.; Wilkinson-Berka, J.; Gilbert, R.E. Tranilast attenuates cardiac matrix deposition in experimental diabetes: Role of transforming growth factor-β. *Cardiovasc. Res.* **2005**, *65*, 694–701. [CrossRef] [PubMed]
118. Jiang, C.; Huang, H.; Liu, J.; Wang, Y.; Lu, Z.; Xu, Z. Adverse Events of Pirfenidone for the Treatment of Pulmonary Fibrosis: A Meta-Analysis of Randomized Controlled Trials. *PLoS ONE* **2012**, *7*, e47024. [CrossRef]
119. Meng, J.; Qin, Y.; Chen, J.; Wei, L.; Huang, X.-R.; Yu, X.; Lan, H.-Y. Treatment of Hypertensive Heart Disease by Targeting Smad3 Signaling in Mice. *Mol. Ther. Methods Clin. Dev.* **2020**, *18*, 791–802. [CrossRef]
120. Chen, K.; Mehta, J.L.; Li, D.; Joseph, L.; Joseph, J. Transforming Growth Factor β Receptor Endoglin Is Expressed in Cardiac Fibroblasts and Modulates Profibrogenic Actions of Angiotensin II. *Circ. Res.* **2004**, *95*, 1167–1173. [CrossRef]
121. Kapur, N.K.; Wilson, S.; Yunis, A.A.; Qiao, X.; Mackey, E.; Paruchuri, V.; Baker, C.; Aronovitz, M.J.; Karumanchi, S.A.; Letarte, M.; et al. Reduced endoglin activity limits cardiac fibrosis and improves survival in heart failure. *Circulation* **2012**, *125*, 2728–2738. [CrossRef] [PubMed]
122. Esnault, C.; Stewart, A.; Gualdrini, F.; East, P.; Horswell, S.; Matthews, N.; Treisman, R. Rho-actin signaling to the MRTF coactivators dominates the immediate transcriptional response to serum in fibroblasts. *Genes Dev.* **2014**, *28*, 943–958. [CrossRef] [PubMed]
123. Hang, P.; Zhao, J.; Cai, B.; Tian, S.; Huang, W.; Guo, J.; Sun, C.; Li, Y.; Du, Z. Brain-Derived Neurotrophic Factor Regulates TRPC3/6 Channels and Protects Against Myocardial Infarction in Rodents. *Int. J. Biol. Sci.* **2015**, *11*, 536–545. [CrossRef]
124. Gallini, R.; Lindblom, P.; Bondjers, C.; Betsholtz, C.; Andrae, J. PDGF-A and PDGF-B induces cardiac fibrosis in transgenic mice. *Exp. Cell Res.* **2016**, *349*, 282–290. [CrossRef] [PubMed]
125. Pontén, A.; Li, X.; Thorén, P.; Aase, K.; Sjöblom, T.; Östman, A.; Eriksson, U. Transgenic Overexpression of Platelet-Derived Growth Factor-C in the Mouse Heart Induces Cardiac Fibrosis, Hypertrophy, and Dilated Cardiomyopathy. *Am. J. Pathol.* **2003**, *163*, 673–682. [CrossRef]
126. Chen, Y.; Surinkaew, S.; Naud, P.; Qi, X.-Y.; Gillis, M.-A.; Shi, Y.-F.; Tardif, J.-C.; Dobrev, D.; Nattel, S. JAK-STAT signalling and the atrial fibrillation promoting fibrotic substrate. *Cardiovasc. Res.* **2017**, *113*, 310–320. [CrossRef]
127. Liao, C.-H.; Akazawa, H.; Tamagawa, M.; Ito, K.; Yasuda, N.; Kudo, Y.; Yamamoto, R.; Ozasa, Y.; Fujimoto, M.; Wang, P.; et al. Cardiac mast cells cause atrial fibrillation through PDGF-A-mediated fibrosis in pressure-overloaded mouse hearts. *J. Clin. Investig.* **2010**, *120*, 242–253. [CrossRef]
128. Koitabashi, N.; Arai, M.; Kogure, S.; Niwano, K.; Watanabe, A.; Aoki, Y.; Maeno, T.; Nishida, T.; Kubota, S.; Takigawa, M.; et al. Increased Connective Tissue Growth Factor Relative to Brain Natriuretic Peptide as a Determinant of Myocardial Fibrosis. *Hypertension* **2007**, *49*, 1120–1127. [CrossRef] [PubMed]
129. Grotendorst, G.R.; Rahmanie, H.; Duncan, M.R. Combinatorial signaling pathways determine fibroblast proliferation and myofibroblast differentiation. *FASEB J.* **2004**, *18*, 469–479. [CrossRef]
130. Panek, A.N.; Posch, M.G.; Alenina, N.; Ghadge, S.K.; Erdmann, B.; Popova, E.; Perrot, A.; Geier, C.; Morano, R.D.I.; Bader, M.; et al. Connective Tissue Growth Factor Overexpression in Cardiomyocytes Promotes Cardiac Hypertrophy and Protection against Pressure Overload. *PLoS ONE* **2009**, *4*, e6743. [CrossRef]
131. Yoon, P.O.; Lee, M.-A.; Cha, H.; Jeong, M.H.; Kim, J.; Jang, S.P.; Choi, B.Y.; Jeong, D.; Yang, D.K.; Hajjar, R.J.; et al. The opposing effects of CCN2 and CCN5 on the development of cardiac hypertrophy and fibrosis. *J. Mol. Cell. Cardiol.* **2010**, *49*, 294–303. [CrossRef] [PubMed]
132. Vainio, L.E.; Szabó, Z.; Lin, R.; Ulvila, J.; Yrjölä, R.; Alakoski, T.; Piuhola, J.; Koch, W.J.; Ruskoaho, H.; Fouse, S.D.; et al. Connective Tissue Growth Factor Inhibition Enhances Cardiac Repair and Limits Fibrosis After Myocardial Infarction. *JACC Basic Transl. Sci.* **2019**, *4*, 83–94. [CrossRef] [PubMed]
133. Gu, J.; Noe, A.; Chandra, P.; Al-Fayoumi, S.; Ligueros-Saylan, M.; Sarangapani, R.; Maahs, S.; Ksander, G.M.; Rigel, D.F.; Jeng, A.Y.; et al. Pharmacokinetics and Pharmacodynamics of LCZ696, a Novel Dual-Acting Angiotensin Receptor-Neprilysin Inhibitor (ARNi). *J. Clin. Pharmacol.* **2010**, *50*, 401–414. [CrossRef] [PubMed]
134. Martens, P.; Beliën, H.; Dupont, M.; Vandervoort, P.; Mullens, W. The reverse remodeling response to sacubitril/valsartan therapy in heart failure with reduced ejection fraction. *Cardiovasc. Ther.* **2018**, *36*, e12435. [CrossRef] [PubMed]
135. Pfau, D.; Thorn, S.L.; Zhang, J.; Mikush, N.; Renaud, J.; Klein, R.; Dekemp, R.A.; Wu, X.; Hu, X.; Sinusas, A.J.; et al. Angiotensin Receptor Neprilysin Inhibitor Attenuates Myocardial Remodeling and Improves Infarct Perfusion in Experimental Heart Failure. *Sci. Rep.* **2019**, *9*, 5791. [CrossRef] [PubMed]
136. Braunwald, E. The Path to an Angiotensin Receptor Antagonist-Neprilysin Inhibitor in the Treatment of Heart Failure. *J. Am. Coll. Cardiol.* **2015**, *65*, 1029–1041. [CrossRef] [PubMed]
137. Liu, J.; Zheng, X.; Zhang, C.; Zhang, C.; Bu, P. Lcz696 Alleviates Myocardial Fibrosis After Myocardial Infarction Through the sFRP-1/Wnt/β-Catenin Signaling Pathway. *Front. Pharmacol.* **2021**, *12*, 724147. [CrossRef] [PubMed]
138. Januzzi, J.L.; Prescott, M.F.; Butler, J.; Felker, G.M.; Maisel, A.S.; McCague, K.; Camacho, A.; Piña, I.L.; Rocha, R.A.; Shah, A.M.; et al. Association of Change in N-Terminal Pro–B-Type Natriuretic Peptide Following Initiation of Sacubitril-Valsartan Treatment with Cardiac Structure and Function in Patients with Heart Failure with Reduced Ejection Fraction. *JAMA* **2019**, *322*, 1085–1095. [CrossRef]

139. Zile, M.R.; O'Meara, E.; Claggett, B.; Prescott, M.F.; Solomon, S.D.; Swedberg, K.; Packer, M.; McMurray, J.J.; Shi, V.; Lefkowitz, M.; et al. Effects of Sacubitril/Valsartan on Biomarkers of Extracellular Matrix Regulation in Patients with HFrEF. *J. Am. Coll. Cardiol.* **2019**, *73*, 795–806. [CrossRef]
140. Solomon, S.D.; Zile, M.; Pieske, B.; Voors, A.; Shah, A.; Kraigher-Krainer, E.; Shi, V.; Bransford, T.; Takeuchi, M.; Gong, J.; et al. The angiotensin receptor neprilysin inhibitor LCZ696 in heart failure with preserved ejection fraction: A phase 2 double-blind randomised controlled trial. *Lancet* **2012**, *380*, 1387–1395. [CrossRef]
141. Solomon, S.D.; McMurray, J.J.V.; Anand, I.S.; Junbo Ge, D.P.; Lam, C.S.P.; Maggioni, A.P.; Martinez, F.; Packer, M.; Pfeffer, M.A.; Pieske, B.; et al. Angiotensin–Neprilysin Inhibition in Heart Failure with Preserved Ejection Fraction. *N. Engl. J. Med.* **2019**, *381*, 1609–1620. [CrossRef] [PubMed]
142. Morimoto, H.; Takahashi, M.; Izawa, A.; Ise, H.; Hongo, M.; Kolattukudy, P.E.; Ikeda, U. Cardiac Overexpression of Monocyte Chemoattractant Protein-1 in Transgenic Mice Prevents Cardiac Dysfunction and Remodeling After Myocardial Infarction. *Circ. Res.* **2006**, *99*, 891–899. [CrossRef] [PubMed]
143. Haudek, S.B.; Cheng, J.; Du, J.; Wang, Y.; Hermosillo-Rodriguez, J.; Trial, J.; Taffet, G.E.; Entman, M.L. Monocytic fibroblast precursors mediate fibrosis in angiotensin-II-induced cardiac hypertrophy. *J. Mol. Cell. Cardiol.* **2010**, *49*, 499–507. [CrossRef] [PubMed]
144. Santamaria, J.G.; Villalba, M.; Busnadiego, O.; López-Olañeta, M.M.; Sandoval, P.; Snabel, J.; López-Cabrera, M.; Erler, J.; Hanemaaijer, R.; Lara-Pezzi, E.; et al. Matrix cross-linking lysyl oxidases are induced in response to myocardial infarction and promote cardiac dysfunction. *Cardiovasc. Res.* **2015**, *109*, 67–78. [CrossRef] [PubMed]
145. Roell, W.; Lewalter, T.; Sasse, P.; Tallini, Y.N.; Choi, B.-R.; Breitbach, M.; Doran, R.; Becher, U.M.; Hwang, S.-M.; Bostani, T.; et al. Engraftment of connexin 43-expressing cells prevents post-infarct arrhythmia. *Nature* **2007**, *450*, 819–824. [CrossRef] [PubMed]
146. Eloff, B.C.; Gilat, E.; Wan, X.; Rosenbaum, D.S. Pharmacological Modulation of Cardiac Gap Junctions to Enhance Cardiac Conduction: Evidence Supporting a Novel Target for Antiarrhythmic Therapy. *Circulation* **2003**, *108*, 3157–3163. [CrossRef] [PubMed]
147. Nagpal, V.; Rai, R.; Place, A.T.; Murphy, S.B.; Verma, S.K.; Ghosh, A.K.; Vaughan, D.E. MiR-125b Is Critical for Fibroblast-to-Myofibroblast Transition and Cardiac Fibrosis. *Circulation* **2016**, *133*, 291–301. [CrossRef] [PubMed]
148. Van Rooij, E.; Sutherland, L.B.; Thatcher, J.E.; DiMaio, J.M.; Naseem, R.H.; Marshall, W.S.; Hill, J.A.; Olson, E.N. Dysregulation of microRNAs after myocardial infarction reveals a role of miR-29 in cardiac fibrosis. *Proc. Natl. Acad. Sci. USA* **2008**, *105*, 13027–13032. [CrossRef] [PubMed]
149. Zhang, Y.; Huang, X.-R.; Wei, L.-H.; Chung, A.C.; Yu, C.-M.; Lan, H.-Y. miR-29b as a Therapeutic Agent for Angiotensin II-induced Cardiac Fibrosis by Targeting TGF-β/Smad3 signaling. *Mol. Ther.* **2014**, *22*, 974–985. [CrossRef]
150. Duisters, R.F.; Tijsen, A.J.; Schroen, B.; Leenders, J.J.; Lentink, V.; van der Made, I.; Herias, V.; van Leeuwen, R.E.; Schellings, M.W.; Barenbrug, P.; et al. miR-133 and miR-30 regulate connective tissue growth factor: Implications for a role of microRNAs in myocardial matrix remodeling. *Circ. Res.* **2009**, *104*, 170–178. [CrossRef]
151. Wang, Y.-S.; Li, S.-H.; Guo, J.; Mihic, A.; Wu, J.; Sun, L.; Davis, K.; Weisel, R.D.; Li, R.-K. Role of miR-145 in cardiac myofibroblast differentiation. *J. Mol. Cell. Cardiol.* **2013**, *66*, 94–105. [CrossRef] [PubMed]
152. Norris, R.A.; Damon, B.; Mironov, V.; Kasyanov, V.; Ramamurthi, A.; Moreno-Rodriguez, R.; Trusk, T.; Potts, J.D.; Goodwin, R.L.; Davis, J.; et al. Periostin regulates collagen fibrillogenesis and the biomechanical properties of connective tissues. *J. Cell. Biochem.* **2007**, *101*, 695–711. [CrossRef] [PubMed]
153. Zhao, S.; Wu, H.; Xia, W.; Chen, X.; Zhu, S.; Zhang, S.; Shao, Y.; Ma, W.; Yang, D.; Zhang, J. Periostin expression is upregulated and associated with myocardial fibrosis in human failing hearts. *J. Cardiol.* **2014**, *63*, 373–378. [CrossRef] [PubMed]
154. Yoshizumi, T.; Zhu, Y.; Jiang, H.; D'Amore, A.; Sakaguchi, H.; Tchao, J.; Tobita, K.; Wagner, W.R. Timing effect of intramyocardial hydrogel injection for positively impacting left ventricular remodeling after myocardial infarction. *Biomaterials* **2015**, *83*, 182–193. [CrossRef]
155. French, K.M.; Maxwell, J.T.; Bhutani, S.; Ghosh-Choudhary, S.; Fierro, M.J.; Johnson, T.D.; Christman, K.L.; Taylor, W.R.; Davis, M.E. Fibronectin and Cyclic Strain Improve Cardiac Progenitor Cell Regenerative PotentialIn Vitro. *Stem Cells Int.* **2016**, *2016*, 8364382. [CrossRef]
156. Traverse, J.H.; Henry, T.D.; Dib, N.; Patel, A.N.; Pepine, C.; Schaer, G.L.; DeQuach, J.A.; Kinsey, A.M.; Chamberlin, P.; Christman, K.L. First-in-Man Study of a Cardiac Extracellular Matrix Hydrogel in Early and Late Myocardial Infarction Patients. *JACC Basic Transl. Sci.* **2019**, *4*, 659–669. [CrossRef]
157. Wang, F.; Li, Z.; Tamama, K.; Sen, C.K.; Guan, J. Fabrication and Characterization of Prosurvival Growth Factor Releasing, Anisotropic Scaffolds for Enhanced Mesenchymal Stem Cell Survival/Growth and Orientation. *Biomacromolecules* **2009**, *10*, 2609–2618. [CrossRef] [PubMed]
158. Pozzobon, M.; Bollini, S.; Iop, L.; De Gaspari, P.; Chiavegato, A.; Rossi, C.A.; Giuliani, S.; Leon, F.F.; Elvassore, N.; Sartore, S.; et al. Human Bone Marrow-Derived CD133$^+$ Cells Delivered to a Collagen Patch on Cryoinjured Rat Heart Promote Angiogenesis and Arteriogenesis. *Cell Transplant.* **2010**, *19*, 1247–1260. [CrossRef] [PubMed]
159. Xiong, Q.; Hill, K.L.; Li, Q.; Suntharalingam, P.; Mansoor, A.; Wang, X.; Jameel, M.N.; Zhang, P.; Swingen, C.; Kaufman, D.S.; et al. A Fibrin Patch-Based Enhanced Delivery of Human Embryonic Stem Cell-Derived Vascular Cell Transplantation in a Porcine Model of Postinfarction Left Ventricular Remodeling. *Stem Cells* **2010**, *29*, 367–375. [CrossRef] [PubMed]

160. Sun, C.-K.; Zhen, Y.-Y.; Leu, S.; Tsai, T.-H.; Chang, L.-T.; Sheu, J.-J.; Chen, Y.-L.; Chua, S.; Chai, H.-T.; Lu, H.-I.; et al. Direct implantation versus platelet-rich fibrin-embedded adipose-derived mesenchymal stem cells in treating rat acute myocardial infarction. *Int. J. Cardiol.* **2014**, *173*, 410–423. [CrossRef]
161. Engler, A.; Krieger, C.; Johnson, C.P.; Raab, M.; Tang, H.-Y.; Speicher, D.W.; Sanger, J.W.; Sanger, J.M.; Discher, D.E. Embryonic cardiomyocytes beat best on a matrix with heart-like elasticity: Scar-like rigidity inhibits beating. *J. Cell Sci.* **2008**, *121 Pt 22*, 3794–3802. [CrossRef]
162. Miyagawa, S.; Saito, A.; Sakaguchi, T.; Yoshikawa, Y.; Yamauchi, T.; Imanishi, Y.; Kawaguchi, N.; Teramoto, N.; Matsuura, N.; Iida, H.; et al. Impaired Myocardium Regeneration with Skeletal Cell Sheets—A Preclinical Trial for Tissue-Engineered Regeneration Therapy. *Transplantation* **2010**, *90*, 364–372. [CrossRef] [PubMed]
163. Miyagawa, S.; Domae, K.; Yoshikawa, Y.; Fukushima, S.; Nakamura, T.; Saito, A.; Sakata, Y.; Hamada, S.; Toda, K.; Pak, K.; et al. Phase I Clinical Trial of Autologous Stem Cell–Sheet Transplantation Therapy for Treating Cardiomyopathy. *J. Am. Heart Assoc.* **2017**, *6*, e003918. [CrossRef] [PubMed]
164. Lagoutte, P.; Bettler, E.; Goff, S.V.-L.; Moali, C. Procollagen C-proteinase enhancer-1 (PCPE-1), a potential biomarker and therapeutic target for fibrosis. *Matrix Biol. Plus* **2021**, *11*, 100062. [CrossRef] [PubMed]
165. Morel, P.S.; Duvivier, V.; Bertin, F.; Provost, N.; Hammoutene, A.; Hubert, E.-L.; Gonzalez, A.; Tupinon-Mathieu, I.; Paradis, V.; Delerive, P. Procollagen C-Proteinase Enhancer-1 (PCPE-1) deficiency in mice reduces liver fibrosis but not NASH progression. *PLoS ONE* **2022**, *17*, e0263828. [CrossRef]
166. Baicu, C.F.; Zhang, Y.; Van Laer, A.O.; Renaud, L.; Zile, M.R.; Bradshaw, A.D. Effects of the absence of procollagen C-endopeptidase enhancer-2 on myocardial collagen accumulation in chronic pressure overload. *Am. J. Physiol. Circ. Physiol.* **2012**, *303*, H234–H240. [CrossRef]
167. Zhou, R.; Wang, C.; Wen, C.; Wang, D. miR-21 promotes collagen production in keloid via Smad7. *Burns* **2017**, *43*, 555–561. [CrossRef] [PubMed]
168. Liu, S.; Li, W.; Xu, M.; Huang, H.; Wang, J.; Chen, X. Micro-RNA 21 Targets Dual Specific Phosphatase 8 to Promote Collagen Synthesis in High Glucose–Treated Primary Cardiac Fibroblasts. *Can. J. Cardiol.* **2014**, *30*, 1689–1699. [CrossRef] [PubMed]
169. Lekgabe, E.D.; Kiriazis, H.; Zhao, C.; Xu, Q.; Moore, X.L.; Su, Y.; Bathgate, R.; Du, X.-J.; Samuel, C.S. Relaxin Reverses Cardiac and Renal Fibrosis in Spontaneously Hypertensive Rats. *Hypertension* **2005**, *46*, 412–418. [CrossRef]
170. Sassoli, C.; Chellini, F.; Pini, A.; Tani, A.; Nistri, S.; Nosi, D.; Zecchi-Orlandini, S.; Bani, D.; Formigli, L. Relaxin Prevents Cardiac Fibroblast-Myofibroblast Transition via Notch-1-Mediated Inhibition of TGF-β/Smad3 Signaling. *PLoS ONE* **2013**, *8*, e63896. [CrossRef] [PubMed]
171. Ponikowski, P.; Metra, M.; Teerlink, J.R.; Unemori, E.; Felker, G.M.; Voors, A.A.; Filippatos, G.; Greenberg, B.; Teichman, S.L.; Severin, T.; et al. Design of the RELAXin in Acute Heart Failure Study. *Am. Heart J.* **2012**, *163*, 149–155. [CrossRef] [PubMed]
172. Spinale, F.G.; Villarreal, F. Targeting matrix metalloproteinases in heart disease: Lessons from endogenous inhibitors. *Biochem. Pharmacol.* **2014**, *90*, 7–15. [CrossRef] [PubMed]
173. Eckhouse, S.R.; Purcell, B.P.; McGarvey, J.R.; Lobb, D.; Logdon, C.B.; Doviak, H.; O'Neill, J.W.; Shuman, J.A.; Novack, C.P.; Zellars, K.N.; et al. Local Hydrogel Release of Recombinant TIMP-3 Attenuates Adverse Left Ventricular Remodeling After Experimental Myocardial Infarction. *Sci. Transl. Med.* **2014**, *6*, 223ra21. [CrossRef]
174. Delinière, A.; Baranchuk, A.; Giai, J.; Bessiere, F.; Maucort-Boulch, D.; Defaye, P.; Marijon, E.; Le Vavasseur, O.; Dobreanu, D.; Scridon, A.; et al. Prediction of ventricular arrhythmias in patients with a spontaneous Brugada type 1 pattern: The key is in the electrocardiogram. *Europace* **2019**, *21*, 1400–1409. [CrossRef] [PubMed]
175. Scridon, A.; Șerban, R.C. Laboratory Monitoring: A Turning Point in the Use of New Oral Anticoagulants. *Ther. Drug Monit.* **2016**, *38*, 12–21. [CrossRef]
176. Khalil, H.; Kanisicak, O.; Vagnozzi, R.J.; Johansen, A.K.; Maliken, B.D.; Prasad, V.; Boyer, J.G.; Brody, M.; Schips, T.; Kilian, K.K.; et al. Cell-specific ablation of Hsp47 defines the collagen-producing cells in the injured heart. *JCI Insight* **2019**, *4*, e128722. [CrossRef] [PubMed]
177. Șerban, R.C.; Scridon, A. Data Linking Diabetes Mellitus and Atrial Fibrillation—How Strong Is the Evidence? From Epidemiology and Pathophysiology to Therapeutic Implications. *Can. J. Cardiol.* **2018**, *34*, 1492–1502. [CrossRef] [PubMed]

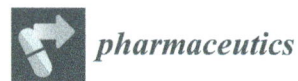

Review

Therapeutic Strategies and Chemoprevention of Atherosclerosis: What Do We Know and Where Do We Go?

Ana Clara Aprotosoaie [1], Alexandru-Dan Costache [2,3,*] and Irina-Iuliana Costache [3,4]

1. Faculty of Pharmacy, Grigore T. Popa University of Medicine and Pharmacy Iasi, 700115 Iasi, Romania; ana.aprotosoaie@umfiasi.ro
2. Department of Cardiovascular Rehabilitation, Clinical Rehabilitation Hospital, 700661 Iasi, Romania
3. Department of Internal Medicine I, Faculty of Medicine, University of Medicine and Pharmacy "Grigore T. Popa", 700115 Iasi, Romania; irina.costache@umfiasi.ro
4. Department of Cardiology, "St. Spiridon" Emergency County Hospital, 700111 Iasi, Romania
* Correspondence: adcostache@yahoo.com; Tel.: +40-758080823

Abstract: Despite progress in understanding the pathogenesis of atherosclerosis, the development of effective therapeutic strategies is a challenging task that requires more research to attain its full potential. This review discusses current pharmacotherapy in atherosclerosis and explores the potential of some important emerging therapies (antibody-based therapeutics, cytokine-targeting therapy, antisense oligonucleotides, photodynamic therapy and theranostics) in terms of clinical translation. A chemopreventive approach based on modern research of plant-derived products is also presented. Future perspectives on preventive and therapeutic management of atherosclerosis and the design of tailored treatments are outlined.

Keywords: atherosclerosis; pharmacotherapy; emergent therapeutics; natural anti-atherosclerotic products

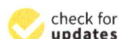

Citation: Aprotosoaie, A.C.; Costache, A.-D.; Costache, I.-I. Therapeutic Strategies and Chemoprevention of Atherosclerosis: What Do We Know and Where Do We Go? *Pharmaceutics* 2022, 14, 722. https://doi.org/10.3390/pharmaceutics14040722

Academic Editor: Maria Teresa Cruz

Received: 25 February 2022
Accepted: 26 March 2022
Published: 28 March 2022

Publisher's Note: MDPI stays neutral with regard to jurisdictional claims in published maps and institutional affiliations.

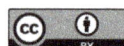

Copyright: © 2022 by the authors. Licensee MDPI, Basel, Switzerland. This article is an open access article distributed under the terms and conditions of the Creative Commons Attribution (CC BY) license (https://creativecommons.org/licenses/by/4.0/).

1. Introduction

Atherosclerosis is currently recognized as a progressive metabolic and immune-inflammatory disease that affects the intimal lining of medium- and large-sized arteries [1–3]. It is considered to be the main cause of atherosclerotic cardiovascular diseases—a category that include coronary artery disease, cerebrovascular disease and peripheral artery disease [4]. Ischemic heart diseases and stroke are the major atherosclerotic cardiovascular events, representing 85% of cardiovascular deaths and 28% of all-cause mortality [5]. According to the Global Burden of Cardiovascular Diseases and Risk Factors Study, 1990–2019, cardiovascular diseases affected 523 million patients globally and were the underlying cause of 18.6 million deaths—approximately one-third of all deaths worldwide [6,7]. Although significant advances have been made in the diagnosis and treatment of atherosclerosis and its pathological mechanisms, subsequent complications and importance in the field of medicine, many aspects are yet to be known and elucidated; in particular, pharmacotherapy of atherosclerosis is a challenging task. The pathogenesis of atherosclerosis is complicated and multifactorial, involving interplay between the cellular structure of the arterial intima, lipid metabolism and inflammatory factors [8–10]. After historically being localized mainly in the Western countries, atherosclerosis has spread worldwide and to younger people, females and all races. Further, in addition to the traditional risk factors (age, males older than 45 years and females older than 55 years, family history of premature cardiovascular diseases, arterial hypertension, hypercholesterolemia, diabetes, smoking and obesity/overweight), new risks factors have been identified, such as genetics, homocysteine, high-sensitivity C-reactive protein (hs-CRP), sleep disorders, sedentary lifestyle, air pollution and environmental stress [4,9,11]. Despite considerable progress in atherosclerosis research, current therapies are insufficient to effectively treat this disease. It is appreciated that the currently available medicines cannot prevent the occurrence of even 70% of clinical events [12]. There is a need for effective preventive strategies and better therapeutic options for atherosclerosis. This review discusses mechanisms, clinical efficacy and limitations and current evidence for atherosclerosis therapy starting from classical pharmacotherapy (statins, fibrates and cholesterol absorption inhibitors) to emerging therapies (antibody-based therapeutics, cytokine-targeting therapy, antisense oligonucleotides, photodynamic therapy and theranostics). Further, alternative chemopreventive strategies based on natural products are explored. Future perspectives on the preventive and therapeutic management of atherosclerosis and the design of tailored treatments are outlined.

2. Pathogenesis of Atherosclerosis

Pathobiology of atherosclerosis involves crosstalk between lipid metabolism imbalance, endothelial dysfunction, inflammatory pathways, oxidative stress and genetic predisposition. Endothelial cells, inflammatory cells and vascular smooth muscle cells (VSMCs) play key roles in disease development and progression. The main events that occur in atherogenesis are illustrated in Figure 1.

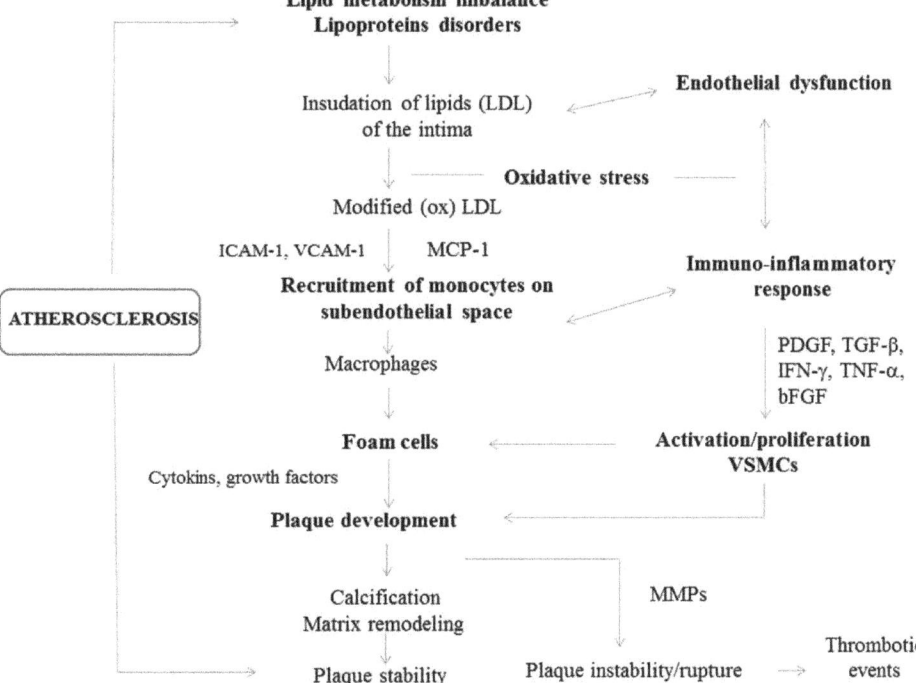

Figure 1. The pathogenesis of atherosclerosis. Atherogenesis is linked to both lipid metabolism and immune-inflammatory pathways. The process which leads to the formation of atherosclerotic plaques is complex and involves multiple steps. Endothelial dysfunction—induced by various noxious stimuli, including cardiovascular risk factors, disturbed hemodynamics and/or high levels of circulating lipids, particularly LDL—is a key component in the onset of atherosclerosis. Subendothelial accumulation of LDL and its oxidative modification to oxLDL promotes endothelial injury and induces a complex picture of immuno-inflammatory responses, starting from monocyte recruitment and macrophage activation, which lead to foam-cell formation and atherosclerotic plaque development. Monocyte chemoattractant protein 1 (MCP-1) and adhesion molecules (vascular cell adhesion molecule-1 (VCAM-1) and intercellular adhesion molecule-1 (ICAM-1)) are mainly responsible for

monocyte chemotaxis and adhesion. Atherogenic activation and phenotypic switching of vascular smooth muscle cells (VSMCs) induced by pro-inflammatory signaling (interferon γ (IFN-γ) and tumor necrosis factor α (TNF-α)) and growth factors (platelet-derived growth factor (PDGF), transforming growth factor β (TGF-β) and basic fibroblastic growth factor (bFGF)) also contribute to foam cell and plaque formation. Calcification and extracellular matrix remodeling may stabilize atherosclerotic plaques. Macrophages and foam cells release matrix metalloproteinases (MMPs) that promote the rupture of plaques and lead to major thrombotic events [13,14].

2.1. Endothelial Cells

Healthy endothelium is a major regulator of vascular homeostasis, releasing a wide spectrum of factors that control vascular tone and permeability, fluid balance, cellular adhesion, thromboresistance and fibro-inflammatory-proliferative responses. Endothelial-derived nitric oxide (NO) is a major factor that promotes vasoprotective and anti-atherosclerotic behavior [15,16]. Classical (hypercholesterolemia, hypertension, diabetes, chronic smoking and aging) and non-classical (ambient air pollution, mental stress and chronic inflammatory diseases) cardiovascular risk factors alter endothelial function, switching from a quiescent phenotype toward one that involves the impairment of NO-dependent signaling and pro-inflammatory and pro-thrombotic maladaptive responses [17]. Damage to endothelial function is an early hallmark of atherosclerosis, but it also has diagnostic and therapeutic significance [17]. Dysfunctional endothelial cells (ECs) exhibit increased permeability, a vasoconstrictive profile and express leukocyte adhesion by releasing adhesion molecules (vascular cell adhesion molecule-1 (VCAM-1), intercellular adhesion molecule-1 (ICAM-1) and E- and P-selectin); also, the pro-inflammatory nuclear factor-κB (NF-κB) and activator protein 1 (AP-1) pathways are activated, and the cytoskeletal and junctional proteins are dysregulated [13,18]. In addition, ECs showed an altered profile of gene expression and repair [19]. This defective endothelial phenotype allows subendothelial accumulation of low-density lipoproteins (LDL) and their atherogenic modification by oxidation and aggregation [20]. Locally reactive oxygen species (ROS) and myeloperoxidase, 15-lipoxygenase and nicotinamide adenine dinucleotide phosphate (NADH/NADPH) oxidases appear to mediate oxidation of LDL [21]. Oxidized LDL (oxLDL) contributes to the development and progression of atherosclerosis through induction of inflammatory and immune cell infiltration into the vascular wall, increase of oxidative stress and upregulation of the renin–angiotensin system [21].

2.2. Inflammatory Cells

Monocytes/macrophages. Recruitment of circulating monocytes within the intima is elicited by the retention of lipoproteins and is one of the earliest atherogenic events; this process continues in subsequent stages of disease progression. Monocyte chemoattractant protein 1 and 3 (MCP-1 and -3) chemokines are implicated in monocytic chemotaxis to damaged vascular areas [22]. In the subendothelial space, monocytes differentiate into macrophages, which engulf the modified LDL via several scavenger receptors (SR-A1, CD36 and LOX1/SR-E1) and lead to the formation of foam cells [23]. Apart from their role as scavengers, the activated macrophages contribute to the release of vasoactive factors (endothelins, eicosanoids, ROS, chemokines, tissue factor (TF) and matrix metalloproteinases (MMP-2, MMP-8, MMP-12)) [14,20,24] that exhibit thrombogenic, inflammatory and plaque-destabilizing properties and accelerate the progression of atherosclerotic lesions [20,25]. Due to their high plasticity, macrophages can adopt different functional phenotypes as a result of their adaptation to the local environment, such as intracellular energy metabolism [26,27]. Genetic and epigenetic variables—including non-coding RNA and gut microbiota—can also influence macrophage function, influencing both inflammatory response and resolution/repair [27]. The traditional model of macrophage polarization includes two phenotypes: M1 and M2. "Classic" M1 macrophages are triggered by Th1 cytokines (interferon-γ (IFN-γ) and tumor necrosis factor α (TNF-α)) and molecular complexes associated with pathogens (lipopolysaccharides). They exhibit an inflammatory behavior, increasing levels of IL-6, IL-12, IL-23, TNF-α and IL-1β cytokines and chemokines involved in Th1 recruitment (CXCL-9, CXCL-10 and CXCL-11). In addition, M1 macrophages produce RSO via NADPH oxidase and stimulate tissue destruction [26]. "Alternative" M2 macrophages are usually polarized by Th2-related cytokines such as IL-4, IL-33 and IL-13. They express immunomodulatory properties, stimulate tissue recovery and secrete anti-inflammatory cytokines (IL-10) and chemokines (CCL17, CCL22, CCL24) [26]. The M1 type is commonly encountered in atherosclerotic areas in patients with coronary heart disease and heart attack, being prevalent in vulnerable plaques [26]. Depending on the stimuli, other macrophage phenotypes have been described in atherosclerosis. Mox macrophages are triggered by oxidized phospholipids and are characterized as a proatherogenic type that is abundant in advanced plaques [23]. Further, the so-called M4 phenotype shows a pro-inflammatory and proatherogenic profile, being polarized by the CXCL4 chemokine. It promotes destabilization of the plaque's fibrous cap and appears to be irreversible in atherosclerotic plaques. Mhem and M(Hb) are bleeding-related phenotypes that exhibit atheroprotective properties, promoting cholesterol outflow and resistance to the formation of foam cells [23,26,28].

Lymphocytes. Immunoregulatory CD4+ and CD8+ T cells are encountered in all stages of atherosclerotic plaque development and progression. On the other hand, B lymphocytes are rare in the intimal plaque [20]. The differentiation of T cells into functional types depends on local metabolic and systemic conditions, such as hypoxia, cellular energy metabolism, cellular cholesterol efflux, hypercholesterolemia and epigenetic changes [27].

CD4+ T-helper (Th) cells represent about 70% of T lymphocytes in atherosclerotic areas, with the Th1 subtype predominant. Th1 cells secrete IFN-γ, TNF-α and IL-2 cytokines, which enhance the atherogenic processes [22,29]. CD8+ T cells are commonly found in severe advanced lesions and appear to exhibit proatherogenic and plaque-destabilizing properties [30]. The Th2 subtype shows both proatherogenic and protective effects. Thus, its related IL-4 cytokines contribute to plaque progression, while IL-5 and IL-33 exhibit anti-atherogenic properties via the production of IgM-type anti-oxLDL antibodies and reduction of the size of the atherosclerotic area. Induction of Th2 cells is pronounced in severe hypercholesterolemia [29].

CD4+ regulatory T cells (Tregs) represent 1–5% of all localized T cells within the atherosclerotic plaque. They exert immunosuppressive effects and are master modulators of inflammatory responses. A prevalent atheroprotective function has been documented for Tregs-related cytokines (IL-10 and transforming growth factor (TGF-β)) [29,31].

The T helper 17 (Th17) cells have been also been identified in atherosclerotic zones. They produce IL-17A that promotes autoimmunity but also induces modification of atherosclerotic plaque. On the one hand, IL-17A can enhance recruitment and activation of myeloid cells, while on the other hand, it stabilizes plaque via stimulation of collagen production. Therefore, its role is controversial [32].

Dendritic cells. Dendritic cells exert both direct and indirect effects in atherogenesis. Direct actions include lipid uptake and transformation in foam cells, antigen presentation and activation/proliferation of T cells and mediation of efferocytosis, a phagocytic clearance of apoptotic cells. Indirect effects are related to regulation of other immune cell functions and recruitment of circulating leucocytes or hematopoietic cells to the vascular area via secretion of pro-inflammatory mediators (TNF-α, IL-1, IL-12, IL-23, IL-27 and IL-33). [33].

2.3. Vascular Smooth Muscle Cells (VSMCs)

VSMCs are involved in the development of atherogenesis through their migration and proliferation and induction of matrix synthesis and foam cell formation. Even VSMC apoptosis and senescence contribute to atherosclerosis [24]. VSMCs are activated in response to various factors (TNF-α, IFN-γ, TGF-β, platelet derived growth factor (PDGF) and basic fibroblastic growth factor (bFGF)), ROS, shear stress, blood flow, matrix stiffness and modified cholesterol); once activated, they switch from a contractile phenotype to a synthetic state that promote extracellular matrix (ECM) production, plaque growth and fibrotic cap formation [18]. The vulnerable thinning of the fibrous cap as a result of defective efferocytosis and cell necrosis can cause rupture of the plaque and thrombosis, which further triggers severe cardiovascular events (unstable angina, myocardial infarction, stroke and sudden cardiac death) [34]. VSMCs genes associated with differentiation, migration and phenotypic switching are transcriptionally regulated by epigenetic mechanisms such as DNA methylation [24].

The role of epigenetics in regulating the atherosclerotic process has been increasingly recognized, with DNA methylation most commonly associated, as methylation levels control the expression of pro- and anti-atherosclerosis genes [35]. Further, non-coding RNA participates in the regulation of apoptosis, pyroptosis, autophagy, proliferation and migration of endothelial cells, monocytes, macrophages and VSMCs, making it a component of the atherosclerotic cycle and a target for future therapy [36].

2.4. Risk Factors

As we mentioned before, atherogenic changes are sustained and magnified by the influence of various classical (conventional) and non-classical (non-traditional) risk factors. A brief description of atherogenic mechanisms induced by the major factors is presented below.

2.4.1. Classical Risk Factors
Hypercholesterolemia

High levels of total cholesterol and triglycerides (TG) plus lipoprotein imbalance (with the prevalence of atherogenic fractions (LDL) and decrease of high-density lipoproteins (HDL)) play a crucial role in atherosclerosis, initiating the pathological processes we previously described. They are associated with the impairment of endothelium-dependent vasodilatation and ECs function and repair, abnormal vasomotor response, disturbed hemodynamics, oxidative stress and inflammation [37,38]. Familial hypercholesterolemia is an inherited hyper-LDL-cholesterolemia caused by deleterious mutations in LDL receptors or genes [39]. Hepatic LDL receptors are important for the removal of plasma cholesterol. The binding of LDL to its receptors is mediated by apolipoprotein B, while proprotein convertase subtilisin-kexin type 9 (PCSK9) is responsible for the degradation of LDL receptors. Mutations of genes that code LDL receptors, apolipoprotein B or PCSK9 may result in minimal cholesterol clearance, leading to extensive accumulation [40].

The control of circulating cholesterol is one of the most-used targets of current anti-atherosclerotic pharmacotherapy and dietary recommendations.

Hypertension. Elevated blood pressure accentuates the progression of atherosclerosis, increasing its severity and expanding lesions. The deleterious effects of arterial hypertension are due to multiple mechanisms, including endothelial dysfunction induced by mechanical and hemodynamic stress, increase of atherogenic lipoprotein uptake into the intima and monocyte adherence to the endothelial line. Further, vascular inflammation, promotion of the synthetic state of VSMCs and the activation of prothrombotic factors via angiotensin (Ang) II and other vasoconstrictive peptides play significant roles [41–43]. In addition to its established role in hypertension, the renin–angiotensin system (RAS) has major implications in atherosclerosis pathogenesis via various cellular and molecular mechanisms. Ang II, the main effector of RAS, induces oxidative stress in the cardiovascular system, significantly alters ECs function, upregulates the expression of adhesion molecules

(ICAM-1, VCAM-1) and inflammatory cytokines (TNF-α, IL-6) and stimulates growth factor expression (insulin-like growth factor and platelet-derived growth factors). Ang II stimulates plaque formation in the early stages and promotes plaque progression; in advanced disease, it destabilization the atherosclerotic plaque by regulating ECM composition and MMP release [44].

Diabetes. Diabetes mellitus increases the incidence of atherosclerosis and accelerates the progression and the clinical manifestation of atherosclerotic pathology. More than 90% of patients with diabetes and atherosclerosis are diagnosed with type 2 diabetes, which is generally known to amplify the risk of cardiovascular complications and mortality. Diabetes-related metabolic abnormalities, such as chronic hyperglycemia, advanced glycation end-products, dyslipidemia, free fatty acid excess and insulin resistance, cause a cascade of modifications that impact multiple cell types and alter vascular homeostasis [45]. They impair endothelial cell function, promote vasoconstriction and thrombosis, increase proinflammatory signaling, enhance foam cell formation and stimulate atherogenic VSMCs behavior [45,46]. Prediabetic patients are also at risk. Hyperglycemia leads to increased hematopoiesis and ROS-producing neutrophils, as well as to the production of extracellular vesicles from vascular endothelial cells and leukocytes, which, in turn, facilitate atherosclerosis via ROS-producing NADPH oxidase and LDL-scavenging CD36. They also carry specific miRNAs that promote hematopoiesis and inflammation [47].

Smoking. Chronic smoking is a major cause of cardiovascular morbidity and mortality. It triggers atherothrombotic events and promotes atherosclerosis and contributes to all of its clinical expressions. Tobacco exposure (even passive smoking) is associated with vasomotor dysfunction and endothelial cell damage, inflammation (elevated levels of TNF-α, IL-6 and CRP), dysfunctional thrombo–hemostatic response via alterations in platelet activity and antithrombotic/prothrombotic factors, impairment of lipid profile and lipid peroxidation and VSMCs proliferation [48,49].

Aging. Atherosclerosis is more frequently encountered in the older population, being linked to changes in both myeloid cell hematopoiesis and vasculature, as these systems share the same inflammatory pathway mediated by IL-6 signaling. This highlights the role of anti-inflammatory therapies in the prevention of atherosclerosis [50]. Aging is an independent risk factor for atherosclerosis and adverse cardiovascular outcomes. All atherogenic events are amplified with increasing age. The most important age-related changes that support and promote atherosclerosis include vascular stiffness and rigidity, endothelial cell injury, persistent vascular inflammation and oxidative stress, increased of atherogenic lipoprotein uptake and leukocyte adhesion, hypertension, alteration of mitochondrial function in vasculature and mitophagy impairment. Elevated DNA damage, extensive telomere shortening, epigenetic alteration and gene transcription dysregulation are characteristic features of both aged cells and atherosclerotic plaques [50,51].

2.4.2. Non-Classical Risk Factors

Hyperhomocysteinemia, defined as homocysteine values higher than 10^{-2} mol/L, is a new, independently important risk factor for atherosclerosis and cardiovascular disease [52]. Elevated levels of plasma homocysteine may arise from abnormalities of enzymes involved in its metabolism or nutritional deficiencies of folate, B6 and/or B12 vitamins. Older age, tobacco use, hypertension and male gender are associated with increased homocysteine levels. Further, patients with renal dysfunction, malignant neoplasm and systemic lupus erythematosus show the same tendency [53]. Hyperhomocysteinemia promotes a proatherogenic and prothrombotic microenvironment via several mechanisms that include oxidative stress, endoplasmic reticulum stress, endothelial dysfunction, increase of platelet aggregation, alteration of fibrinolysis, activation of proinflammatory cytokine production and stimulation of VSMCs proliferation [52,53]. It is important to mention that hyperhomocysteinemia reinforces the effects of other risk factors, such as smoking, hypertension and lipid metabolism imbalance [54].

Bacterial and viral infections.

Infection with a variety of pathogens (*Chlamydia pneumoniae*, periodontal pathogens, *Helicobacter pylori*, Human Immunodeficiency Virus, Influenza virus and Cytomegalovirus) may contribute to the development of atherosclerosis triggering and enhancing the systemic inflammatory response. Elevated CRP levels as a marker for predictive atherosclerotic risk have been reported in these patients. Besides, other mechanisms that promote atherogenesis can be also involved, such as: endothelial damage, altered cell metabolism, monocyte and macrophage activation, dysregulated lipid metabolism and hyperhomocysteinemia [48]. Severe Acute Respiratory Syndrome Coronavirus-2 (SARS-CoV-2), responsible for the 2019 coronavirus pandemic (COVID-19) is also strongly associated with atherosclerotic cardiovascular diseases and their complications. The suggested mechanisms include cytokine storm (TNF-α, IL-1β, IL-2, IL-6 and CRP) and thrombotic microangiopathy [55].

Environmental Pollutants.

Epidemiological studies show a consistent relationship between atmospheric pollutants (particulate matter and gaseous products) exposure and atherosclerotic cardiovascular diseases. Air pollutants generated by anthropogenic activities (fossil fuels, refining and construction) and natural sources (volcanic eruptions and wildfires) can induce atherogenic responses via several mechanisms, such as: endothelial dysfunction, alteration of systemic micro- and macrovascular tone, hyperlipidemia, tissue inflammation, increase of thrombogenicity, oxidative and neuroendocrine stress, tissue damage and plaque instability. It is important to mention that air pollution exposure amplifies the effects of other cardiovascular risk factors (hypertension, insulin resistance and aging) [48,56].

Some autoimmune disorders (psoriasis, rheumatoid arthritis, systemic lupus erythematous and antiphospholipid syndrome), mental health disorders (chronic depression), sleep disorders and polycystic ovarian syndrome have also been linked to an increased atherosclerotic and cardiovascular risk. Although the mechanisms are not fully understood, chronic inflammation, oxidative stress and neuro-endocrine abnormalities may contribute significantly [48].

Given the higher prevalence of atherosclerosis in men as compared to women in the pre-menopause age, plus the sudden rise of incidence in women after menopause, together with the abundance of sex hormone receptors in the vascular endothelium, sex hormones also play a role in atherosclerosis development, and the onset of menopause represents another risk factor [57].

2.5. Groups Prone to Atherosclerosis

Several population groups are at a higher risk of developing atherosclerosis or a disease associated with it. These include: familial dyslipidemia, women, older people, type 2 diabetes mellitus, metabolic syndrome, patients with acute coronary syndromes, stroke, chronic kidney disease, transplantation, peripheral artery disease, chronic immune-mediated inflammatory diseases, patients with Human Immunodeficiency Virus (HIV) and patients with severe mental illness. Familial dyslipidemias are associated with genetic syndromes, the most frequent and studied being familial hypercholesterolemia. Usually, they imply the alteration of lipid metabolism and a similar lipid profile in many members of the same family. Women have a lower risk than men before the onset of menopause; however, after the age of 55, the risk is equal in both genders, and cardiovascular mortality tends to be higher in women. The use of statins has not been fully studied in patients >75 years old and thus there is no full recommendation for treatment to be initiated. Further, given the lower treatment adherence in this group and high likelihood of other comorbidities, cardiovascular risk is also higher. Type 2 diabetes mellitus is associated with organ damage (nephropathy and retinopathy neuropathy), dyslipidemia, obesity and hypertension, which significantly increase the risk for atherosclerotic cardiovascular disease. Patients who have already suffered major events such as coronary syndromes or strokes (which also have a major atherosclerotic etiology) are at a higher risk of reoccurrence plus have more difficulty reaching and maintaining LDL target values. Chronic kidney disease is itself a major cardiovascular risk factor, and it is associated with increased atherosclerosis. From the early stages, TG levels rise and HDL levels are low, while small, dense LDL particles become predominant with disease progression. Post-transplant patients (especially heart, lung, liver, kidney or allogenic hematopoietic stem cell transplantation) as well as those who have undergone immunosuppressive therapy have an altered lipid profile, with increased total cholesterol, very-low-density lipoprotein (VLDL) and TG levels. Further, interactions between immunosuppressive medication and lipid-lowering drugs should be taken into consideration. Peripheral artery disease is already a manifestation of atherosclerosis, yet it is always associated with an increased risk for major events, such as strokes or coronary atherosclerotic syndromes [58].

3. Current Pharmacotherapy in Atherosclerosis

Currently available anti-atherosclerotic pharmacotherapy includes mainly lipid-lowering agents, namely statins, fibrates, cholesterol-absorption inhibitors and proprotein convertase subtilisin/kexin type 9 (PCSK-9) inhibitors [59]. Antiplatelet and antihypertensive drugs are also prescribed.

3.1. Statins

Statins are the most-commonly prescribed drugs, being first-line therapy for atherosclerosis and clinical management of the cardiovascular risk. They are effective both in primary and secondary prevention of cardiovascular disease [60]. The atheroprotective activity of statins involves both potent LDLc-lowering properties and multiple non-lipid-related pleiotropic effects, including enhancement of nitric oxide (NO) bioavailability, alleviation of endothelial dysfunction, anti-inflammatory, immunomodulatory and antioxidant abilities, stabilization of atherosclerotic plaques and inhibition of cardiac hypertrophy [61]. The major mechanism of statins is competitive and reversible inhibition of 3-hydroxy-3-methyl glutaryl coenzyme A (HMG-CoA) reductase, a rate-limiting enzyme in the cholesterol biosynthesis pathway. The decrease of cholesterol levels leads to upregulation of LDL-receptor expression and increased bloodstream LDLc clearance, reducing circulating LDLc by 20–55% [60]. Further, statins inhibit hepatic synthesis of apolipoprotein B100 and decrease production of triglyceride-rich lipoprotein [62]. They can alter plaque biology and reduce foam cell formation via suppression of oxLDL uptake by CD36, scavenger receptor A and LOX-1 receptor and inhibition of macrophage oxidative activity [62,63]. Other beneficial effects of statins include inhibition of endothelial nitric oxide synthase (eNOS), decrease of CRP levels, reduction of adhesion molecules (E-selectin and ICAM-1), suppression of myeloperoxidase-derived and nitric oxide-derived oxidants, upregulation of key antioxidant enzymes (glutathione peroxidase and superoxide dismutase) and recruitment of endothelial progenitor cells (useful in repairing ischemic injuries) [61,64]. Clinical statins are simvastatin, lovastatin, pravastatin, fluvastatin, atorvastatin, rosuvastin and pitavastatin [62]. The most important side effects of statin therapy are muscle symptoms (myalgia and rhabdomyolysis), liver dysfunction and renal failure. [60,65].

3.2. Fibrates

These lipid-lowering agents attenuate premature atherosclerosis and cardiovascular risk in atherogenic dyslipidemias, including those from type II diabetes and metabolic syndrome [66]. Fibrates are considered an effective therapeutic strategy in patients with moderate to high residual cardiovascular risk, mainly those with hypertriglyceridemia and low high-density lipoprotein cholesterol (HDLc) values [67]. They decrease plasma triglycerides (TG) and TG-rich lipoproteins and increase HDLc, primarily through the activation of peroxisome proliferator-activated receptor α (PPARα), a master transcription factor that regulates lipid and carbohydrate metabolism, impacting fatty acid uptake and activation, TG turnover, lipid droplet biology and gluconeogenesis [68,69]. Additional anti-atherogenic activity of fibrates includes anti-inflammatory effects and the decrease of vascular cell adhesion molecule (VCAM) and MCP-1 levels [67]. The best-known fibrates are fenofibrate, gemfibrozil and bezafibrate. Common adverse effects associated with fibrates are gastro-intestinal, liver and musculoskeletal disturbances [59].

3.3. Cholesterol Absorption Inhibitors

Ezetimibe is the commonly used drug of this type. It inhibits intestinal absorption of dietary and biliary cholesterol and related phytosterols, preventing transport of cholesterol through the intestinal wall [70]. Its association with simvastatin enhances the lipid-lowering effect of ezetimibe. The molecular target of the drug is Niemann–Pick C1-Like 1 protein, a critical cholesterol-trafficking factor [59,71].

3.4. Proprotein Convertase Subtilisin/Kexin Type 9 (PCSK-9) Inhibitors

PCSK-9 is another relevant cholesterol-lowering target that is involved in the regulation of LDL receptors. The gene that encodes PCSK-9 is implicated in familial hypercholesterolemia, and their gain- and loss-of-function mutations lead to high and low levels of LDLc, respectively. Alirocumab and evolocumab are two human monoclonal antibodies that act as PCSK-9 inhibitors. They are approved in the treatment of familial hypercholesterolemia and in patients with atherosclerotic cardiovascular disease who require additional LDLc reduction.

Further, inclisiran is a small interfering RNA molecule (siRNAs) that suppresses PCSK-9 synthesis in hepatocytes. It specifically binds to PCSK-9 mRNA, inhibits its translation and switches off PCSK-9 synthesis, resulting in a substantial and long-lasting decrease of serum LDLc levels. Analysis of data from three clinical trials showed that inclisiran decreased LDLc concentration by 51%, total cholesterol by 37%, ApoB by 41% and lowered the incidence of significant negative cardiovascular events by 24% [12]. The main therapeutic indications of inclisiran are primary hypercholesterolemia and mixed dyslipidemia in monotherapy or combined with statins or other lipid-lowering agents in patients who cannot achieve LDLc goals. Although the drug has an acceptable side effects–benefits profile, it should be noted that the potential pro-thrombotic activity of inclisiran can become clinically relevant after a long period of use in patients with high cardiovascular risk [72].

3.5. Renin–Angiotensin System (RAS) Inhibitors

RAS can be inhibited using three main types of agents: direct renin inhibitors (e.g., Aliskiren), angiotensin converting enzyme (ACE) inhibitors (captopril, enalapril and perindopril) and angiotensin receptor blockers (ARBs) (losartan, candesartan and irbesartan). Apart from their main activity, these drug classes can also have a hypolipemic effect, as atherosclerosis is linked to the renin–angiotensin system, as previously mentioned. Prevention of post-vascular injury myointimal proliferation, inhibition of Ang II-induced vascular proliferation or simply the lowering of blood pressure can decrease atherosclerosis formation. Further, compared to other blood-pressure-lowering classes (beta-blockers and calcium channel blockers), only RAS inhibitors exhibit anti-atherosclerotic properties. However, it should be noted that these drug classes are foremost blood-pressure-lowering medication, and the lipid-lowering properties are only potential additional effects [73–77].

4. Emerging Therapies

4.1. Cytokine-Targeting Therapy

Since atherosclerosis is no longer considered just a lipid-derived disease, and the role of inflammation in the atherosclerotic process has been revealed, strategies targeting inflammatory pathways were developed as promising new avenues to treat this pathology. The most-investigated inflammatory targets have been IL-1β, IL-6, CRP, TNF-α and IFN-γ, and the promising therapeutics are presented below [78].

4.1.1. Anti-IL-1β Agents

Cytokine IL-1β is involved in all stages of atherosclerosis, being a major pathogenic factor in plaque instability. It increases expression of chemokines (MCP-1) and adhesion molecules (ICAM-1, VCAM-1), stimulates proliferation and differentiation of vascular smooth muscle cells, and induces the activation of macrophages and the secretion of different proinflammatory mediators (IL-6) and MMPs [79]. Canakinumab is a recombinant human monoclonal antibody that was approved for the treatment of cryopyrin-associated periodic syndrome, adult-onset Still's disease, systemic juvenile idiopathic arthritis or familial Mediterranean fever. It binds to IL-1β and blocks its interaction with the IL-1 receptor, neutralizing IL-1β signaling [80]. In the CANTOS study (Canakinumab Anti-inflammatory Thrombosis Outcome Study), involving patients with a history of myocardial infarction and a high-sensitivity CRP level ($\geq$2 mg/L), canakinumab therapy led to a 15% reduction in major cardiovascular events (nonfatal myocardial infarction, nonfatal stroke and cardiovascular death). Furthermore, in a pre-specified secondary analysis of trial results, all-cause and cardiovascular mortality decreased by 31% in treated patients, regardless of the reduction in lipid levels. The safety profile of canakinumab is favorable, but it can increase the risk of infections and could promote plaque instability [79,81]. Another known IL-1β blocker is anakinra, a recombinant IL-1 receptor antagonist used in therapy of rheumatoid arthritis and neonatal-onset multisystem inflammatory disease [80]. In clinical trials in patients with acute coronary syndrome, anakinra significantly reduced the acute inflammatory response and subsequent cardiovascular events and hospitalizations. Due to side effects related to frequent administration, however, the drug is not appropriate for chronic disease management [79].

4.1.2. Anti-IL-6 Agents

IL-6 is a pleiotropic and potent cytokine, being a marker of inflammation related to cardiovascular risk. Elevated IL-6 levels are associated with increased cardiovascular events and mortality. Pro-atherogenic effects of IL-6 include increase of amyloid protein, fibrinogen, adhesion molecules (ICAM-1, VCAM) and CRP expression, activation of endothelial cells and platelets, stimulation of vascular smooth muscle proliferation and macrophage lipid accumulation. In addition, IL-6 promotes progression of coronary artery disease [82,83]. There are also data that support some atheroprotective properties of IL-6 via upregulation of ATP binding cassette transporter (ABC)A1, a protein that mediates cholesterol efflux from cells to apolipoproteins and prevents foam cell formation. Tocilizumab is a recombinant humanized monoclonal antibody that interferes with the binding of IL-6 to its specific receptors on different cell types. It prevents inflammatory responses and is recommended in moderate to severe rheumatoid arthritis, systemic juvenile idiopathic arthritis and in COVID patients. Clinical studies have shown some cardiovascular benefits of tocilizumab. In patients with non-ST-segment elevation myocardial infarction (NSTEMI), tocilizumab reduced CRP levels by up to 50%. Further, it decreased troponin T values in patients who underwent percutaneous coronary intervention (PCI) and improved myocardial salvage after STEMI (ASSAIL-MI trial) [84]. Unfortunately, tocilizumab causes adverse changes in the lipid profile, raising LDL and TG via reductions in LDL receptor levels. Currently, ziltivekimab, a novel human monoclonal antibody targeting the IL-6 ligand, is being developed for atherosclerosis treatment. Phase 2 of the RESCUE trial reported that subcutaneous administration of ziltivekimab in patients with high cardiovascular risk significantly reduced biomarkers of systemic inflammation and thrombosis known to promote the atherothrombotic process (hsCRP, fibrinogen, serum amyloid A, secretory phospholipase A2 and LP(a)). Treatment was well-tolerated and had no influence on the total cholesterol to HDLc ratio [12,85].

4.1.3. Anti-TNF-α Agents

TNF-α is a master regulator of inflammatory events and immune responses and a major player in atherogenesis. It induces endothelial barrier dysfunction by increasing vascular permeability, decreases NO bioavailability, stimulates vascular ROS generation (primarily anion superoxide), promotes endothelial expression of cell adhesion molecules (E-selectin, VCAM-1 and ICAM-1) and stimulates the recruitment and migration of leukocytes in the vascular wall. Moreover, TNF-α alters smooth muscle cell function by stimulating their proliferation and inducing a proatherogenic phenotype [86]. Several TNF-α inhibitors, such as monoclonal antibodies (infliximab, adalimumab, golimumab and certolizumab pegol) and etanercept, a dimeric fusion protein produced by recombinant DNA technology, have been developed and introduced against inflammatory and autoimmune disorders. Studies have shown that anti-TNF-α medicines improve endothelial function, aortic stiffness and vascular wall properties and decrease the risk of cardiovascular events in rheumatological patients or those with psoriasis. However, in patients with severe cardiovascular disease, TNF-α inhibitors failed to show clinical benefits. To the best of our knowledge, currently there are no ongoing clinical trials focused on the use of anti-TNF-α agents in patients with high cardiovascular risk [87,88].

4.2. Anti-P-Selectin Therapy

P-selectin is another interesting therapeutic target in atherosclerosis and vascular diseases. It is an inflammatory adhesion molecule strongly expressed on the surface of activated platelets and endothelial cells. P-selectin facilitates recruitment and attachment of circulating leukocytes to vascular walls and promotes proinflammatory cytokine release and thrombus formation [89]. Therapeutics targeting P-selectin are being intensively investigated in preclinical and clinical studies. Among them, inclacumab, a fully human IgG4 monoclonal antibody, is a very promising agent. It inhibits P-selectin activity and showed anti-cell adhesion, anti-inflammatory and antithrombotic effects in patients with cardiovascular diseases. The SELECT-ACS trial found that inclacumab significantly reduced myocardial damage after PCI in NSTEMI patients [12]. The drug appears to be well-tolerated, and new clinical trials with inclacumab are planned [90].

4.3. Angiopoietin Like (ANGPTL3) Targeting Agents

ANGPTL3 is a secretory protein belonging to the angiopoietin-like protein family. Due to its crucial role in human lipoprotein metabolism by inhibition of lipoprotein and endothelial lipases, ANGPTL3 has emerged as a promising target in cardiovascular and metabolic therapy [91]. Inhibition of ANGPTL3 activity leads to an important reduction in all major lipoprotein types, and loss-of-function (LOF) variants of ANGPTL3 were associated with a protective role against cardiovascular disorders, decreasing the risk of coronary heart disease by 34% [92]. Evinacumab is a recombinant human monoclonal antibody that inactivates circulating ANGPTL3 via the formation of complexes with the protein. It reduces plasma TG, LDLc and very-low-density lipoprotein cholesterol (VLDLc) levels, augmenting the clearance of TG-rich lipoproteins. In 2021, evinacumab was approved by the FDA for treatment of homozygous familial hypercholesterolemia [12,93]. An intensive therapy based on evinacumab, alirocumab and atorvastatin, targeting all apoB-containing lipoproteins, may provide an improved anti-atherosclerotic approach. This combination inhibited the progression of atherosclerotic lesions, reducing the area, size and proliferation of macrophages in plaque [94].

Alongside evinacumab, a similar reduction in atherogenic lipoproteins was obtained in human subjects with vupanorsen (AKCEA/IONIS-ANGPTL3-L_{RX}), a N-acetyl galactosamine-conjugated second generation antisense oligonucleotide. It targets hepatic ANGPTL-3mRNA interacting with the asialoglycoprotein receptor and can develop favorable cardiometabolic effects in patients with atherosclerosis [95]. Although the product met the primary endpoint of the Phase IIb TRANSLATE-TIMI 70 clinical trial (that included statin-treated subjects with dyslipidemia), some current programs of clinical development for vupanorsen have been discontinued due to safety issues related to hepatic side effects [96].

4.4. Photodynamic Therapy (PDT)

PDT is an emerging minimally invasive procedure used to treat various oncologic, infectious and non-oncologic diseases. In recent years, PDT has attracted attention as an interesting therapeutic option in atherosclerosis. It induces the stabilization and regression of atherosclerotic plaques and promotes vascular healing. Macrophage depletion, decrease in foam cell content and repopulation of plaques with non-proliferating smooth muscle cells contribute to the plaque stabilizing effects induced by PDT. Besides, PDT can prevent restenosis following clinical coronary angioplasty. The procedure involves three components: photosensitizer, light with a specific wavelength and molecular oxygen. The photosensitizer specifically accumulates in the atherosclerotic plaques and, after light activation, triggers a photochemical response that includes the generation of ROS and interference of cell survival and remodeling processes [97–100]. A number of conventional photosensitizers, namely porphyrins (hematoporphyrin derivative, Verteporfin), phtalocyanine derivatives, chlorins (Talaporfin sodium), 5-aminolevulinic acid and motexafin lutetium showed phototherapeutic properties in atherosclerosis in preclinical studies [101–110]. However, translation of PDT to clinical use warrants further studies with experimental models similar to human coronary atherosclerosis, clarification of some issues related to the appropriate type, toxicity and dosage of photosensitizer, light hypersensitivity and cutaneous photosensitivity, interference with arterial calcification and lipid-lowering/antiplatelet drugs and selective delivery in the atherosclerotic area [97–99]. Novel nanotechnology-based delivery systems and intravascular administration (balloon catheters) of photosensitizers allow targeted, selective therapy and minimization of side effects. Polymer nanoparticles, self-assembled protein nanostructures and liposome-based formulations were suggested as possible delivery strategies. Further, photosensitizer targeting could be increased by conjugation with various ligands for class A scavenger receptors or dextran receptors localized on macrophage surfaces. Significant improvements in laser technology may also support the optimization of PDT and its translation to clinical settings [97,99].

4.5. Theranostics

Theranostics constitute an innovative strategy integrating diagnosis and therapy in a single delivery agent. Although the application of theranostics in cardiovascular diseases is still in its infancy, the field has attracted increasing attention, and research on the development of these agents is growing. Theranostic medicine allows targeted therapy, enhances drug effectiveness and provides efficient, image-guided and personalized treatment of diseases [111,112].

Advanced imaging techniques (magnetic resonance imaging (MRI), computed tomography (CT), photoacoustic imaging, positron emission tomography (PET), optical coherence tomography (OCT) and laser device imaging (LDI)) and various nanocarriers (inorganic particles (metal oxides, gold, silver and silica), lipid-based nanoparticles, polymeric nanoparticles, dendrimers or carbon nanotubes) have been studied in theranostic therapy of atherosclerosis and vascular diseases [113–115]. Macrophages are the most-used target for theranostics, and nanomaterials are conjugated with binding ligands such as peptides or antibodies for this purpose [115].

Iron oxide nanoparticles, paramagnetic perfluorocarbon nanoparticles conjugated with fumagillin, cerium oxide and iron oxide nanocomposites, solid lipid nanoparticles and HDL-like magnetic nanostructures were designed mainly as MRI contrast agents [116–122]. Among them, iron oxide nanoparticles appear to be the most promising materials for MRI treatment. Their conjugation with antibodies targeting macrophages proved their ability to visualize atherosclerotic plaques [115,123,124]. An intrinsic affinity of the atherosclerotic plaque for macrophages and the lack of immunoreactions were noticed for HDL-like nanoparticles. They stimulated cholesterol efflux and regression of the atherosclerotic plaque. Theranostic systems comprised of MRI, solid lipid nanoparticles and ultrasmall superparamagnetic iron oxide particles loaded with prostacyclin inhibited platelet aggregation, and iron nanocomposites quenched ROS in inflammatory macrophages [122].

Gold nanoparticles were mostly used as CT contrast agents, damaging inflammatory macrophages. Further, copper sulfide nanoparticles conjugated with monoclonal antibody targeting transient receptor potential cation channel subfamily V member (TRPV1) provided feasible agents for photoacoustic imaging in atherosclerosis. They are able to detect and reduce lipid storage and atherosclerotic lesions in vivo [125]. For improved detection and visualization of atherosclerotic plaques, hybrid nanosystems combining imaging techniques (PET-MRI, PET-CT) and different associated nanoparticles with multimodal properties (such as magneto-fluorescent nanoparticles with high affinity for endothelial cells, dextran-coated magnetofluorescent iron oxide nanoparticles labeled with PET tracer ^{64}Cu and HDL-mimicking nanoparticles) have been suggested [125–127].

Although theranostics provides rapid and noninvasive diagnosis of atherosclerosis in animal models, development of clinically acceptable theranostics implies further research to solve some drawbacks related to design, systemic toxicity and stability of nanomaterials, the use of experimental models closer to human atherosclerosis and industrial production [115].

5. Natural Products with Anti-Atherosclerotic Properties

Medicinal plants and their bioactive compounds are considered as alternative preventive and therapeutic strategies in atherosclerosis as well as a valuable resource for pharmaco-research. Many plant products found in the daily human diet promote normal cardiovascular physiology and reduce the impact of conventional cardiovascular risk factors. There is also strong preclinical and clinical evidence that some plant products are capable of exerting significant anti-atherosclerotic effects. They can attenuate oxidative stress, protect against lipid peroxidation, positively modulate HDLc function, develop lipid-lowering effects, suppress proinflammatory signaling pathways and mediators, improve endothelial function, inhibit foam cell formation and reduce the severity and progression of atherosclerotic lesions (Table 1) [128]. In addition, plant products can modulate human gut microbiota to a healthier phenotype by revitalizing beneficial phylotypes (*Bacteroides*, *Lactobacillus*, *Bifidobacterium* and *Akkermansia*) and reducing proatherogenic commensals (*Clostridium*, *Prevotella* and *Desulfovibrio*) [129]. The mechanisms of action are multiple and versatile, and the same product can exert pleiotropic effects. The most-promising medicinal plants and phytocompounds with anti-atherosclerotic properties are presented in Table 1.

Table 1. Natural products and their anti-atherosclerotic effects.

Plant Products	Bioactives/Chemical Class	Anti-Atherosclerotic Effects	Putative Mechanisms	Clinical Studies	References
Allium sativum, garlic	Organo-sulfur derivatives	Lipid-lowering LDLc oxidation inhibition VSMC antiproliferative CIMT inhibition Inhibition of cholesterol accumulation in arterial wall Endothelial protective Anti-inflammatory Antithrombotic Antihypertensive	↓ACC, ACAT, HMGR, (SREBP)-1c, G6PD ↓TNF-α, IL-1β, COX-2 ↓CAM-1, HLA-DR ↓TXB2, PGE2, leukotriene C4 ↓GPIIb/IIIa receptor, fibrinogen binding ↓sialidase Regulation of NO synthesis ↓AngII receptor	Heterogeneous results on blood lipid profile Reduction in LDLc, TC in patients with hypercholesterolemia if it is used for longer than 2 months Reduction (by 38%) in risk of coronary events Decrease of blood pressure in hypertensive subjects Decrease of CIMT and regression of plaque in patients with carotid atherosclerosis, coronary heart disease	[128,130,131]
Berberine	Isoquinoline alkaloid	Endothelial protective Lipid regulator Plaque-stabilizing Decrease of foam cell formation Increase of macrophage autophagy Anti-inflammatory Gut microbiota modulation	↑LDL receptors, apoE expression ↓HMGR ↓NF-κB, TNF-α, MCP-1, IL-6, MMP-9 ↓p38-MPK ↑LXR-α, ABCA1 ↑AMPK-SIRT1-PPARγ ↑AMPK/mTOR ↓PI3/Akt/mTOR	Reduction in serum cholesterol in patients with hypercholesterolemia Decrease of atherosclerotic area	[129,132,133]
Curcuma	Diarylheptanoids	Anti-inflammatory Endothelial protective Lipid-lowering and regulation of lipid metabolism Plaque stabilizing Reduction of foam cell formation Decrease of macrophage infiltration Modulation of macrophage polarization Decrease of atherosclerotic lesions Decrease of carotid artery neointima formation VSMC antiproliferative Antioxidant Antiplatelet	↑cholesterol efflux ↑LXR-ABCA1/SR-BI ↓CD36 ↑TLR4 expression ↓oxLDL ↓NF-κB, TNF-α, IL-1β, IL-6, MCP-1, MMP-9, -13 ↓ICAM-1, VCAM-1 ↓Ang II ↑PPARγ ↑Nrf2 ↓PAF	Reduction of LDLc, TC in patients with acute coronary syndrome Decrease of hCRP, TG, TC and LDLc in patients with type 2 diabetes	[134–137]

Table 1. Cont.

Plant Products	Bioactives/Chemical Class	Anti-Atherosclerotic Effects	Putative Mechanisms	Clinical Studies	References
Green tea catechins	Polyphenols	Antioxidant Endothelial protective Anti-inflammatory Lipid lowering Inhibition of oxLDL VSMC antiproliferative Decrease of plaque formation	↑Nrf2/HO-1 ↓NF-κB, TNF-α, IL-6 ↓CRP ↓TLR4 ↑IL-10 ↑AMPK/PPARγ ↑PPARα ↑markers of autophagy Regulation of LXRα, FAS, SIRT-1, Insig-1-SREBP-SCAP ↑Notch receptor ↓AngII receptor 1	Improvement of blood lipid profile (↓TC, ↓LDLc, ↓TG) in patients with mild hypercholesterolemia Improvement of endothelial function in prehypertensive subjects	[138]
Morus alba, mulberry	Phenolic acids Flavonoids Iminosugar alkaloids	Antihyperlipidemic LDL oxidation inhibition Decrease of lipid accumulation in foam cells Decrease of plaque volume Anti-inflammatory Antioxidant VSMC antiproliferative Antiplatelet	Regulation of FAS, GPAT, SREBP-1c, LXR ↑AMPK, PPARα AP-1, STAT3 signaling modulation ↓NF-κB, TNF-α, IL-1β, IL-6, COX-2 ↑SOD, GPx, glutathione-S-transferase ↓lipid peroxidation ↓sVCAM-1 ↓integrin α$_{IIb}$β$_3$ secretion ↓TXA2	Improvement of serum lipid profile (↓TC, ↓LDLc, ↓TG, ↑HDLc) in patients with early stage of dyslipidemia, type 2 diabetes and dyslipidemia, heart disease Reduction of atherosclerotic lesions and CIMT in patients with coronary heart disease ↓CRP levels in mild dyslipidemia	[129,139,140]
Panax ginseng	Triterpenes (ginsenosides)	Enhancement of plaque stability Decrease of foam cell formation Reduction of plaque formation Increase of macrophage autophagy Decrease of monocyte adhesion events Decrease of vascular calcification Attenuation of neointimal hyperplasia VSMC antiproliferative Antioxidant	↑AMPK/mTOR ↑GPER, p-PI3K ↓p38/JNK-MAPK ↑IL-4, STAT6 ↓oxLDL uptake ↑LXRα, ABCGA1 ↓NF-κB, TNF-α, MMP-2,-9 ↓VCAM-1, ICAM-1, E-selectin ↑Nrf2/HO-1, SOD	Attenuation of endothelial dysfunction in hypertensive patients Improvement of lipid profile in type 2 diabetic patients Inconsistent results in most of the studies	[129,140–143]

Table 1. Cont.

Plant Products	Bioactives/Chemical Class	Anti-Atherosclerotic Effects	Putative Mechanisms	Clinical Studies	References
Punica granatum, pomegranate	Tannins, Anthocyanins, Flavonoids	Antioxidant Anti-inflammatory Lipid-lowering Modulation of gut microbiota	↑LXRα, ABCA1 ↓NF-κB, TNF-α ↑IL-10	Blood lipid-lowering effects in hyperlipidemic, overweight and obese subjects but also discordant results in other studies Decrease (up to 30%) of CIMT in patients with carotid artery stenosis Reduction of blood pressure in hypertensive patients with mild/high cardiovascular risk	[129,144,145]
Resveratrol	Stilbene	Antioxidant Anti-inflammatory Lipid regulator Decrease of LDLc oxidation Decrease of foam cell formation Reduction of plaque formation Vasoprotective Antiproliferative/antimineralizing	↓NADPH oxidase ↓NF-κB, TNF-α, MCP-1, IL-6, IL-8 ↓ICAM-1, VCAM-1 ↓oxLDL uptake ↑LDL receptors expression ↑CYP7A1 expression ↓HMGR ↓LOX1 ↑AMPK-PPAR ↑PPARγ ↑LXRα, ABCA1	Reduction in plasma TG in obese patients/smokers Reduction of LDLc in type 2 diabetes patients Reduction (20%) in oxLDL in patients with statins and high cardiovascular risk	[146]
Salvia miltiorrhiza, Chinese sage, Danshen	Tanshinones Salvianolic acids	Antioxidant Endothelial protective Anti-inflammatory Lipid regulator Reduction of foam cell formation Inhibition of progression of atherosclerotic plaque Antithrombotic Antihypertensive	↑SOD ↑NO ↓NF-κB, TNF-α, IL-1β, IL-6, MCP-1 ↓ICAM-1, VCAM-1, (MMP)-2,-3,-9 ↓oxLDL ↓CD36, PPARγ ↑ERK/Nrf2/HO-1 ↓CCL-20 ↓p38MAPKK ↑Prdx1/ABCA1 signaling ↓PI3K signaling	Improvement of blood lipid profile in patients with hyperlipidemia Reduction of blood pressure and pulse rate in hypertensive subjects Recovery of cardiac function in patients with myocardial infarction undergoing PCI	[129,147]

ABCA1, ATP-binding cassette transporter A1; ACAT, acyl-CoA cholesterol acyltransferase; ACC, acetyl-CoA carboxylase; Akt, protein kinase B; AMPK, adenosine monophosphate protein kinase; AngII, angiotensin II; AP-1, activator protein 1; Apo E, apolipoprotein E; CD36, cluster of differentiation 36, platelet membrane glycoprotein IV, scavenger receptor class B, member 3; CIMT, carotid intima-media thickness; COX, cyclooxygenase; ERK, extracellular signal-regulated kinase; FAS, fatty acid synthase; CYP7A1, cytochrome P450 family 7 subfamily A member 1; GAPT, glycerol-3-phosphate acyltransferase; G6PD, glucose-6-phosphate dehydrogenase; GPER, G protein-coupled estrogen receptor 1; GPx, glutathione peroxidase; GPIIb/IIIa, glycoprotein IIb/IIIa; hCRP, human C-reactive protein; HDLc, high-density lipoprotein cholesterol; HLA-DR, human leucocyte antigen-DR isotype; HMGR, 3-hydroxy-3-methyl-glutaryl-coenzyme A reductase; HO-1, heme oxygenase 1; ICAM-1, intercellular adhesion molecule 1; IL, interleukin; Insig-1, insulin-induced gene 1; JNK, c-Jun N-terminal kinase; LDLc, low-density lipoprotein cholesterol; LOX-1, receptor of oxLDL; LXRα, liver X receptor α; mTOR, mammalian target of rapamycin; MCP-1, monocyte chemoattractant protein-1; MMP (-2, -3, -9, -13), matrix metalloproteinase; NADPH oxidase, nicotinamide adenine dinucleotide phosphate oxidase; NF-κB, nuclear factor-κB; NO, nitric oxide; Nrf2, nuclear factor erythroid 2-related factor 2; oxLDL, oxidized LDL; p38/MAPK, p38 mitogen-activated protein kinase; PAF-2, platelet-activating factor acetylhydrolase homolog 2; PCI, percutaneous coronary intervention; PGE2, prostaglandin E2; PI3K, phosphoinositide 3-kinase; PPAR (-α, -γ), peroxisome proliferator-activated receptor; Prdx1, peroxiredoxin 1; SCAP, SREBP cleavage-activating protein; SR-BI, scavenger receptor class B type I; SIRT1, sirtuin 1; SOD, superoxide dismutase; SREBP-1c, sterol regulatory element-binding protein-1c; STAT (-3, -6) signal transducer and activator of transcription (-3, -6); TC, total cholesterol; TG, triglycerides; TLR4, Toll-like receptor 4; TNF-α, tumor necrosis factor α; TXA2, TXB2, thromboxane A2, thromboxane B2; VCAM-1, vascular cell adhesion molecule 1; VSMC, vascular smooth muscle cells; ↑, upregulation/increase of levels; ↓, downregulation/decrease of levels.

Among plant bioactives, phenolic compounds (flavonoids, stilbenes, anthocyanins and phenolic acids) appear to more potently modulate simultaneous signaling and mechanistic pathways in atherosclerosis. Further, dietary intervention trials support their protective effect in cardiovascular risk [148]. Daily intake of more than 29 mg of flavonoids may lead to a 68% reduction in the occurrence of major cardiovascular events (after correction of some known cardiovascular risk factors, such as smoking, sedentary lifestyle, obesity and high blood pressure) [149]. Garlic and Chinese sage preparations have been intensively studied and showed the most obvious atheroprotective properties. Despite strong preclinical evidence, clinical trials reported heterogeneous or inconsistent results for some plant products. This can be explained by great interindividual variability, methodological shortcomings, product diversity in terms of botanical origins, chemical characterization and lack of standardization, dosage, study period and short follow-up. Genetic polymorphisms and functionality of gut microbiota also contribute to variability of clinical outcomes. Controlled and multicentric trials of plant-derived products with large sample size and robust criteria for selection of subjects, as well as long-term evaluation, are needed to substantiate their potential clinical use in atherosclerosis.

6. Conclusions and Future Perspectives

Our review provides updated information on atherosclerosis and current pharmacotherapeutic approaches. In spite of remarkable progress achieved in understanding the mechanisms underlying the complex pathogenesis of atherosclerosis, the development of successful anti-atherosclerotic therapies remains a challenging task. Current therapeutic interventions are focused on improving lipoprotein metabolism and on modulation of atherosclerosis progression. Apart from statins, emerging therapies based on some cytokine-targeted agents (mainly, monoclonal antibodies) are also included in clinical practice. Another interesting emerging strategy is theranostics, which allows simultaneous treatment and imaging, promising an efficient approach to atherosclerosis and cardiovascular diseases. However, theranostics needs additional research, especially encompassing systemic toxic effects and the nanomaterial manufacturing process prior to clinical use. The establishment of chemopreventive strategies in atherosclerosis is also of paramount importance since prophylaxis is more beneficial than trying to reduce atherosclerotic lesions and plaque. The inclusion of documented and well-characterized plant products as components of these preventive programs could be a valuable intervention. Besides the effect of standardized plant products as an add-on therapy to conventional medicines, they could be an interesting avenue for the development of new therapeutics. The design of personalized treatments based on the concept of so-called "network medicine"—that includes the analysis and integration of genetic, metabolic and epigenetic factors—has been suggested as a more effective and appropriate therapeutic strategy in atherosclerosis [12].

Author Contributions: Conceptualization A.C.A., A.-D.C. and I.-I.C.; Methodology A.C.A., A.-D.C. and I.-I.C.; Writing—original draft preparation A.C.A. and A.-D.C.; writing—review and editing, A.C.A., A.-D.C. and I.-I.C.; visualization A.C.A. and A.-D.C.; supervision A.C.A. and I.-I.C. All authors have read and agreed to the published version of the manuscript.

Funding: This research received no external funding.

Institutional Review Board Statement: Not applicable.

Informed Consent Statement: Not applicable.

Data Availability Statement: Not applicable.

Conflicts of Interest: The authors declare no conflict of interest.

References

1. Moriya, J. Critical roles of inflammation in atherosclerosis. *J. Cardiol.* **2019**, *73*, 22–27. [CrossRef] [PubMed]
2. Glass, C.K.; Witztum, J.L. Atherosclerosis: The road ahead. *Cell* **2001**, *104*, 503–516. [CrossRef]
3. Mota, R.; Homeister, J.W.; Willis, M.S.; Bahnson, E.M. Atherosclerosis: Pathogenesis, genetics and experimental models. In *Encyclopedia of Life Sciences*; Cooper, D., Ed.; John Wiley, Ltd.: Chichester, UK, 2017; pp. 1–10.
4. Pahwa, R.; Jialal, I. *Atherosclerosis*; StatPearls Publishing: Treasure Island, FL, USA, 2022. Available online: https://www.ncbi.nlm.nih.gov/books/NBK507799/ (accessed on 15 February 2022).
5. Garcia, C.; Blesso, C.N. Antioxidant properties of anthocyanins and their mechanism of action in atherosclerosis. *Free. Radic. Biol. Med.* **2021**, *172*, 152–166. [CrossRef] [PubMed]
6. Surma, S.; Banach, M. Fibrinogen and atherosclerotic cardiovascular diseases-review of the literature and clinical studies. *Int. J. Mol. Sci.* **2022**, *23*, 193. [CrossRef]
7. Roth, G.A.; Mensah, G.A.; Johnson, C.O.; Addolorato, G.; Ammirati, E.; Baddour, L.M.; Barengo, N.C.; Beaton, A.Z.; Benjamin, E.J.; Benziger, C.P.; et al. Global Burden of Cardiovascular Diseases and Risk Factors, 1990–2019: Update from the GBD 2019 Study. *J. Am. Coll. Cardiol.* **2020**, *76*, 2982–3021. [CrossRef] [PubMed]
8. Libby, P. The biology of atherosclerosis comes full circle: Lessons for conquering cardiovascular disease. *Nat. Rev. Cardiol.* **2021**, *18*, 683–684. [CrossRef] [PubMed]
9. Ilias, N.; Hamzah, H.; Ismail, I.S.; Mohidin, T.B.M.; Idris, M.F.; Ajat, M. An insight on the future therapeutic application potential of Stevia rebaudiana Bertoni for atherosclerosis and cardiovascular diseases. *Biomed. Pharmacother.* **2021**, *143*, 112207. [CrossRef]
10. Duan, H.; Zhang, Q.; Liu, J.; Li, R.; Wang, D.; Peng, W.; Wu, C. Suppression of apoptosis in vascular endothelial cell, the promising way for natural medicines to treat atherosclerosis. *Pharmacol. Res.* **2021**, *168*, 105599. [CrossRef]
11. Libby, P. The changing landscape of atherosclerosis. *Nature* **2021**, *592*, 524–533. [CrossRef] [PubMed]
12. Gluba-Brzózka, A.; Franczyk, B.; Rysz-Górzyńska, M.; Ławiński, J.; Rysz, J. Emerging anti-atherosclerotic therapies. *Int. J. Mol. Sci.* **2021**, *22*, 12109. [CrossRef] [PubMed]
13. Gopalan, C.; Kirk, E. Atherosclerosis. In *Biology of Cardiovascular and Metabolic Diseases*; Gopalan, C., Kirk, E., Eds.; Academic Press: Cambridge, MA, USA, 2022; pp. 85–101.
14. Wang, T.; Butany, J. Pathogenesis of atherosclerosis. *Diagn. Histopathol.* **2017**, *23*, 473–478. [CrossRef]
15. Deanfield, J.E.; Halcox, J.P.; Rabelink, T.J. Endothelial function and dysfunction. Testing and clinical relevance. *Circulation* **2007**, *115*, 1285–1295. [CrossRef] [PubMed]
16. Gimbrone, M.A., Jr.; García-Cardeña, G. Endothelial cell dysfunction and the pathobiology of atherosclerosis. *Circ. Res.* **2016**, *118*, 620–636. [CrossRef]
17. Daiber, A.; Chlopicki, S. Revisiting pharmacology of oxidative stress and endothelial dysfunction in cardiovascular disease: Evidence for redox-based therapies. *Free Radic. Biol. Med.* **2020**, *157*, 15–37. [CrossRef]
18. Wang, T.; Palucci, D.; Law, K.; Yanagawa, B.; Yam, J.; Butany, J. Atherosclerosis: Pathogenesis and pathology. *Diagn. Histopathol.* **2012**, *18*, 461–467. [CrossRef]
19. Raggi, P.; Genest, J.; Giles, J.T.; Rayner, K.J.; Dwivedi, G.; Beanlands, R.S.; Gupta, M. Role of inflammation in the pathogenesis of atherosclerosis and therapeutic interventions. *Atherosclerosis* **2018**, *276*, 98–108. [CrossRef] [PubMed]
20. Falk, E. Pathogenesis of atherosclerosis. *J. Am. Coll. Cardiol.* **2006**, *47* (Suppl. S8), C7–C12. [CrossRef] [PubMed]
21. Alfarisi, H.A.H.l.; Mohamed, Z.B.H.; Ibrahim, M.B. Basic pathogenic mechanisms of atherosclerosis. *Egypt J. Basic Appl. Sci.* **2020**, *7*, 116–125. [CrossRef]
22. Mehu, M.; Narasimhulu, C.A.; Singla, D.K. Inflammatory Cells in Atherosclerosis. *Antioxidants* **2022**, *11*, 233. [CrossRef] [PubMed]
23. Farahi, L.; Sinha, S.K.; Lusis, A.J. Roles of macrophages in atherogenesis. *Front Pharmacol.* **2021**, *12*, 785220. [CrossRef] [PubMed]
24. Hai, Z.; Zuo, W. Aberrant DNA methylation in the pathogenesis of atherosclerosis. *Clin. Chim. Acta* **2016**, *456*, 69–74. [CrossRef] [PubMed]
25. Fukuda, D.; Sata, M. Role of bone marrow renin-angiotensin system in the pathogenesis of atherosclerosis. *Pharmacol. Ther.* **2008**, *118*, 268–276. [CrossRef] [PubMed]
26. Poznyak, A.V.; Nikiforov, N.G.; Starodubova, A.V.; Popkova, T.V.; Orekhov, A.N. Macrophages and foam cells: Brief overview of their role, linkage, and targeting potential in atherosclerosis. *Biomedicines* **2021**, *9*, 1221. [CrossRef]
27. Tabas, I.; Lichtman, A.H. Monocyte-Macrophages and T Cells in Atherosclerosis. *Immunity* **2017**, *47*, 621–634. [CrossRef] [PubMed]
28. Bobryshev, Y.V.; Ivanova, E.A.; Chistiakov, D.A.; Nikiforov, N.G.; Orekhov, A.N. Macrophages and their role in atherosclerosis: Pathophysiology and transcriptome analysis. *BioMed Res. Int.* **2016**, *2016*, 9582430. [CrossRef] [PubMed]
29. Pedicino, D.; Giglio, A.F.; Ruggio, A.; Massaro, G.; D'Aiello, A.; Trotta, F.; Lucci, C.; Graziani, F.; Biasucci, L.M.; Crea, F.; et al. Inflammasome, T lymphocytes and innate-adaptive immunity crosstalk: Role in cardiovascular disease and therapeutic perspectives. *Thromb. Haemost.* **2018**, *118*, 1352–1369. [CrossRef] [PubMed]
30. Ilhan, F.; Kalkanli, S.T. Atherosclerosis and the role of immune cells. *World J. Clin. Cases.* **2015**, *3*, 345–352. [CrossRef] [PubMed]
31. Malat, Z.; Taleb, S.; Ait-Oufella, H.L.; Tegdui, A. The role of adaptative T cell immunity in atherosclerosis. *J. Lipid Res.* **2009**, *50*, S364–S369. [CrossRef] [PubMed]
32. Van Bruggen, N.; Ouyang, W. Th17 cells at the crossroads of autoimmunity, inflammation, and atherosclerosis. *Immunity* **2014**, *40*, 10–12. [CrossRef]

33. Zhao, Y.; Zhang, J.; Zhang, W.; Xy, Y. A myriad of roles of dendritic cells in atherosclerosis. *Clin. Exp. Immunol.* **2021**, *206*, 12–27. [CrossRef] [PubMed]
34. Subramanian, M.; Tabas, I. Dendritic cells in atherosclerosis. *Semin. Immunopathol.* **2014**, *36*, 93–102. [CrossRef] [PubMed]
35. Hou, H.; Zhao, H. Epigenetic factors in atherosclerosis: DNA methylation, folic acid metabolism, and intestinal microbiota. *Clin. Chim. Acta* **2021**, *512*, 7–11. [CrossRef] [PubMed]
36. Yuan, Y.; Xu, L.; Geng, Z.; Liu, J.; Zhang, L.; Wu, Y.; He, D.; Qu, P. The role of non-coding RNA network in atherosclerosis. *Life Sci.* **2021**, *265*, 118756. [CrossRef] [PubMed]
37. Frolich, J.; Lear, S.A. Old and new risk factors for atherosclerosis and development of treatment recommendations. *Clin. Exp. Pharmacol. Physiol.* **2002**, *29*, 838–842. [CrossRef] [PubMed]
38. Fruchart, J.C.; Nierman, M.C.; Stroes, E.S.; Kastelein, J.J.; Duriez, P. New risk factors for atherosclerosis and patient risk assessment. *Circulation* **2004**, *109*, III15–III19. [CrossRef] [PubMed]
39. Tada, H.; Takamura, M.; Kawashiri, M. Familial hypercholesterolemia: A narrative review on diagnosis and management strategies for children and adolescents. *Vasc. Health Risk Manag.* **2021**, *17*, 59–67. [CrossRef] [PubMed]
40. Turgeon, R.D.; Barry, A.R.; Pearson, G.J. Familial hypercholesterolemia. Review of diagnosis, screening, and treatment. *Can. Fam. Physician* **2016**, *62*, 32–37. [PubMed]
41. Vogel, R.A. Coronary risk factors, endothelial function, and atherosclerosis: A review. *Clin Cardiol.* **1997**, *20*, 426–432. [CrossRef] [PubMed]
42. Chobanian, A.V.; Alexander, R.W. Exacerbation of atherosclerosis by hypertension: Potential mechanisms and clinical implications. *Arch. Intern. Med.* **1996**, *156*, 1952–1956. [CrossRef]
43. Kirabo, A.; Harrison, D.G. Hypertension as a risk factor for atherosclerosis. In *Atherosclerosis: Risks, Mechanisms, and Therapies*; Wang, H., Patterson, C., Eds.; John Wiley & Sons, Inc.: New York, NY, USA, 2015; pp. 63–75.
44. Poznyak, A.V.; Bharadwaj, D.; Prasad, G.; Grechko, A.V.; Sazonova, M.A.; Orekhov, A.N. Renin-angiotensin system in pathogenesis of atherosclerosis and treatment of CVD. *Int. J. Mol. Sci.* **2021**, *22*, 6702. [CrossRef] [PubMed]
45. Poznyak, A.; Grechko, A.V.; Poggio, P.; Myasoedova, V.A.; Alfieri, V.; Orekhov, A.N. The diabetes mellitus-atherosclerosis connection: The role of lipid and glucose metabolism and chronic inflammation. *Int. J. Mol. Sci.* **2020**, *21*, 1835. [CrossRef] [PubMed]
46. Beckman, J.A.; Creager, M.A.; Libby, P. Diabetes and atherosclerosis: Epidemiology, pathophysiology, and management. *JAMA* **2002**, *287*, 2570–2581. [CrossRef]
47. Liang, Y.; Wang, M.; Wang, C.; Liu, Y.; Naruse, K.; Takahashi, K. The mechanisms of the development of atherosclerosis in prediabetes. *Int. J. Mol. Sci.* **2021**, *22*, 4108. [CrossRef] [PubMed]
48. Kuk, M.; Ward, N.C.; Dwivedi, G. Extrinsic and intrinsic responses in the development and progression of atherosclerosis. *Heart Lung Circ.* **2021**, *30*, 807–816. [CrossRef] [PubMed]
49. Ambrose, J.A.; Barua, R.S. The pathophysiology of cigarette smoking and cardiovascular disease: An update. *J. Am. Coll. Cardiol.* **2004**, *43*, 1731–1737. [CrossRef]
50. Tyrrell, D.J.; Goldstein, D.R. Ageing and atherosclerosis: Vascular intrinsic and extrinsic factors and potential role of IL-6. *Nat. Rev. Cardiol.* **2021**, *18*, 58–68. [CrossRef]
51. Wang, J.C.; Bennett, M. Aging and atherosclerosis: Mechanisms, functional consequences, and potential therapeutics for cellular senescence. *Circ. Res.* **2012**, *111*, 245–259. [CrossRef]
52. Zhao, J.; Chen, H.; Liu, N.; Chen, J.; Gu, Y.; Chen, J.; Yang, K. Role of hyperhomocysteinemia and hyperuricemia in pathogenesis of atherosclerosis. *J. Stroke Cerebrovasc. Dis.* **2017**, *26*, 2695–2699. [CrossRef]
53. Stein, J.H.; McBride, P.E. Hyperhomocysteinemia and atherosclerotic vascular disease: Pathophysiology, screening, and treatment. *Arch. Intern. Med.* **1998**, *158*, 1301–1306. [CrossRef]
54. Ganguly, P.; Alam, S.F. Role of homocysteine in the development of cardiovascular disease. *Nutr. J.* **2015**, *14*, 6. [CrossRef]
55. Szwed, P.; Gąsecka, A.; Zawadka, M.; Eyileten, C.; Postuła, M.; Mazurek, T.; Szarpak, Ł.; Filipiak, K.J. Infections as novel risk factors of atherosclerotic cardiovascular diseases: Pathophysiological links and therapeutic implications. *J. Clin. Med.* **2021**, *10*, 2539. [CrossRef]
56. Bevan, G.H.; Al-Kindi, S.G.; Brook, R.D.; Münzel, T.; Rajagopalan, S. Ambient air pollution and atherosclerosis: Insights into dose, time, and mechanisms. *Arterioscler. Thromb. Vasc. Biol.* **2021**, *41*, 628–637. [CrossRef] [PubMed]
57. Nasser, S.A.; Afify, E.A.; Kobeissy, F.; Hamam, B.; Eid, A.H.; El-Mas, M.M. Inflammatory basis of atherosclerosis: Modulation 678 by sex hormones. *Curr. Pharm. Des.* **2021**, *27*, 2099–2111. [CrossRef] [PubMed]
58. Mach, F.; Baigent, C.; Catapano, A.L.; Koskinas, K.C.; Casula, M.; Badimon, L.; Chapman, M.J.; De Backer, G.G.; Delgado, V.; Ference, B.A.; et al. ESC Scientific Document Group. 2019 ESC/EAS Guidelines for the management of dyslipidaemias: Lipid modification to reduce cardiovascular risk. *Eur. Heart J.* **2020**, *41*, 111–188. [CrossRef] [PubMed]
59. Gupta, K.K.; Ali, S.; Sanghera, R.S. Pharmacological options in atherosclerosis: A review of the existing evidence. *Cardiol. Ther.* **2019**, *8*, 5–20. [CrossRef] [PubMed]
60. Ward, N.C.; Watts, G.F.; Eckel, R.H. Statin toxicity mechanistic insights and clinical implications. *Circ. Res.* **2019**, *124*, 328–350. [CrossRef] [PubMed]
61. Davignon, J. Beneficial cardiovascular pleiotropic effects of statins. *Circulation* **2004**, *109* (Suppl. SIII), III39–III43. [CrossRef] [PubMed]

62. McFarland, A.J.; Anoopkumar-Dukie, S.; Arora, D.S.; Grant, G.D.; McDermott, C.; Perkins, A.V.; Davey, A.K. Molecular mechanisms underlying the effects of statins in the central nervous system. *Int. J. Mol. Sci.* **2014**, *15*, 20607–20637. [CrossRef]
63. Libby, P.; Aikawa, M. Mechanisms of plaque stabilization with statins. *Am. J. Cardiol.* **2003**, *91*, 4B–8B. [CrossRef]
64. Zinellu, A.; Mangoni, A.A. A systematic review and meta-analysis of the effect of statins on glutathione peroxidase, superoxide dismutase, and catalase. *Antioxidants* **2021**, *10*, 1841. [CrossRef]
65. Cai, T.; Abel, L.; Langford, O.; Monaghan, G.; Aronson, J.K.; Stevens, R.J.; Lay-Flurrie, S.; Koshiaris, C.; McManus, R.J.; Hobbs, R.D.F.; et al. Associations between statins and adverse events in primary prevention of cardiovascular disease: Systematic review with pairwise, network, and dose-response meta-analyses. *BMJ* **2021**, *374*, n1537. [CrossRef]
66. Chapman, M.J. Fibrates in 2003: Therapeutic action in atherogenic dyslipidaemia and future perspectives. *Atherosclerosis* **2003**, *171*, 1–13. [CrossRef]
67. Kim, N.H.; Kim, S.G. Fibrates revisited: Potential role in cardiovascular risk reduction. *Diabetes Metab. J.* **2020**, *44*, 213–221. [CrossRef] [PubMed]
68. Kersten, S. Integrated physiology and systems biology of PPARα. *Mol. Metab.* **2014**, *3*, 354–371. [CrossRef]
69. Inaba, T.; Yagyu, H.; Itabashi, N.; Tazoe, F.; Fujita, N.; Nagashima, S.; Okada, K.; Okazaki, M.; Furukawa, Y.; Ishibashi, S. Cholesterol reduction and atherosclerosis inhibition by bezafibrate in low-density lipoprotein receptor knockout mice. *Hypertens. Res.* **2008**, *31*, 999–1005. [CrossRef] [PubMed]
70. Catapano, A.L. Ezetimibe: A selective inhibitor of cholesterol absorption. *Eur. Heart J.* **2001**, *3* (Suppl. SE), E6–E10. [CrossRef]
71. Jia, L.; Betters, J.L.; Yu, L. Niemann-pick C1-like 1 (NPC1L1) protein in intestinal and hepatic cholesterol transport. *Annu. Rev. Physiol.* **2011**, *73*, 239–259. [CrossRef] [PubMed]
72. Dyrbuś, K.; Mariusz, G.; Penson, P.; Ray, K.K.; Banach, M. Inclisiran new hope in the management of lipid disorders? *J. Clin. Lipidol.* **2019**, *14*, 16–27. [CrossRef]
73. Lu, H.; Balakrishnan, A.; Howatt, D.A.; Wu, C.; Charnigo, R.; Liau, G.; Cassis, L.A.; Daugherty, A. Comparative effects of different modes of renin angiotensin system inhibition on hypercholesterolaemia-induced atherosclerosis. *Br. J. Pharmacol.* **2012**, *165*, 2000–2008. [CrossRef] [PubMed]
74. Ferrario, C.M. Use of angiotensin II receptor blockers in animal models of atherosclerosis. *Am. J. Hypertens.* **2002**, *15*, 9S–13S. [CrossRef]
75. Lonn, E. Angiotensin-converting enzyme inhibitors and angiotensin receptor blockers in atherosclerosis. *Curr. Atheroscler. Rep.* **2002**, *4*, 363–372. [CrossRef] [PubMed]
76. Ambrosioni, E.; Bacchelli, S.; Degli Esposti, D.; Borghi, C. ACE-inhibitors and atherosclerosis. *Eur. J. Epidemiol.* **1992**, *8*, 129–133. [CrossRef] [PubMed]
77. Curzen, N.P.; Fox, K.M. Do ACE inhibitors modulate atherosclerosis? *Eur. Heart J.* **1997**, *18*, 1530–1535. [CrossRef]
78. Poznyak, A.V.; Bharadwaj, D.; Prasad, G.; Grechko, A.V.; Sazonova, M.A.; Orekhov, A.N. Anti-inflammatory therapy for atherosclerosis: Focusing on cytokines. *Int. J. Mol. Sci.* **2021**, *22*, 7061. [CrossRef] [PubMed]
79. Mai, W.; Liao, Y. Targeting IL-1β in the treatment of atherosclerosis. *Front Immunol.* **2020**, *11*, 589654. [CrossRef] [PubMed]
80. Gram, H. The long and winding road in pharmaceutical development of canakinumab from rare genetic autoinflammatory syndromes to myocardial infarction and cancer. *Pharmacol. Res.* **2020**, *154*, 104139. [CrossRef] [PubMed]
81. Soehnlein, O.; Libby, P. Targeting inflammation in atherosclerosis-from experimental insights to the clinic. *Nat. Rev.* **2021**, *20*, 589–610. [CrossRef] [PubMed]
82. Lindmark, E.; Diderholm, E.; Wallentin, L.; Siegbahn, A. Relationship between interleukin 6 and mortality in patients with unstable coronary artery disease: Effects of an early invasive or noninvasive strategy. *JAMA* **2001**, *286*, 2107–2113. [CrossRef] [PubMed]
83. Reiss, A.B.; Siegart, N.M.; De Leon, J. Interleukin-6 in atherosclerosis: Atherogenic or atheroprotective? *Clin. Lipidol.* **2017**, *12*, 14–23.
84. Broch, K.; Anstensrud, A.K.; Woxholt, S.; Sharma, K.; Tøllefsen, I.M.; Bendz, B.; Aakhus, S.; Ueland, T.; Amundsen, B.H.; Damås, J.K.; et al. Randomized trial of interleukin-6 receptor inhibition in patients with acute ST-Segment Elevation Myocardial Infarction. *J. Am. Coll. Cardiol.* **2021**, *77*, 1845–1855. [CrossRef] [PubMed]
85. Ridker, P.M.; Devalaraja, M.; Baeres, F.M.M.; Engelmann, M.D.M.; Hovingh, G.K.; Ivkovic, M.; Lo, L.; Kling, D.; Pergola, P.; Raj, D.; et al. IL-6 inhibition with ziltivekimab in patients at high atherosclerotic risck (RESCUE): A double-blind, randomized, placebo-controlled, phase 2 trial. *Lancet* **2021**, *397*, 2060–2069. [CrossRef]
86. Urschel, K.; Cicha, I. TNF-α in the cardiovascular system: From physiology to therapy. *Int. J. Interferon Cytokine Mediat. Res.* **2015**, *7*, 9–25.
87. Ji, E.; Lee, S. Antibody-based therapeutics for atherosclerosis and cardiovascular diseases. *Int. J. Mol. Sci.* **2021**, *22*, 5770. [CrossRef] [PubMed]
88. Tousoulis, D.; Oikonomou, E.; Economou, E.E.; Crea, F.; Kaski, J.C. Inflammatory cytokines in atherosclerosis: Current therapeutic approaches. *Eur. Heart J.* **2016**, *37*, 1723–1735. [CrossRef] [PubMed]
89. Woollard, K.J.; Chin-Dusting, J. Therapeutic targeting of p-selectin in atherosclerosis. *Inflamm. Allergy Drug Targets* **2007**, *6*, 69–74. [CrossRef] [PubMed]

90. Geng, X.; Mihaila, R.; Yuan, Y.; Strutt, S.; Benz, J.; Tang, T.; Mayer, C.; Oksenberg, D. Inclacumab, a fully human anti-P-selectin antibody, directly binds to PSGL-1 binding region and demonstrates robust and durable inhibition of cell adhesion. *Blood* **2020**, *136* (Suppl. S1), 10–11. [CrossRef]
91. Ruhanen, H.; Haridas, P.A.N.; Jauhiainen, M.; Olkkonen, V.M. Angiopoietin-like protein 3, an emerging cardiometabolic therapy target with systemic and cell-autonomous functions. *Biochim. Biophys. Acta Mol. Cell. Biol. Lipids* **2020**, *1865*, 158791. [CrossRef] [PubMed]
92. Stitziel, N.O.; Khera, A.V.; Wang, X.; Bierhals, A.J.; Vourakis, A.C.; Sperry, A.E.; Natarajan, P.; Klarin, D.; Emdin, C.A.; Zekavat, S.M.; et al. PROMIS and Myocardial Infarction Genetics Consortium Investigators. ANGPTL3 deficiency and protection against coronary artery disease. *J. Am. Coll. Cardiol.* **2017**, *69*, 2054–2063. [CrossRef]
93. European Medicines Agency. Available online: https://www.ema.europa.eu/en/medicines/human/EPAR/evkeeza (accessed on 8 February 2022).
94. Pouwer, M.G.; Pieterman, E.J.; Worms, N.; Keijzer, N.; Jukema, J.W.; Gromada, J.; Gusarova, V.; Princen, H.M.G. Alirocumab, evinacumab, and atorvastatin triple therapy regresses plaque lesions and improves lesion composition in mice. *J. Lipid Res.* **2020**, *61*, 365–375. [CrossRef]
95. Gaudet, D.; Karwatowska-Prokopczuk, E.; Baum, S.J.; Hurh, E.; Kingsbury, J.; Bartlet, V.J.; Figueroa, A.L.; Piscitelli, P.; Singleton, W.; Witztum, J.L.; et al. Vupanorsen, an N-acetyl galactosamine-conjugated antisense drug to ANGPTL3 mRNA, lowers triglycerides and atherogenic lipoproteins in patients with diabetes, hepatic steatosis, and hypertriglyceridaemia. *Eur. Heart J.* **2020**, *41*, 3936–3945. [CrossRef]
96. Pharmaceutical INN. Available online: https://investingnews.com/pfizer-and-ionis-announce-discontinuation-of-vupanorsen-clinical-development-program/ (accessed on 8 February 2022).
97. Jain, M.; Zellweger, M.; Wagnières, G.; van den Bergh, H.; Cook, S.; Giraud, M.N. Photodynamic therapy for the treatment of atherosclerotic plaque: Lost in translation? *Cardiovasc. Ther.* **2017**, *35*, 12238. [CrossRef] [PubMed]
98. Benov, L. Photodynamic therapy: Current status and future directions. *Med. Princ. Pract.* **2015**, *24* (Suppl. S1), 14–28. [CrossRef] [PubMed]
99. Houthoofd, S.; Vuylsteke, M.; Mordon, S.; Fourneau, I. Photodynamic therapy for atherosclerosis. The potential of indocyanine green. *Photodiagn. Photodyn. Ther.* **2020**, *29*, 101568. [CrossRef] [PubMed]
100. Correaia, J.H.; Rodrigues, J.A.; Pimenta, S.; Dong, T.; Yang, Z. Photodynamic therapy review: Principles, photosensitizers, applications, and future directions. *Pharmaceutics* **2021**, *13*, 1332. [CrossRef] [PubMed]
101. Hsiang, Y.N.; Fragoso, M.; Tsang, V.; Schereiber, W.E. Determining the optimal dose of Photofrin in miniswine atherosclerotic plaque. *Photochem. Photobiol.* **1993**, *57*, 518–525. [CrossRef] [PubMed]
102. Spokojni, A.M.; Serur, J.R.; Skilman, J.; Spears, J.R. Uptake of hematoporphyrin-derivative by atheromatous plaques: Studies in human in vitro and rabbit in vivo. *J. Am. Coll. Cardiol.* **1986**, *8*, 1386–1392. [CrossRef]
103. Hsiang, Y.N.; Crespo, M.T.; Richter, A.M.; Jain, A.K.; Fragoso, M.; Levy, J.G. In vitro and in vivo uptake of benzoporphyrin derivative into human and miniswine atherosclerotic plaque. *Photochem. Photobiol.* **1993**, *5*, 670–674. [CrossRef] [PubMed]
104. Jain, M.; Zellweger, M.; Frobert, A.; Valentin, J.; van den Bergh, H.; Wagnières, G.; Cook, S.; Giraud, M.N. Intra-arterial drug and light delivery for photodynamic therapy using Visudyne®: Implication for atherosclerotic plaque treatment. *Front. Physiol.* **2016**, *7*, 400. [CrossRef]
105. Nyamekye, I.; Buonaccorsi, G.; McEwan, J.; MacRobert, A.; Bown, S.; Bishop, C. Inhibition of intimal hyperplasia in balloon injured arteries with adjunctive phthalocyanine sensitised photodynamic therapy. *Eur. J. Vasc. Endovasc. Surg.* **1996**, *11*, 19–28. [CrossRef]
106. Nagae, T.; Aizawa, K.; Uchimura, N.; Tani, D.; Abe, M.; Fujishima, K.; Wilson, S.E.; Ishimaru, S. Endovascular photodynamic therapy using mono-L-aspartyl-chlorin e6 to inhibit intimal hyperplasia in balloon-injured rabbit arteries. *Lasers Surg. Med.* **2001**, *28*, 381–388. [CrossRef] [PubMed]
107. Jenkins, M.P.; Buonaccorsi, G.; MacRobert, A.; Bishop, C.C.; Bown, S.G.; McEwan, J.R. Intra-arterial photodynamic therapy using 5-ALA in a swine model. *Eur. J. Vasc. Endovasc. Surg.* **1998**, *16*, 284–291. [CrossRef]
108. Jenkins, M.P.; Buonaccorsi, G.A.; Mansfield, R.; Bishop, C.C.R.; Bown, S.G.; McEwan, J.R. Reduction in the response to coronary and iliac artery injury with photodynamic therapy using 5-aminolaevulinic acid. *Cardiovasc. Res.* **2000**, *45*, 478–485. [CrossRef]
109. Hayase, M.; Woodbum, K.W.; Perlroth, J.; Miller, R.A.; Baumgardner, W.; Yock, P.G.; Yeung, A. Photoangioplasty with local motexafin lutetium delivery reduces macrophages in a rabbit post-balloon injury model. *Cardiovasc. Res.* **2001**, *49*, 449–455. [CrossRef]
110. Yamaguchi, A.; Woodburn, K.W.; Hayase, M.; Robbins, R.C. Reduction of vein graft disease using photodynamic therapy with motexafin lutetium in a rodent isograft model. *Circulation* **2000**, *102*, III275–III280. [CrossRef] [PubMed]
111. Geetha Bai, R.; Muthoosamy, K.; Manickam, S. Nanomedicine in theranostics. In *Nanotechnology Applications for Tissue Engineering*; Thomas, S., Grohens, Y., Ninan, N., Eds.; William Andrew Publishing: Norwich, CT, USA, 2015; pp. 195–213.
112. Zhang, Y.; Koradia, A.; Kamato, D.; Popat, A.; Little, P.J.; Ta, H.T. Treatment of atherosclerotic plaque: Perspectives on theranostics. *J. Pharm. Pharmacol.* **2019**, *71*, 1029–1043. [CrossRef]
113. Bejarano, J.; Navarro-Marquez, M.; Morales-Zavala, F.; Morales, J.O.; Garcia-Carvajal, I.; Araya-Fuentes, E.; Flores, Y.; Verdejo, H.E.; Castro, P.F.; Lavandero, S.; et al. Nanoparticles for diagnosis and therapy of atherosclerosis and myocardial infarction: Evolution toward prospective theranostic approaches. *Theranostics* **2018**, *8*, 4710–4732. [CrossRef] [PubMed]

114. Agrawal, S.; Nooti, S.K.; Singh, H.; Rai, V. Nanomaterial-mediated theranostics for vascular diseases. *J. Nanotheranostics* **2021**, *2*, 1–15. [CrossRef]
115. Wu, Y.; Vazquez-Prada, K.X.; Liu, Y.; Whittaker, A.K.; Zhang, R.; Ta, H.T. Recent advances in the development of theranostic nanoparticles for cardiovascular diseases. *Nanotheranostics* **2021**, *5*, 499–514. [CrossRef]
116. Evans, R.J.; Lavin, B.; Phinikaridou, A.; Chooi, K.Y.; Mohri, Z.; Wong, E.; Boyle, J.J.; Krams, R.; Botnar, R.; Long, N.J. Targeted molecular iron oxide contrast agents for imaging atherosclerotic plaque. *Nanotheranostics* **2020**, *4*, 184–194. [CrossRef]
117. Vazquez-Prada, K.X.; Lam, J.; Kamato, D.; Xu, Z.P.; Little, P.J.; Ta, H.T. Targeted molecular imaging of cardiovascular diseases by iron oxide nanoparticles. *Arterioscler. Thromb. Vasc. Biol.* **2021**, *41*, 601–613. [CrossRef] [PubMed]
118. Wang, Y.-X.J. Supermagnetic iron oxide based MRI contrast agents: Current status of clinical application. *Quant. Imaging Med. Surg.* **2011**, *1*, 35–44. [PubMed]
119. Winter, P.M.; Neubauer, A.M.; Caruthers, S.D.; Harris, T.D.; Robertson, J.D.; Williams, T.A.; Schmieder, A.H.; Hu, G.; Allen, J.S.; Lacy, E.K.; et al. Endothelial αvβ3 integrin–targeted fumagillin nanoparticles inhibit angiogenesis in atherosclerosis. *Arterioscler. Thromb. Vasc. Biol.* **2006**, *26*, 2103–2109. [CrossRef] [PubMed]
120. Wu, Y.; Yang, Y.; Zhao, W.; Xu, Z.P.; Little, P.J.; Whittaker, A.K.; Zhang, R.; Ta, H.T. Novel iron oxide-cerium oxide core-shell nanoparticles as a potential theranostic material for ROS related inflammatory diseases. *J. Mater. Chem. B* **2018**, *6*, 4937–4951. [CrossRef] [PubMed]
121. Kim, C.W.; Hwang, B.H.; Moon, H.; Kang, J.; Park, E.H.; Ihm, S.H.; Chang, K.; Hong, K.S. In vivo MRI detection of intraplaque macrophages with biocompatible silica-coated iron oxide nanoparticles in murine atherosclerosis. *J. Appl. Biomater. Funct. Mater.* **2021**, *19*, 1014751. [CrossRef] [PubMed]
122. Oumzil, K.; Ramin, M.A.; Lorenzato, C.; Hémadou, A.; Laroche, J.; Jacobin-Valat, M.J.; Mornet, S.; Roy, C.E.; Kauss, T.; Gaudin, K.; et al. Solid lipid nanoparticles for image-guided therapy of atherosclerosis. *Bioconjug. Chem.* **2016**, *27*, 569–575. [CrossRef] [PubMed]
123. Chen, J.; Zhang, X.; Millican, R.; Creutzmann, J.E.; Martin, S.; Jun, H.W. High density lipoprotein mimicking nanoparticles for atherosclerosis. *Nano. Converg.* **2020**, *7*, 6. [CrossRef]
124. Nandwana, V.; Ryoo, S.-R.; Kanthala, S.; McMahon, K.M.; Rink, J.S.; Li, Y.; Venkatraman, S.S.; Thaxton, C.S.; Dravid, V.P. High-density lipoprotein-like magnetic nanostructures (HDL-MNS): Theranostic agents for cardiovascular disease. *Chem. Mater.* **2017**, *29*, 2276–2282. [CrossRef]
125. Kelly, K.A.; Allport, J.R.; Tsourkas, A.; Shinde-Patil, V.R.; Josephson, L.; Weissleder, R. Detection of vascular adhesion molecule-1 expression using a novel multimodal nanoparticle. *Circ. Res.* **2005**, *96*, 327–336. [CrossRef] [PubMed]
126. Nahrendorf, M.; Zhang, H.; Hembrador, S.; Panizzi, P.; Sosnovik, D.E.; Aikawa, E.; Libby, P.; Swirski, F.K.; Weissleder, R. Nanoparticle PET-CT imaging of macrophages in inflammatory atherosclerosis. *Circulation* **2008**, *117*, 379–387. [CrossRef] [PubMed]
127. Cormode, D.P.; Skajaa, T.; van Schooneveld, M.M.; Koole, R.; Jarzyna, P.; Lobatto, M.E.; Calcagno, C.; Barazza, A.; Gordon, R.E.; Zanzonico, P.; et al. Nanocrystal core high-density lipoproteins: A multimodal molecular imaging contrast agent platform. *Nano Lett.* **2008**, *8*, 3715–3723. [CrossRef] [PubMed]
128. Kirichenko, T.V.; Sukhorukov, V.N.; Markin, A.M.; Nikiforov, N.G.; Liu, P.-Y.; Sobenin, I.A.; Tarasov, V.V.; Orekhov, A.N.; Aliev, G. Medicinal plants as a potential and successful treatment option in the context of atherosclerosis. *Front. Pharmacol.* **2020**, *11*, 403. [CrossRef]
129. Zhao, X.; Oduro, P.K.; Tong, W.; Wang, Y.; Gao, X.; Wang, Q. Therapeutic potential of natural products against atherosclerosis: Targeting on gut microbiota. *Pharmacol. Res.* **2021**, *163*, 105362. [CrossRef] [PubMed]
130. Sobenin, I.A.; Myasoedova, V.A.; Iltchuk, M.I.; Zhang, D.-W.; Orekhov, A.N. Therapeutic effects of garlic in cardiovascular atherosclerotic disease. *Chin. J. Nat. Med.* **2019**, *17*, 721–728. [CrossRef]
131. Aviello, G.; Abenavoli, L.; Borrelli, F.; Capasso, R.; Izzo, A.A.; Lembo, F.; Romano, B.; Capasso, F. Garlic: Empiricism or science? *Nat. Prod. Commun.* **2009**, *4*, 1785–1796. [CrossRef]
132. Wu, M.; Yang, S.; Wang, S.; Cao, Y.; Zhao, R.; Li, X.; Xing, Y.; Liu, L. Effect of berberine on atherosclerosis and gut microbiota modulation and their correlation in high-fat diet-fed ApoE$^{-/-}$ mice. *Front. Pharmacol.* **2020**, *11*, 223. [CrossRef] [PubMed]
133. Rui, R.; Yang, H.; Liu, Y.; Zhou, Y.; Xy, X.; Li, C.; Liu, S. Effects of berberine on atherosclerosis. *Front. Pharmacol.* **2021**, *12*, 764175. [CrossRef] [PubMed]
134. Jian, X.; Liu, Y.; Zhao, Z.; Zhao, L.; Wang, D.; Liu, Q. The role of traditional Chinese medicine in the treatment of atherosclerosis through the regulation of macrophage activity. *Biomed. Pharmacother.* **2019**, *118*, 109375. [CrossRef] [PubMed]
135. Pagliaro, B.; Santolamazza, C.; Simonelli, F.; Rubattu, S. Phytochemical compounds and protection from cardiovascular diseases: A state of the art. *Biomed. Res. Int.* **2015**, *2015*, 918069. [CrossRef] [PubMed]
136. Stamenkovska, M.; Hadzi-Petrushev, N.; Nikodinovski, A.; Gagov, H.; Atanasova-Panchevska, N.; Mitrokhin, V.; Kamkin, A.; Mladenov, M. Application of curcumine and its derivatives in the treatment of cardiovascular diseases: A review. *Int. J. Food Prop.* **2021**, *24*, 1510–1528. [CrossRef]
137. Cox, F.F.; Misiou, A.; Vierkant, A.; Ale-Agha, N.; Grandoch, M.; Haendeler, J.; Altschmied, J. Protective effects of curcumin in cardiovascular diseases—Impact on oxidative stress and mitochondria. *Cells* **2022**, *11*, 342. [CrossRef] [PubMed]

138. Cao, S.-Y.; Zhao, C.-N.; Gan, R.-Y.; Xu, X.-Y.; Wei, X.-L.; Corke, H.; Atanasov, A.G.; Li, H.-B. Effects and mechanisms of tea and its bioactive compounds for the prevention and treatment of cardiovascular diseases: An updated review. *Antioxidants* **2019**, *8*, 166. [CrossRef] [PubMed]
139. Thaipitakwong, T.; Numhom, S.; Aramwit, P. Mulberry leaves and their potential effects against cardiometabolic risks: A review of chemical compositions, biological properties and clinical efficacy. *Pharm. Biol.* **2018**, *56*, 109–118. [CrossRef] [PubMed]
140. Aramwit, P.; Supasyndh, O.; Siritienthong, T.; Bang, N. Mulberry leaf reduces oxidation and C-reactive protein level in patients with mild dyslipidemia. *Biomed. Res. Int.* **2013**, *2013*, 787981. [CrossRef] [PubMed]
141. Xue, Q.; He, N.; Wang, Z.; Fu, X.; Aung, L.H.H.; Liu, Y.; Li, M.; Cho, J.Y.; Yang, Y.; Yu, T. Functional roles and mechanisms of ginsenosides from Panax ginseng in atherosclerosis. *J. Ginseng Res.* **2021**, *45*, 22–31. [CrossRef]
142. Aminifard, T.; Razavi, B.M.; Hosseinzadeh, H. The effects of ginseng on the metabolic syndrome: An updated review. *Food Sci. Nutr.* **2021**, *9*, 5293–5311. [CrossRef]
143. Buettner, C.; Yeh, G.Y.; Phillips, R.S.; Mittleman, M.A.; Kaptchuk, T.J. Systematic review of the effects of ginseng on cardiovascular risk factors. *Ann. Pharmacother.* **2006**, *40*, 83–95. [CrossRef]
144. Aviram, M.; Rosenblat, M.; Gaitini, D.; Nitecki, S.; Hoffman, A.; Dornfeld, L.; Volkova, N.; Presser, D.; Attias, J.; Liker, H.; et al. Pomegranate juice consumption for 3 years by patients with carotid artery stenosis reduces common carotid intima-media thickness, blood pressure and LDL oxidation. *Clin. Nutr.* **2004**, *23*, 423–433. [CrossRef]
145. Giménez-Bastida, J.A.; Ávila-Gálvez, M.A.; Espín, J.C.; González-Sarrías, A. Evidence for health properties of pomegranate juices and extracts beyond nutrition: A critical systematic review of human studies. *Trends Food Sci. Technol.* **2021**, *114*, 410–423. [CrossRef]
146. Zordoky, B.N.; Robertson, I.M.; Dyck, J.R. Preclinical and clinical evidence for the role of resveratrol in the treatment of cardiovascular diseases. *Biochim. Biophys. Acta* **2015**, *1852*, 1155–1177. [CrossRef]
147. Ren, J.; Fu, L.; Nile, S.H.; Zhang, J.; Kai, G. Salvia miltiorrhiza in treating cardiovascular diseases: A review on its pharmacological and clinical applications. *Front. Pharmacol.* **2019**, *10*, 753. [CrossRef]
148. Santhakumar, A.B.; Battino, M.; Alvarez-Suarez, J.M. Dietary polyphenols: Structures, bioavailability and protective effects against atherosclerosis. *Food Chem. Toxicol.* **2018**, *113*, 49–65. [CrossRef] [PubMed]
149. Grassi, D.; Desideri, G.; Di Giosia, P.; De Feo, M.; Fellini, E.; Cheli, P.; Ferri, L.; Ferri, C. Tea, flavonoids, and cardiovascular health: Endothelial protection. *Am. J. Clin. Nutr.* **2013**, *98* (Suppl. S6), 1660S–1666S. [CrossRef] [PubMed]

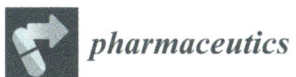 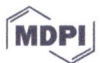

Review

Oxidative Stress in Arterial Hypertension (HTN): The Nuclear Factor Erythroid Factor 2-Related Factor 2 (Nrf2) Pathway, Implications and Future Perspectives

Daniela Maria Tanase [1,2,†], Alina Georgiana Apostol [3,4], Claudia Florida Costea [5,6,†], Claudia Cristina Tarniceriu [7,8,†], Ionut Tudorancea [9,10,*], Minela Aida Maranduca [9,†], Mariana Floria [1,11,†] and Ionela Lacramioara Serban [9]

1. Department of Internal Medicine, "Grigore T. Popa" University of Medicine and Pharmacy, 700115 Iasi, Romania; tanasedm@gmail.com (D.M.T.); floria_mariana@yahoo.com (M.F.)
2. Internal Medicine Clinic, "St. Spiridon" County Clinical Emergency Hospital, 700115 Iasi, Romania
3. Department of Neurology, "Grigore T. Popa" University of Medicine and Pharmacy, 700115 Iasi, Romania; georgianaapostol07@gmail.com
4. Neurology Clinic, Clinical Rehabilitation Hospital, 700661 Iasi, Romania
5. Department of Ophthalmology, Faculty of Medicine, "Grigore T. Popa" University of Medicine and Pharmacy, 700115 Iasi, Romania; costea10@yahoo.com
6. 2nd Ophthalmology Clinic, "Prof. Dr. Nicolae Oblu" Emergency Clinical Hospital, 700309 Iasi, Romania
7. Department of Morpho-Functional Sciences I, Discipline of Anatomy, "Grigore T. Popa" University of Medicine and Pharmacy, 700115 Iasi, Romania; cristinaghib@yahoo.com
8. Hematology Clinic, "St. Spiridon" County Clinical Emergency Hospital, 700111 Iasi, Romania
9. Department of Morpho-Functional Sciences II, Discipline of Physiology, "Grigore T. Popa" University of Medicine and Pharmacy, 700115 Iasi, Romania; minela.maranduca@umfiasi.ro (M.A.M.); ionela.serban@umfiasi.ro (I.L.S.)
10. Cardiology Clinic "St. Spiridon" County Clinical Emergency Hospital, 700111 Iasi, Romania
11. Internal Medicine Clinic, Emergency Military Clinical Hospital, 700483 Iasi, Romania
* Correspondence: ionut.tudorancea@umfiasi.ro
† These authors contributed equally to this work.

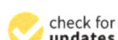

Citation: Tanase, D.M.; Apostol, A.G.; Costea, C.F.; Tarniceriu, C.C.; Tudorancea, I.; Maranduca, M.A.; Floria, M.; Serban, I.L. Oxidative Stress in Arterial Hypertension (HTN): The Nuclear Factor Erythroid Factor 2-Related Factor 2 (Nrf2) Pathway, Implications and Future Perspectives. *Pharmaceutics* **2022**, *14*, 534. https://doi.org/10.3390/pharmaceutics14030534

Academic Editor: Yasumasa Ikeda

Received: 2 February 2022
Accepted: 25 February 2022
Published: 27 February 2022

Publisher's Note: MDPI stays neutral with regard to jurisdictional claims in published maps and institutional affiliations.

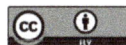

Copyright: © 2022 by the authors. Licensee MDPI, Basel, Switzerland. This article is an open access article distributed under the terms and conditions of the Creative Commons Attribution (CC BY) license (https://creativecommons.org/licenses/by/4.0/).

Abstract: Arterial hypertension (HTN) is one of the most prevalent entities globally, characterized by increased incidence and heterogeneous pathophysiology. Among possible etiologies, oxidative stress (OS) is currently extensively studied, with emerging evidence showing its involvement in endothelial dysfunction and in different cardiovascular diseases (CVD) such as HTN, as well as its potential as a therapeutic target. While there is a clear physiological equilibrium between reactive oxygen species (ROS) and antioxidants essential for many cellular functions, excessive levels of ROS lead to vascular cell impairment with decreased nitric oxide (NO) availability and vasoconstriction, which promotes HTN. On the other hand, transcription factors such as nuclear factor erythroid factor 2-related factor 2 (Nrf2) mediate antioxidant response pathways and maintain cellular reduction–oxidation homeostasis, exerting protective effects. In this review, we describe the relationship between OS and hypertension-induced endothelial dysfunction and the involvement and therapeutic potential of Nrf2 in HTN.

Keywords: arterial hypertension; HTN; nuclear factor erythroid factor 2-related factor 2; Nrf2; oxidative stress; antioxidant

1. Introduction

Arterial hypertension (HTN) represents a persistent increase in blood pressure (BP), measuring at least 140/90 mmHg according to the European Society of Hypertension (ESH) and European Society of Cardiology (ESC), and it is one of the major risk factors for cardiovascular diseases (CVD) [1]. It is estimated that 1.13 billion people suffer from hypertension worldwide, making it the main cause of strokes and coronary heart disease

(CHD). Therefore, approximately 8.5 million deaths per annum are attributed to raised BP [2]. Considering the context of the COVID-19 pandemic, it is worth mentioning that almost all available evidence up to this date suggests that HTN can be a risk factor of severe COVID-19 disease and can also become a serious sequela [3–6]. The etiology of hypertension, as it is complex and involves a myriad of varied factors, continues to remain one of the top scientific subjects of interest. While the role of inflammation and oxidative stress (OS) in HTN is currently extensively explored [7–10], the precise deleterious effect of HTN on endothelial integrity and the involvement of molecules such as the nuclear factor erythroid 2-related factor 2 (Nrf2) in the pathogenesis and evolution of raised BP remain elusive [11,12].

In this narrative review, we aim to describe the relationship between OS and hypertension-induced endothelial dysfunction and the role and therapeutic potential of Nrf2 in HTN.

2. Oxidative Stress in Hypertension

Oxidative stress is a process that takes place inside the cells and occurs in situations where there is an increased number of reactive oxygen species (ROS) or a low antioxidant response towards cell aggression [13–15]. There are several endogenous sources of ROS within cardiac myocytes, especially enzymes such as mitochondrial enzymes, nicotinamide adenine dinucleotide phosphate (NADPH) oxidase, xanthine oxidoreductase (XOR), and uncoupled endothelial nitric oxide synthase (eNOS) [16–18]. OS exerts its harmful effects on tissues by causing endothelial lesions and enlargement and thickening of the heart's walls, mainly of the left ventricle, thus serving as one of the main processes that lead to HTN and other CVDs [19]. Endothelial dysfunction is characterized by decreased NO, with or without an imbalance between endothelium-derived relaxing and contracting factors combined with a prothrombotic and a proinflammatory state [20].

An immense variety of enzymes work to keep the balance inside the cells. In addition, molecules such as glutathione and ascorbate act as direct antioxidants in increased blood pressure conditions [21]. For a long time, researchers have been investigating the precise role of OS as a generator or potential therapeutic target, not only in the pathophysiology of HTN [22], or in pulmonary hypertension [23,24], but also in endothelial dysfunction associated with other cardiovascular and metabolic diseases [25]. Therefore, we will briefly discuss the main precursors of OS and their involvement in HTN.

2.1. ROS and Nitric Oxide

ROS following OS have extremely harmful cardiac effects because the heart is a big consumer of oxygen (~8–15 mL O_2/min/100 g tissue while resting, and it can go up to more than >70 mL O_2/min/100 g tissue while exercising) [26,27]. During sustained physical activity, molecular O_2 is no longer reduced to water, but to superoxide O_2-. This free radical is the precursor to most of the other ROS: hydrogen peroxide (H_2O_2), hydroxyl radical ($\cdot OH$), singlet oxygen ($1O_2$), and alpha-oxygen (α-O). ROS are also known to have benefits such as defense against pathogens, but increased levels can lead to cardiovascular apoptosis and ischemic injuries [28–30]. The main harmful processes exerted on cardiac myocytes are DNA and RNA damage, lipid peroxidation, deactivation of specific enzymes, and oxidation of amino acids [31]. Enhanced levels of ROS have been associated with HTN; however, new generations of protein targets that include ROS-forming or toxifying enzymes that could act as pharmacological agents are needed [32,33].

Nitric oxide (NO) is a colorless gas, a molecule produced by the myocardium in physiological conditions, and its major function is to dilate vessels. Decreased levels of NO are associated with cardiovascular diseases [34,35]. There are four known NOS isoforms: endothelial NOS (eNOS), found in cardiac and coronary endothelium; neuronal NOS (nNOS), found in cardiac cells; inducible NOS (iNOS), derived from neutrophils or myocytes in conditions of inflammation; and mitochondrial NOS (mtNOS), present in cardiac mitochondria [36,37]. The beneficial roles of NOS are mediating heart protection, improving endothelial integrity, and decreasing injuries of reperfusion caused by ischemia [38]. In ischemic situations, NO accumulates and produces ROS, leading to cardiac insults [36]. Usually, eNOS is the main source of endothelium-derived NO [39]. In order to synthesize NO from eNOS, a series of cofactors are involved, and its disruption leads to a monomeric form of the enzyme, which is uncoupled, and instead of NO, superoxide is formed. Uncoupled eNOS has been observed in patients with essential hypertension and atherosclerosis [40,41]. Endogenously activated Nrf2 and eNOS are thought to play a role in OS induced by myocardial infarction [36]. Higashi et al. [42] studied deficiency of tetrahydrobiopterin (BH4), a cofactor for NO synthase, and concluded that BH4 restores endothelium-dependent vasodilation in hypertensive patients.

2.2. Mitochondria

Mitochondria have multiple functions, being a variable source of ROS under physiological conditions and maintaining the redox status inside cells [43]. The small amount of ROS produced during respiration is not dangerous, and it is detoxified by endogenous means. However, in hypoxic or ischemic conditions, mitochondria generate elevated levels of ROS, which increase the chances of apoptosis and even myocardial infarction (MI) [44]. An increasing number of studies have emphasized that mitochondria can produce high levels of ROS in hypertensive animal models [45–47]. Dikalov et al. [48] have shown in their study that endothelial tissue treated with angiotensin II increased mitochondrial ROS generation and the damage caused to the cells and the body systems, such as decreased membrane potential and decreased respiratory control ratio, respectively. Aside from the peripheral effects, ROS can regulate blood pressure via central mechanisms. Mitochondrial superoxide is overproduced in conditions of activated renin–angiotensin system (RAS) in the central nervous system (CNS) [49]. More than that, the mitochondrial ROS activate Nrf2 and promote the expression of genes involved in the control of mitochondrial and antioxidant genes via various protein kinases [50]. Taking into consideration the mitochondrial implications in cardiovascular pathophysiology, further studies could lead to new treatment strategies in hypertension.

2.3. NADPH Oxidase (Nox)

NADPH oxidase (Nox) is a membrane-bound enzyme complex considered an important source of ROS in cardiac cells. This is the only known category of enzymes specialized in producing ROS, and it was first described in immune cells such as macrophages and neutrophils as molecules with antimicrobial properties. The Nox family is comprised of Nox 1, Nox 2, Nox 3, Nox 4, Nox 5, dual oxidase 1 (Duox 1), and Duox 2 which in states of hyperactivity produce excessive levels of ROS, contributing to endothelial dysfunction, inflammation, and cardiovascular remodeling. Angiotensin II regulates Nox function in vessels [51–54]. Mice and rats treated with this peptide hormone expressed increased generation of ROS and enhanced activity of Nox 1, Nox 2, and Nox 4 [21]. In order to establish how Nox-produced ROS influence blood pressure, many researchers conducted genetic studies. Their results noted that in mice with Nox 1 deletion, hypertension cannot be induced by angiotensin II. Overexpression of human Nox 1 in experimental animals revealed increased blood pressure and aortic superoxide production as a result of angiotensin II action in vascular smooth muscle cells, ventricular hypertrophy, and oxidative stress [55]. In fibroblast-specific deficiency of Nox 2 knockout mice, the response to angiotensin II was considerably decreased. This resulted in a decreased hypertensive response and an inhibited vascular smooth muscle growth [56]. On the other hand, Nox 4 knockout mice infused with angiotensin II showed no change in blood pressure. However, in these mice, vascular inflammation, thickening of the media, and endothelial dysfunction have been noted, showing that Nox 4 exerts beneficial effects on the cardiovascular system. The experimental animals which developed hypertension were treated with nonspecific Nox inhibitors (apocynin or diphenylene iodonium) and the specific inhibitor gp91 ds-tat. Consequently, both the blood pressure and the vascular OS in those animals were lowered [21].

As is known, the glucose metabolism is altered in hypertension. The pentose phosphate pathway (PPP), also called the phosphogluconate pathway and the hexose monophosphate (HMP) shunt, acts as an essential element of cellular metabolism. The HMP shunt pathway plays a key role in NADPH2 and in ribose-5-phosphate formation and is involved in metabolic control by interacting with other metabolic pathways such as glycolysis, gluconeogenesis, and glucuronic acid. This pathway occurs in two phases that are illustrated by many reactions. The oxidative phase reactions are catalyzed by prostaglandin (PGD) and by the glucose-6-phosphate dehydrogenase (G6PD), both known to be controlled by Nrf2 [57,58]. G6PD is involved in the pathogenesis of pulmonary artery remodeling and occlusive lesion formation within the hypertensive lungs [59]. In the nonoxidative phase, NRF2 positively regulates the expression of transaldolase 1 (TALDO1) and transketolase (TKT) [58]. As deficiency in the HMP pathway can lead to different disorders, research data suggest the HMP shunt may have potential as a therapeutic target.

2.4. XOR

Xanthine oxidoreductase is an important source of superoxide and hydrogen peroxide in conditions of heart ischemia, inflammation, and OS. Its catalytic properties transform hypoxanthine to the end-product uric acid [60]. Mervaala et al. [61] studied the involvement of XOR in vascular damage induced by angiotensin II using double-transgenic rats (dTGRs) harboring human renin and human angiotensin genes. They showed that these rats presented overactivity of XOR in kidneys in contrast with control rats. The activity of the enzyme was successfully decreased using valsartan, an angiotensin II type 1 receptor antagonist. Moreover, valsartan, 30 mg/kg for three weeks, reduced not only blood pressure, but also cardiac hypertrophy and 24 h proteinuria. In the same study, oxypurinol, an XOR inhibitor, was used to preincubate renal arteries, resulting in an endothelium-dependent vascular relaxation by 20%. However, it has been proven that ROS generated by XOR are not the major factors responsible for endothelial dysfunction in dTGRs and that other enzymes might play a major role in angiotensin II-induced vascular dysfunction in these rats [62].

Data so far show that OS and endothelial dysfunction are causes or consequences of HTN. Dysfunctional endothelium secondary to OS and its derivative molecules and pathways loses its capacity to protect the vessel wall, with the subsequent possibility of smooth muscle cell proliferation, monocyte adhesion, raised adhesion molecule expression, and finally development of atherosclerosis. Therefore, in order to prevent this vicious chain of events, researchers focus their attention on different pathways or molecules which contribute to OS-induced HTN.

3. Nrf2

Nrf2 was first discovered in 1994 by Moi et al. [63], and it is a nuclear transcription factor that plays a major role in regulating the cellular adaptive antioxidant response. It is a master regulator of cytoprotective responses [64]. Nrf2 does not have antioxidative functions but exerts antioxidant effects by activating the transcription of target antioxidant genes: HMOX-1, NQ01, MT1A, superoxide dismutase (SOD), catalase (CAT), glutathione peroxidase (GPx), glutathione-S-transferase (GST), and γ-glutamylcysteine synthase (γGCS) [65,66]. Nrf2 is a polypeptide composed of 605 amino acids and 7 domains (Neh1, Neh2, Neh3, Neh4, Neh5, Neh6, Neh7). Kelch-like ECH-associated protein 1 (Keap1) inhibits Nrf2's transcriptional action by keeping it bound to itself under physiological conditions [67]. Keap1 is a polypeptide composed of 624 amino acid residues and 5 domains: NTR (N-terminus), IVR, BTB/POZ DGR, and CTR (C-terminus). Scientific research established in cell lines and animal models that Nrf2/Keap1 pathway activation exerts protective effects in ischemia–reperfusion injury in vessels [68].

Under oxidative stress conditions, Nrf2 can be phosphorylated by several enzymatic pathways. Protein kinase C phosphorylates Nrf2 on Ser40 and allows Nrf2 to detach from Keap1 [69]. Other kinases that can modulate Nrf2's activity include extracellular signal-regulated kinase (ERK) [70], phosphoinositide 3-kinases (PI3K) [71], AMP-activated protein kinase (AMPK) [72], and mitogen-activated protein kinase (MAPK) [73]. Phosphorylated Nrf2 (p-Nrf2) then binds to antioxidant response elements (AREs) in the nucleus, triggering the transcription of various genes which encode antioxidants, detoxifying enzymes, proteasomes, and antiapoptotic proteins aiming to scavenge excessive ROS. Nrf2 can also be activated through the canonical mechanism, where ROS oxidize part of the cysteine residues in Keap1, which in turn decreases Nrf2 ubiquitination and increases Nrf2 translocation to the nucleus, where the antioxidant transcription process can be initiated [74,75]. More than that, in Nrf2's activity, phosphorylation by kinases plays a vital role in its posttranslational regulation. Notably, glycogen synthase kinase-3 (GSK-3) regulates negatively, whereas AMP-activated kinase, casein kinase 2, and protein kinase C positively modulate Nrf2 activity via phosphorylation of various sites [76]. Nrf2 is the key activator of AREs [77] (Figure 1).

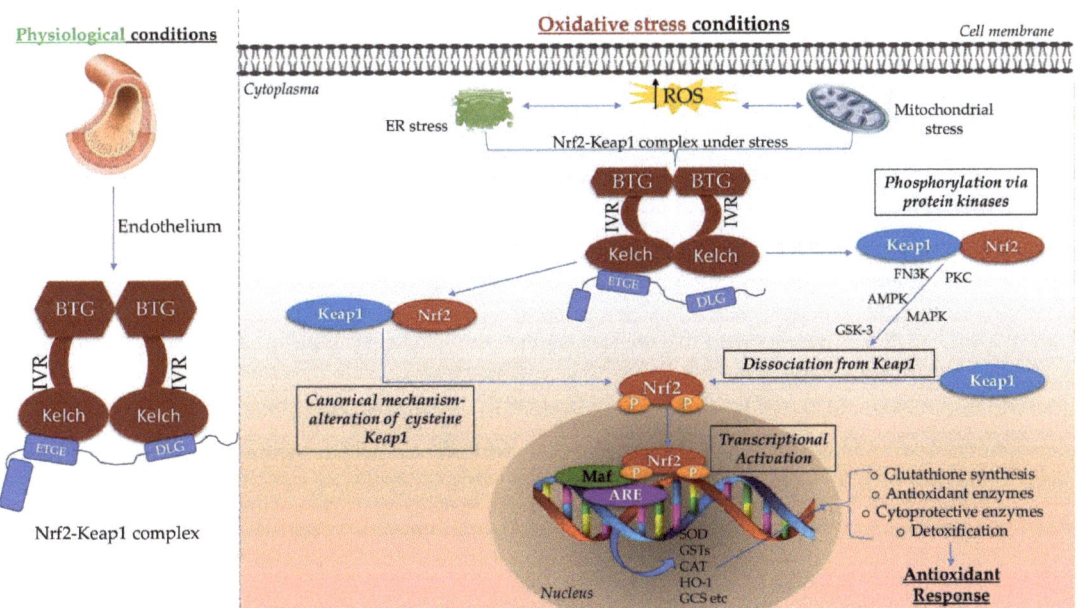

Figure 1. Role of the nuclear factor erythroid factor 2-related factor 2 (Nrf2) in oxidative stress. In physiological conditions, Nrf2 is bound to Keap1 (the key negative regulator and the inhibitory protein of Nrf2) and is secured to the actin cytoskeleton. This limits its transcriptional activity in the nucleus. Under OS conditions, the IVR domain leads to conformational alterations. Nrf2 is activated via canonical mechanism and/or via phosphorylation with secondary dissociation of Nrf2 from Keap1, which translocates into the nucleus and combines with the Maf protein to compose a heterodimer, capable of identifying the suitable ARE sequence. This activated ARE-mediated gene transcription is the Nrf2/Keap1–ARE pathway, which exerts antioxidant cellular functions via regulating the expression of antioxidant genes such as SOD, GST, CAT, and NQO1. Kelch-like ECH-associated protein 1 (Keap1); intervening region (IVR); endoplasmic reticulum (ER); reactive oxygen species (ROS); antioxidant response element (ARE); musculoaponeurotic fibrosarcoma (Maf); superoxide dismutase (SOD); glutathione S-transferases (GSTs), catalase (CAT); heme oxygenase-1 (HO-1); glutamylcysteine synthetase (GCS); protein kinase C (PKC); fructosamine-3-kinase (FN3K); AMP-activated protein kinase (AMPK); mitogen-activated protein kinase (MAPK).

Although Nrf2 has been portrayed as an effective agent to protect the heart, its destructive side has been of current interest [78]. Kannan et al. [79] noted in 2013 that sustained activation of Nrf2 can also lead to cardiac dysfunction. Others have stressed the protective role of Nrf2 in the first phase of pressure overload-induced adaptation of the heart, while the Nrf2 KO showed a decreased rate of cardiac hypertrophy and recovery of cardiac function by eight weeks after transverse aortic arch constriction in rodents [80]. Considering both sides of Nrf2, it is clear that further research regarding how this transcription factor can affect the heart and blood vessels at a molecular level is needed.

Nrf2 in Hypertension

A gamut of evidence displays the key role of Nrf2 in cardiovascular diseases [81]; in metabolic disorders [82], diabetes [83,84], or obesity [85–87]; and even in autoimmune, gastrointestinal, and neurodegenerative diseases or cancer [88].

Endothelial dysfunction represents a crucial step in the development of atherosclerosis. As it needs to be prevented by means of antioxidative processes, Nrf2 may represent a modality to protect cells against endogenous and exogenous oxidants and thus prevent endothelial dysfunction onset [89].

Associated with Nrf2, peroxisome proliferator-activated receptor gamma (PPARγ) is a nuclear receptor and a nutritional factor that is involved in inflammation response and homeostatic control by stimulating the expression of antioxidant genes together with the retinoid X receptor (RXR) [90]. It acts as a modulator of different pathways, such as Nrf2, RAS, and P13/Akt/NOS [91]. Blood pressure regulation, improved lipid profile and anti-inflammatory response, and ameliorated sensitivity to insulin are amongst the beneficial effects of PPARγ [92].

ROS produced during inflammation can activate Nrf2 and the nuclear factor kappa-light-chain-enhancer of activated B cells (NF-kB). Once activated, Nrf2 attenuates ROS and consequently NF-kB activity [88]. Therefore, Nrf2 and NF-kB are both transcription factors that mediate the cellular response under conditions of OS and inflammation. NF-kB plays an important role in inducing the expression of multiple proinflammatory genes, such as those encoding chemokines and cytokines [93,94]. As a consequence, disrupted NF-kB activation contributes to the pathogenesis of multiple inflammatory diseases. Bhandari et al. [95] proposed a potential interplay between Nrf2 and NF-kB, where each pathway could inhibit the transcription activity of the other factor. Moreover, this crosstalk appears to work both ways, with Nrf2 having the ability to inhibit NF-kb and the other way around. Other transcription factors that activate Nrf2 are the aryl hydrocarbon receptor (AhR), specificity protein 1 (Sp-1), myocyte-specific enhancer factor 2 D (MEF2D), p53, c-Myc, c-Jun, and breast cancer 1 (BRCA1) [78]. Additionally, recent evidence displays the major role of Nrf2 in protecting against OS and inflammation by stimulating phase II antioxidant enzymes such as glutathione S-transferase (GST), UDP-glucuronosyltransferase (UGT), UDP-glucuronic acid synthesis enzymes, and HO-1 [96,97]. Nrf2 also exerts its anti-inflammatory effect by binding to the promoter sequence of the key proinflammatory cytokines (IL-1β, IL-6) and by reducing the activity of RNA polymerase II, which will result in the suppression of gene expression [98].

The link between OS and HTN has already been proven in several animal models, but there is still room for research to also prove this in humans. Lopes et al. [99] used male Wistar Kyoto rats (WKY) and stroke-prone spontaneously hypertensive rats (SHRSP) to study how the vascular Nrf2 system influences vascular function and redox signaling. Nrf2 was downregulated in SHRSP in conditions of increased vascular OS which was connected with vascular dysfunction. However, Nrf2 activators, bardoxolone and L-sulforaphane, blocked the formation of angiotensin II-induced ROS, resulting in restored endothelial dysfunction and decreased inflammation in both WKY and SHRSP cells. Therefore, the author stresses the vasoprotective function of Nrf2 in HTN.

Another study performed by Banday and Lokhandwala [100] also investigated the role of Nrf2 in decreasing OS and BP in rats. Rats treated with L-buthionine-sulfoximine (BSO) were used to test whether sulforaphane could lower OS, decrease BP, and repair renal dopamine receptors (D1Rs). The study has successfully demonstrated the hypothesis that by activating Nrf2, the phase II antioxidant enzymes are generated, which leads to decreased OS and a well-functioning D1R system. These findings confirm that the use of sulforaphane helps in keeping BP in a normal range.

Tan et al. [69] have recently studied how the Nrf2 pathway decreases OS in the rostral ventrolateral medulla (RVLM) and whether Nrf2 intervenes in β-arrestin1's antihypertensive action. RVLM is one of the key areas involved in the regulation of BP and sympathetic activity. β-Arrestin1 is a cytosolic protein acting as a cofactor in the desensitization of β-adrenergic receptors [101]. The results confirmed the antihypertensive role of the overexpression of β-arrestin1 in the RVLM by activating the Nrf2 pathway and increasing the generation of antioxidant enzymes. All these reactions lead to a decreased sympathetic outflow and a reduced BP value.

High BP caused by kidney diseases is often called renal HTN or renovascular HTN. It is important to mention that HTN could be both a cause and an effect of chronic kidney disease [102]. The renin–angiotensin–aldosterone (RAAS) system is responsible for regulating BP and electrolyte and fluid balance in the kidneys. The activation of this hormone system generates angiotensin II, which stimulates in turn the production of aldosterone. Aldosterone is the main mineral corticosteroid hormone, and its main function is to preserve sodium and water in the kidneys, thus causing the BP to increase [103–105]. Xiao et al. [106] discovered that in mice suffering from chronic heart failure which overexpressed angiotensin-converting enzyme 2 (ACE2), the sympathetic output was remarkably low. Others studied the hypothesis that ACE2 could decrease ROS generation using a pathway involving Nrf2 and antioxidant enzymes in the RVLM. The study succeeded in proving that both ACE2 and Nrf2 have the ability to inhibit sympathetic activity in HTN and chronic heart failure when they are administered in the RVLM [107]. Others noted in hypertensive rodent models that via OS and endothelial dysfunction, HTN could be one of the causes of Nrf2 transcriptional misregulations and not the other way around [99,108]. By cause of raised levels of Nrf2 repressors in hypertensive models, these results imply that the Nrf2 antioxidant defense system is insufficient to counteract the effects of OS.

Current scientific research focuses more on discovering specific factors linked to an inadequate Nrf2 signaling system, rather than on the Nrf2 antioxidant adaptative responses [108]. Nonetheless, perhaps amplifying Nrf2 activity may hold therapeutic potential for ameliorating HTN.

4. Therapeutic Options in HTN

The pharmacological Nrf2 activators are electrophilic compounds that can modify cysteine residues in Keap1 and ultimately its conformation through oxidation/alkylation. This process induces inhibition of Keap1-mediated degradation of Nrf2, with a consequently raised load of newly synthesized Nrf2, which augments Nrf2 transcription functions [109]. As follows, these "Nrf2 activators" actually represent Keap1 inhibitors [110].

The antioxidant defense system represented by the Nrf2 activators may include a wide range of compounds and derivatives with great potential in chronic diseases; however, few are explored in hypertension. Examples include the following: phenolic compounds (butylated hydroxyanisole, butylated hydroxytoluene, and tert-butyl hydroquinone), isopropyl sulfur cyanogen compounds (sulforaphane), 1,2-mercapto-3-sulfur ketone derivatives (oltipraz), hydrogen peroxide compounds (hydrogen peroxide, isopropyl benzene hydrogen peroxide, and 4-butyl hydroperoxide), natural compounds from plants (curcumin, resveratrol, plumbagin, tanshinone, luteolin, oleanolic acid, etc.), and compounds that are rich in arsenic, selenium, trace elements, and heavy metal ions [109,111]. Registered drugs such as statins and metformin also have the ability to activate Nrf2 [91].

4.1. Nrf2 Activators: Bardoxolone Methyl, Sulforaphane, and Dimethyl Fumarate

Bardoxolone methyl (BM), a semisynthetic triterpenoid, is an Nrf2 activator and NF-kB pathway inhibitor, reducing OS, inflammation, and excessive RAS activation and promoting mitochondrial functions within the cells [112,113]. It has been proven that BM can be used as a powerful antiviral treatment option in hepatocyte cultures of hepatitis B and C viruses and also in herpes simplex virus type 1 [114,115]. Due to the current pandemic situation, studies regarding the use of BM in treating SARS-CoV-2 infections are still ongoing. There are currently two clinical phase III trials ongoing that investigate the safety of bardoxolone (CDD0-ME) therapy in patients with pulmonary hypertension: the Ranger trial (NCT03068130) and the CATALYST trial (NCT02657356). As we are at the inception of exploring the Nrf2–HTN relationship, it is not unexpected that we could not identify a specific clinical trial that explores therapy with Nrf2 in HTN.

Taking this into consideration, it is necessary to understand Nrf2's mediator role and the additional contribution of BM in the anti-inflammatory processes which take place throughout the body systems.

Sulforaphane (SFN), an isothiocyanate, is also a potent natural Nrf2 activator, which was first isolated from red cabbage and hoary cress and later from broccoli [116]. Its direct interaction with Keap1 allows Nrf2 to accumulate in the nucleus and to activate cytoprotective mechanisms in order to protect cells from ROS [117]. SFN has the ability to activate over 500 genes by means of the Nrf2/ARE signaling pathway. SFN is known as a natural compound that can induce phase II enzymes in vivo and in vitro. These enzymes play a role in inactivating and eliminating toxic substances accumulated during periods of OS within the vascular smooth muscle cells [118]. Senanayake et al. [119] studied the effect of SFN on SHRSP and Sprague Dawley (SD) rats. The research demonstrated that this Nrf2 activator decreased the three used parameters (systolic blood pressure, diastolic blood pressure, and mean arterial pressure) by 9%, 12%, and 11%, respectively, in SHRSP, while there was no effect on SD rats. Moderate activation of Nrf2 by SFN, which is basically a dietary factor, may emphasize the mild protective role of Nrf2 through a healthy diet, which could amplify the therapeutic benefits of this antioxidant-gene-modulated system.

Dimethyl fumarate (DMF) (Tecfidera), named after the earth smoke plant (Fumaria officinalis), is the methyl ester of fumaric acid. DMF has been reported to be one of the most potent Nrf2 activators, having antioxidant and anti-inflammatory properties [92]. This drug was approved in 2013 by the US Food and Drug Administration (FDA) as first-line treatment of relapsing–remitting multiple sclerosis [120] and in 2017 was approved by the European Medicines Agency (EMA) for the treatment of moderate-to-severe chronic plaque psoriasis [121].

DMF exerts potential neuroprotective, immunomodulating, antifibrotic, and radiosensitizing activities, which are dependent on Nrf2 antioxidant pathways. After oral administration, DMF is converted into its active metabolite monomethyl fumarate (MMF). MMF reacts with C151 in Keap1, thereby activating Nrf2 which subsequently translocates to the nucleus and binds to the AREs. This induces the expression of a number of cytoprotective genes, including NAD(P)H quinone oxidoreductase 1 (NQO1), sulfiredoxin 1 (Srxn1), heme oxygenase-1 (HO1, HMOX1), superoxide dismutase 1 (SOD1), gamma-glutamylcysteine synthetase (gamma-GCS), thioredoxin reductase-1 (TXNRD1), GST, and glutamate-cysteine ligase catalytic subunit (Gclc). It increases the synthesis of the antioxidant glutathione (GSH), and via inhibition of the NF-kB-mediated pathway, DMF modulates the production of certain cytokines [120]. Additionally, DMF activates the Nrf2/Keap1 pathway by S-alkylating Keap1 and by forcing BACH1, an Nrf2 inhibitor, to leave the nucleus [122].

Little attention has been given to the relation between DMF and CVDs, especially HTN. Experimental studies show that DMF reduces inflammation, oxidative damage, and fibrosis in mouse models of pulmonary arterial hypertension [123] and can attenuate aberrant remodeling after acute vascular injury in rodent carotid arteries [124]. Hsu et al. [125] studied male rats which were exposed prenatally to dexamethasone and postnatally to a diet rich in fats in order to develop HTN. After maternal DMF therapy in offspring, programmed HTN was prevented from developing. Via AKT/Nrf2 pathway, DMF reduces ROS generation and stimulates the expression of antioxidative genes regulated by Nrf2, having a protective role in pulmonary HTN or in diabetic cardiomyopathy [126]. Other researchers noted that fumaric acid and succinic acid may treat gestational hypertension by downregulating the expression of ten-eleven translocation 1 (TET1) and calcium-activated potassium channel subunit β1 (KCNMB1) [127].

Although DMF demonstrated efficacy in diverse clinical trials in other diseases, hypertension-related studies failed to show therapeutic efficacy and were dropped, terminated, or withdrawn. A double-blinded, placebo-controlled study of DMF (NCT02981082) in systemic sclerosis–pulmonary hypertension (SSc-PAH) patients was terminated due to low recruitment numbers. In a small-size pilot study, patients with pulmonary arterial hypertension-associated systemic sclerosis tolerated DMF poorly and did not provide power to suggest efficacy. Still, authors suggest that Nrf2 remains a valid therapeutic target and should be tested in future trials by using better Nrf2 agonists [128].

Considering this emerging evidence, we may consider that fumaric acid esters might be beneficial for patients with vascular diseases [129]; however, more research that could expand the treatment area of DMF to other diseases such as hypertension, with clinical utility and favorable safety profiles, is desired.

4.2. Natural Nrf2 Activators

A myriad of ingredients that are used daily and have the ability to promote the nuclear translocation of Nrf2 are reported in Table 1. Among these, spices were demonstrated to have potential as natural Nrf2 pathway activators that can be used in disorders caused by OS [130,131].

Table 1. Salient effects of natural Nrf2 activators. Kelch-like ECH-associated protein 1 (Keap1); nuclear factor erythroid factor 2-related factor 2 (Nrf2); glycogen synthase kinase-3 (GSK-3); malondialdehyde (MDA); superoxide dismutase (SOD); nuclear factor kappa-light-chain-enhancer of activated B cells (NF-κB); heme oxygenase-1 (HO-1); plasma glutathione peroxidase (GSH-Px).

Authors and Ref.	Natural Compound	Organic Compound	Species and/or Cells Researched	Meaningful Findings
Kim et al. [132]	Pepper	Methysticin	Murine cell cultures murine RAW 264.7 cell line	- Oxidation or alkylation of the Keap1 proteins; - Inhibited binding of Nrf2 to Keap1; - Phosphorylation of Nrf2 by GSK-3 and subsequent proteasomal degradation.
Wafi et al. [133]	Turmeric	Curcumin	Sixty male C57BL/6 mice 10 weeks of age	- Decreased MDA and SOD levels; - Suppression of the Bax/Bcl-2-caspase-3 pathway-mediated cell death; - Diminished inflammation, fibrosis, and hypertrophy.
Ji et al. [134]	Ginger	6-Dehydrogingerdione	Human mesenchymal stem cells	- Inhibition of NF-κB activation.
Mimura et al. [135]	Rosemary	Carnosic acid	U373MG cells (human glioblastoma astrocytoma cells)	- Keap1 inactivation.
Mohan Manu et al. [136]	Water hyssop (Bacopa monnieri)	Dammarane-type triterpenoid saponins	Adult male Wistar rats	- Restored expression of Nrf2, NQO1 gene, and HO-1 followed by increased antioxidant enzymes and total glutathione levels.

Table 1. *Cont.*

Authors and Ref.	Natural Compound	Organic Compound	Species and/or Cells Researched	Meaningful Findings
He et al. [137]	Thyme	Thymol	Zebrafish	- Activated Nrf2/Keap1 pathway (signifcant downregulation of Keap1 expression and upregulation of Nrf2 expression).
Korenori et al. [138]	Wasabi	Allyl isothiocyanate	HepG2 (human hepatoma)	- Increased Keap1 modification and diminished Nrf2 degradation.
Kanlaya et al. [139]	Green tea	Catechins	Madin–Darby Canine Kidney (MDCK) renal tubular cells	- Increased antioxidative activity of phase II enzymes.
Paul et al. [140]	Ashwagandha	Triterpene lactones	Coronary artery occlusion in rats; myocardial infarction in rats	- Abrogated apoptosis in an Nrf2-dependent manner; - Increased phase II detoxification enzymes.
Farkhondeh et al. [141]	Grapes, berries, cranberries, nuts, cocoa, and dark chocolate	Resveratrol	Adult male Sprague-Dawley rats	- Significant increase in GSH-Px and SOD.
Yang et al. [142]	Tomatoes, watermelons, red carrots, grapefruits, and papayas	Lycopene	Human umbilical vein cell line	- Inhibited NF-κB nuclear translocation and transactivation.
Ramyaa et al. [143]	Apples, citrus fruits, onions, green leafy vegetables, honey	Quercetin	Vero cells (African green monkey kidney epithelial cells)	- Nuclear Nrf2 translocation.

The experimental studies from Table 1 demonstrated that modulating natural products via Nrf2 pathways exerts beneficial antioxidant and anti-inflammatory effects [132,137,140] in severe heart failure [133], in radiation-induced OS [134], in induced-cardiac stress [136], in renal impairment [139], in atherosclerosis [142], and in ochratoxin-induced toxicity [143] and also shows cytoprotective and antimicrobial properties [135]; cytoprotective and cancer chemopreventive effects [138]; and anti-inflammatory, antioxidant, hepatoprotective, neuroprotective, cardioprotective, renoprotective, antiobesity, antidiabetic, and anticancer effects [141] in other chronic diseases. Although the studies mentioned did not directly explore the effect of natural products in hypertension, the administration of these natural products leads to an Nrf2 response with subsequent activation of various protective pathways which can be linked to vascular protection.

These elements bring new scientific ideas and opportunities for future researchers to explore the association between these natural Nrf2 activators and HTN and the potential therapeutic targets of these natural Nrf2 activators in this disease.

4.3. Other Therapeutic Options via Nrf2

Antioxidants consist of a group of enzymes and molecules that counteract the harmful effects of ROS, and their main role is to keep a balance between these two systems, not to fully reduce oxidants, as they can also protect against pathogens [144]. Antioxidants can be produced endogenously, but their level might be inadequate. Therefore, the body needs additional exogenous sources of antioxidants, usually obtained from plants or drugs [145]. Plants have been used for their antioxidant properties for a long period of time, and they have proved to be able to effectively restore the balance between oxidation and antioxidation by removing ROS. They have few side effects, decrease ROS production, and stop oxidation by restricting the beginning and spreading of redox reactions [146].

Thioredoxin (Trx), glutaredoxin (Grx), and peroxiredoxin (Prx) belong to the thioredoxin family and can be found in all organisms. They function as antioxidants and are implicated in a myriad of CVDs, including HTN, atherosclerosis, ischemic heart diseases, and cardiac hypertrophy [147]. Ahsan et al.'s review article [148] emphasized how Trx serum levels can work as biomarkers in identifying cardiac adaptive reactions. Moreover, mesenchymal stem cells genetically modified to express Trx1 showed an increased ability to proliferate and divide into cardiomyocytes, smooth muscle cells, and endothelial cells, making them a potential therapy for cardiac failure [149,150].

Inhibition of G6PD with a competitive inhibitor (6-aminonicotinamide) and with noncompetitive inhibitors (dehydroepiandrosterone and epiandrosterone) relaxes pulmonary arteries and precontracted aorta [151]. Dehydroepiandrosterone reduces pulmonary vascular resistance in pulmonary hypertensive rats [152], and researchers reported in humans that low levels of dehydroepiandrosterone sulfate are associated with increased severity of pulmonary hypertension [153]. A double-blind, randomized, placebo-controlled phase III study (NCT00581087) demonstrated that dehydroepiandrosterone improves pulmonary hypertension in chronic obstructive pulmonary disease (COPD) [154].

Additionally, researchers demonstrated that fructosamine 3-kinase (FN3K) triggers protein deglycation influencing Nrf2 activity. Sanghvi et al. [155] noted that FN3K is absent in certain cell stress such as cancer, and via Keap1, this can lead to extensively glycated Nrf2, which affects the ability of Nrf2 to bind proteins and interact with transcription cofactors. FN3K may represent a novel target of Nrf2 activity in cancer [155,156]. Even if the role of FN3K in arterial hypertension remains unclear, polymorphisms of the FN3K gene in patients with diabetes display a protective role against severe microangiopathy and macroangiopathy diabetes complications [157]. These data suggest that the FN3K–Nrf2 pathway is involved in different vascular alterations that may lead to hypertension and could represent a new therapeutic target.

Currently, multiple drugs are being used in the treatment of HTN, but they do not act via the Nrf2/Keap1 pathway. Among promising redox drugs for CVD therapy are antioxidants targeted against mitochondria (mitoQ) and Nrf2 activators (SFN, BM, DMF) [158]. There is strong evidence for resveratrol's antioxidant and anti-inflammatory properties and its beneficial role for patients with CVD, but it was found to be less effective in obese individuals [159]. Anyway, further research into resveratrol's properties and bioavailability is desirable.

As hypertension is a multifactorial disease, its clinical management usually includes lifestyle approaches and multiple-drug administration. So far, the efforts to find redox-based therapies are still ongoing as there is still no evidence of a fully efficient Nrf2-targeted drug in CVD, and implicitly HTN [8,109]. Further investigation and validation through clinical trials of a single Nrf2 activator via a certain pathway or a combination with another antioxidant are needed [150]. These results may provide enough scientific proof to implement a novel Nrf2–HTN therapeutic approach with practicability in clinical settings.

5. Conclusions and Future Directions

Arterial hypertension continues to remain an incremental and significant worldwide medical issue. The complex heterogeneity behind HTN also includes the imbalance and misregulation of OS factors. Even if HTN pathogenesis cannot be explained by only one mechanism, present-day data exhibit the deleterious effects of enhanced OS activity and excessive ROS products which perpetuate endothelial dysfunction and hypertension via different pathways. Nonetheless, research continuously brings us new molecules and transcriptional factors such as Nrf2, which in addition to its involvement in cardiovascular pathogenesis holds potential as a novel therapeutic approach in chronic diseases such as HTN. Preclinical studies support the anti-OS and anti-inflammatory effects of Nrf2 in

HTN through regulation via various pathways. The pharmaceutical modulation of Nrf2 activity using natural and synthetic compounds enhances cell survival and sets in motion the endogenous defense antioxidant system. Biopharmaceutical companies are currently working on developing new drugs that target the Keap1–Nrf2 system, being challenged however by off-target effects and lack of a precise monitoring panel.

These results should encourage scientists to continue their research in this field. We hope for new discoveries which could help further demonstrate the key role of Nrf2 in HTN and its potential as a novel therapeutic target. Therefore, more research on this subject is essential for translating the OS concept into clinical practice.

Author Contributions: Conceptualization, D.M.T., A.G.A., M.A.M. and M.F.; methodology, C.F.C. and C.C.T.; software, I.T. and A.G.A.; validation, D.M.T., I.L.S. and M.A.M.; formal analysis, M.F.; investigation, I.T., A.G.A., C.F.C., C.C.T. and I.L.S.; resources, I.T.; data curation, D.M.T.; writing—original draft preparation, M.A.M. and I.L.S.; writing—review and editing I.T.; visualization, C.F.C.; supervision, C.C.T.; project administration, D.M.T.; funding acquisition, A.G.A. All authors have read and agreed to the published version of the manuscript.

Funding: This research received no external funding.

Conflicts of Interest: The authors declare no conflict of interest.

References

1. Williams, B.; Mancia, G.; Spiering, W.; Rosei, E.A.; Azizi, M.; Burnier, M.; Clement, D.L.; Coca, A.; De Simone, G.; Dominiczak, A.; et al. 2018 ESC/ESH Guidelines for Themanagement of Arterial Hypertension: The Task Force for the management of arterial hypertension of the European Society of Cardiology (ESC) and the European Society of Hypertension (ESH). *Eur. Heart J.* **2018**, *39*, 3021–3104. [CrossRef]
2. Zhou, B.; Carrillo-Larco, R.M.; Danaei, G.; Riley, L.M.; Paciorek, C.J.; Stevens, G.A.; Gregg, E.W.; Bennett, J.E.; Solomon, B.; Singleton, R.K.; et al. Worldwide trends in hypertension prevalence and progress in treatment and control from 1990 to 2019: A pooled analysis of 1201 population-representative studies with 104 million participants. *Lancet* **2021**, *398*, 957–980. [CrossRef]
3. Batiha, G.E.-S.; Gari, A.; Elshony, N.; Shaheen, H.M.; Abubakar, M.B.; Adeyemi, S.B.; Al-kuraishy, H.M. Hypertension and its management in COVID-19 patients: The assorted view. *Int. J. Cardiol. Cardiovasc. Risk Prev.* **2021**, *11*, 200121. [CrossRef]
4. Chen, G.; Li, X.; Gong, Z.; Xia, H.; Wang, Y.; Wang, X.; Huang, Y.; Barajas-Martinez, H.; Hu, D. Hypertension as a sequela in patients of SARS-CoV-2 infection. *PLoS ONE* **2021**, *16*, e0250815. [CrossRef]
5. Savoia, C.; Volpe, M.; Kreutz, R. Hypertension, a moving target in COVID-19: Current views and perspectives. *Circ. Res.* **2021**, *128*, 1062–1079. [CrossRef]
6. Muhamad, S.A.; Ugusman, A.; Kumar, J.; Skiba, D.; Hamid, A.A.; Aminuddin, A. COVID-19 and Hypertension: The What, the Why, and the How. *Front. Physiol.* **2021**, *12*, 1–11. [CrossRef]
7. Patrick, D.M.; Van Beusecum, J.P.; Kirabo, A. The role of inflammation in hypertension: Novel concepts. *Curr. Opin. Physiol.* **2021**, *19*, 92–98. [CrossRef]
8. Griendling, K.K.; Camargo, L.L.; Rios, F.J.; Alves-Lopes, R.; Montezano, A.C.; Touyz, R.M. Oxidative Stress and Hypertension. *Circ. Res.* **2021**, *128*, 993–1020. [CrossRef]
9. Janczura, M.; Rosa, R.; Dropinski, J.; Gielicz, A.; Stanisz, A.; Kotula-Horowitz, K.; Domagala, T. The associations of perceived and oxidative stress with hypertension in a cohort of police officers. *Diabetes Metab. Syndr. Obes.* **2021**, *14*, 1783–1797. [CrossRef]
10. Touyz, R.M.; Rios, F.J.; Alves-Lopes, R.; Neves, K.B.; Camargo, L.L.; Montezano, A.C. Oxidative Stress: A Unifying Paradigm in Hypertension. *Can. J. Cardiol.* **2020**, *36*, 659–670. [CrossRef]
11. Theofilis, P.; Sagris, M.; Oikonomou, E.; Antonopoulos, A.S.; Siasos, G.; Tsioufis, C.; Tousoulis, D. Inflammatory mechanisms contributing to endothelial dysfunction. *Biomedicines* **2021**, *9*, 781. [CrossRef]
12. Chaudhary, P.; Pandey, A.; Azad, C.S.; Tia, N.; Singh, M.; Gambhir, I.S. Association of oxidative stress and endothelial dysfunction in hypertension. *Anal. Biochem.* **2020**, *590*, 113535. [CrossRef]
13. Forman, H.J.; Zhang, H. Targeting oxidative stress in disease: Promise and limitations of antioxidant therapy. *Nat. Rev. Drug Discov.* **2021**, *20*, 689–709. [CrossRef]
14. Serra, A.J.; Pinto, J.R.; Prokić, M.D.; Arsa, G.; Vasconsuelo, A. Oxidative Stress in Muscle Diseases: Current and Future Therapy 2019. *Oxid. Med. Cell. Longev.* **2020**, *2020*, 4–7. [CrossRef]
15. Sies, H. Oxidative eustress: On constant alert for redox homeostasis. *Redox Biol.* **2021**, *41*, 101867. [CrossRef]
16. Qiu, D.; Wu, J.; Li, M.; Wang, L.; Zhu, X.; Chen, Y. Impaction of factors associated with oxidative stress on the pathogenesis of gestational hypertension and preeclampsia: A Chinese patients based study. *Medicine* **2021**, *100*, e23666. [CrossRef]
17. Sharifi-Rad, M.; Anil Kumar, N.V.; Zucca, P.; Varoni, E.M.; Dini, L.; Panzarini, E.; Rajkovic, J.; Tsouh Fokou, P.V.; Azzini, E.; Peluso, I.; et al. Lifestyle, Oxidative Stress, and Antioxidants: Back and Forth in the Pathophysiology of Chronic Diseases. *Front. Physiol.* **2020**, *11*, 1–21. [CrossRef]

18. Snezhkina, A.V.; Kudryavtseva, A.V.; Kardymon, O.L.; Savvateeva, M.V.; Melnikova, N.V.; Krasnov, G.S.; Dmitriev, A.A. ROS generation and antioxidant defense systems in normal and malignant cells. *Oxid. Med. Cell. Longev.* **2020**, *2019*, 6175804. [CrossRef]
19. Liu, Q.Q.; Ren, K.; Liu, S.H.; Li, W.M.; Huang, C.J.; Yang, X.H. MicroRNA-140-5p aggravates hypertension and oxidative stress of atherosclerosis via targeting Nrf2 and Sirt2. *Int. J. Mol. Med.* **2019**, *43*, 839–849. [CrossRef]
20. Masi, S.; Georgiopoulos, G.; Chiriacò, M.; Grassi, G.; Seravalle, G.; Savoia, C.; Volpe, M.; Taddei, S.; Rizzoni, D.; Virdis, A. The importance of endothelial dysfunction in resistance artery remodelling and cardiovascular risk. *Cardiovasc. Res.* **2020**, *116*, 429–437. [CrossRef]
21. Pinheiro, L.C.; Oliveira-Paula, G.H. Sources and Effects of Oxidative Stress in Hypertension. *Curr. Hypertens. Rev.* **2019**, *16*, 166–180. [CrossRef] [PubMed]
22. Sousa, T.; Reina-Couto, M.; Gomes, P. Role of Oxidative Stress in the Pathophysiology of Arterial Hypertension and Heart Failure. In *Oxidative Stress in Heart Diseases*; Chakraborti, S., Dhalla, N.S., Ganguly, N.K., Dikshit, M., Eds.; Springer: Singapore, 2019; pp. 509–537. ISBN 978-981-13-8273-4. [CrossRef]
23. Wu, Y.; Ding, Y.; Ramprasath, T.; Zou, M.H. Oxidative Stress, GTPCH1, and Endothelial Nitric Oxide Synthase Uncoupling in Hypertension. *Antioxid. Redox Signal.* **2021**, *34*, 750–764. [CrossRef] [PubMed]
24. Rudyk, O.; Aaronson, P.I. Redox Regulation, Oxidative Stress, and Inflammation in Group 3 Pulmonary Hypertension. *Adv. Exp. Med. Biol.* **2021**, *1303*, 209–241. [CrossRef] [PubMed]
25. Incalza, M.A.; D'Oria, R.; Natalicchio, A.; Perrini, S.; Laviola, L.; Giorgino, F. Oxidative stress and reactive oxygen species in endothelial dysfunction associated with cardiovascular and metabolic diseases. *Vascul. Pharmacol.* **2018**, *100*, 1–19. [CrossRef]
26. Narasimhan, M.; Rajasekaran, N.S. Exercise, Nrf2 and antioxidant signaling in cardiac aging. *Front. Physiol.* **2016**, *7*, 1–8. [CrossRef] [PubMed]
27. Powers, S.K.; Deminice, R.; Ozdemir, M.; Yoshihara, T.; Bomkamp, M.P.; Hyatt, H. Exercise-induced oxidative stress: Friend or foe? *J. Sport Health Sci.* **2020**, *9*, 415–425. [CrossRef] [PubMed]
28. Li, H.; Zhou, X.; Huang, Y.; Liao, B.; Cheng, L.; Ren, B. Reactive Oxygen Species in Pathogen Clearance: The Killing Mechanisms, the Adaption Response, and the Side Effects. *Front. Microbiol.* **2021**, *11*, 3610. [CrossRef]
29. Maldonado, E.; Rojas, D.A.; Morales, S.; Miralles, V.; Solari, A. Dual and Opposite Roles of Reactive Oxygen Species (ROS) in Chagas Disease: Beneficial on the Pathogen and Harmful on the Host. *Oxid. Med. Cell. Longev.* **2020**, *2020*, 8867701. [CrossRef]
30. Di Meo, S.; Reed, T.T.; Venditti, P.; Victor, V.M. Role of ROS and RNS Sources in Physiological and Pathological Conditions. *Oxid. Med. Cell. Longev.* **2016**, *2016*, 1245049. [CrossRef]
31. D'Oria, R.; Schipani, R.; Leonardini, A.; Natalicchio, A.; Perrini, S.; Cignarelli, A.; Laviola, L.; Giorgino, F. The Role of Oxidative Stress in Cardiac Disease: From Physiological Response to Injury Factor. *Oxid. Med. Cell. Longev.* **2020**, *2020*, 5732956. [CrossRef]
32. Casas, A.I.; Dao, V.T.-V.; Daiber, A.; Maghzal, G.J.; Di Lisa, F.; Kaludercic, N.; Leach, S.; Cuadrado, A.; Jaquet, V.; Seredenina, T.; et al. Reactive Oxygen-Related Diseases: Therapeutic Targets and Emerging Clinical Indications. *Antioxid. Redox Signal.* **2015**, *23*, 1171–1185. [CrossRef] [PubMed]
33. Dubois-Deruy, E.; Peugnet, V.; Turkieh, A.; Pinet, F. Oxidative Stress in Cardiovascular Diseases. *Antioxidants* **2020**, *9*, 864. [CrossRef] [PubMed]
34. Farah, C.; Michel, L.Y.M.; Balligand, J.-L. Nitric oxide signalling in cardiovascular health and disease. *Nat. Rev. Cardiol.* **2018**, *15*, 292–316. [CrossRef] [PubMed]
35. Tejero, J.; Shiva, S.; Gladwin, M.T. Sources of vascular nitric oxide and reactive oxygen species and their regulation. *Physiol. Rev.* **2019**, *99*, 311–379. [CrossRef]
36. Kosutova, M.; Pechanova, O.; Barta, A.; Franova, S.; Cebova, M. Different adaptive NO-dependent Mechanisms in Normal and Hypertensive Conditions. *Molecules* **2019**, *24*, 1682. [CrossRef]
37. Costa, E.D.; Rezende, B.A.; Cortes, S.F.; Lemos, V.S. Neuronal nitric oxide synthase in vascular physiology and diseases. *Front. Physiol.* **2016**, *7*, 1–8. [CrossRef]
38. Bondonno, C.P.; Croft, K.D.; Hodgson, J.M. Dietary Nitrate, Nitric Oxide, and Cardiovascular Health. *Crit. Rev. Food Sci. Nutr.* **2016**, *56*, 2036–2052. [CrossRef]
39. Mónica, F.Z.; Bian, K.; Murad, F. Chapter One—The Endothelium-Dependent Nitric Oxide–cGMP Pathway. In *Endothelium*; Khalil, R.A., Ed.; Academic Press: Cambridge, MA, USA, 2016; Volume 77, pp. 1–27. ISBN 1054-3589. [CrossRef]
40. Gao, L.; Siu, K.L.; Chalupsky, K.; Nguyen, A.; Chen, P.; Weintraub, N.L.; Galis, Z.; Cai, H. Role of Uncoupled eNOS in Abdominal Aortic Aneurysm Formation: Treatment with Folic Acid. *Hypertension* **2012**, *59*, 158–166. [CrossRef]
41. Fleming, I. Chapter 23—NO Signaling Defects in Hypertension. In *Nitric Oxide: Biology and Pathobiology*, 3rd ed.; Ignarro, L.J., Freeman, B.A., Eds.; Academic Press: Cambridge, MA, USA, 2017; pp. 301–311. ISBN 978-0-12-804273-1. [CrossRef]
42. Higashi, Y.; Sasaki, S.; Nakagawa, K.; Fukuda, Y.; Matsuura, H.; Oshima, T.; Chayama, K. Tetrahydrobiopterin enhances forearm vascular response to acetylcholine in both normotensive and hypertensive individuals. *Am. J. Hypertens.* **2002**, *15*, 326–332. [CrossRef]
43. Zhang, Y.; Wong, H.S. Are mitochondria the main contributor of reactive oxygen species in cells. *J. Exp. Biol.* **2021**, *224*, jeb221606. [CrossRef]
44. Xin, T.; Lv, W.; Liu, D.; Jing, Y.; Hu, F. Opa1 Reduces Hypoxia-Induced Cardiomyocyte Death by Improving Mitochondrial Quality Control. *Front. Cell Dev. Biol.* **2020**, *8*, 1–13. [CrossRef] [PubMed]

45. Dikalov, S.I.; Dikalova, A.E. Contribution of mitochondrial oxidative stress to hypertension. *Curr. Opin. Nephrol. Hypertens.* **2016**, *25*, 73. [CrossRef] [PubMed]
46. Tirichen, H.; Yaigoub, H.; Xu, W.; Wu, C.; Li, R.; Li, Y. Mitochondrial Reactive Oxygen Species and Their Contribution in Chronic Kidney Disease Progression Through Oxidative Stress. *Front. Physiol.* **2021**, *12*, 1–12. [CrossRef]
47. Togliatto, G.; Lombardo, G.; Brizzi, M.F. The future challenge of reactive oxygen species (ROS) in hypertension: From bench to bed side. *Int. J. Mol. Sci.* **2017**, *18*, 1988. [CrossRef] [PubMed]
48. Dikalov, S.I.; Nazarewicz, R.R. Angiotensin II-induced production of mitochondrial reactive oxygen species: Potential mechanisms and relevance for cardiovascular disease. *Antioxid. Redox Signal.* **2013**, *19*, 1085–1094. [CrossRef]
49. García-Navas, R.; Liceras-Boillos, P.; Gómez, C.; Baltanás, F.C.; Calzada, N.; Nuevo-Tapioles, C.; Cuezva, J.M.; Santos, E. Critical requirement of SOS1 RAS-GEF function for mitochondrial dynamics, metabolism, and redox homeostasis. *Oncogene* **2021**, *40*, 4538–4551. [CrossRef]
50. Kasai, S.; Shimizu, S.; Tatara, Y.; Mimura, J.; Itoh, K. Regulation of Nrf2 by Mitochondrial Reactive Oxygen Species in Physiology and Pathology. *Biomolecules* **2020**, *10*, 320. [CrossRef]
51. Emmerson, A.; Trevelin, S.C.; Mongue-Din, H.; Becker, P.D.; Ortiz, C.; Smyth, L.A.; Peng, Q.; Elgueta, R.; Sawyer, G.; Ivetic, A.; et al. Nox2 in regulatory T cells promotes angiotensin II–induced cardiovascular remodeling. *J. Clin. Investig.* **2018**, *128*, 3088–3101. [CrossRef]
52. Hashad, A.M.; Sancho, M.; Brett, S.E.; Welsh, D.G. Reactive Oxygen Species Mediate the Suppression of Arterial Smooth Muscle T-type Ca2+ Channels by Angiotensin II. *Sci. Rep.* **2018**, *8*, 1–11. [CrossRef]
53. Gray, S.P.; Shah, A.M.; Smyrnias, I. NADPH oxidase 4 and its role in the cardiovascular system. *Vasc. Biol.* **2019**, *1*, H59–H66. [CrossRef]
54. Birk, M.; Baum, E.; Zadeh, J.K.; Manicam, C.; Pfeiffer, N.; Patzak, A.; Helmstädter, J.; Steven, S.; Kuntic, M.; Daiber, A.; et al. Angiotensin ii induces oxidative stress and endothelial dysfunction in mouse ophthalmic arteries via involvement of at1 receptors and nox2. *Antioxidants* **2021**, *10*, 1238. [CrossRef] [PubMed]
55. Zhang, Y.; Murugesan, P.; Huang, K.; Cai, H. NADPH oxidases and oxidase crosstalk in cardiovascular diseases: Novel therapeutic targets. *Nat. Rev. Cardiol.* **2020**, *17*, 170–194. [CrossRef]
56. Harrison, C.B.; Trevelin, S.C.; Richards, D.A.; Santos, C.X.C.; Sawyer, G.; Markovinovic, A.; Zhang, X.; Zhang, M.; Brewer, A.C.; Yin, X.; et al. Fibroblast Nox2 (NADPH Oxidase-2) Regulates ANG II (Angiotensin II)-Induced Vascular Remodeling and Hypertension via Paracrine Signaling to Vascular Smooth Muscle Cells. *Arterioscler. Thromb. Vasc. Biol.* **2021**, *2*, 698–710. [CrossRef] [PubMed]
57. Akram, M.; Ali Shah, S.M.; Munir, N.; Daniyal, M.; Tahir, I.M.; Mahmood, Z.; Irshad, M.; Akhlaq, M.; Sultana, S.; Zainab, R. Hexose monophosphate shunt, the role of its metabolites and associated disorders: A review. *J. Cell. Physiol.* **2019**, *9*, 14473–14482. [CrossRef] [PubMed]
58. Song, M.-Y.; Lee, D.-Y.; Chun, K.-S.; Kim, E.-H. The Role of NRF2/KEAP1 Signaling Pathway in Cancer Metabolism. *Int. J. Mol. Sci.* **2021**, *22*, 4376. [CrossRef]
59. Hashimoto, R.; Gupte, S. Pentose Shunt, Glucose-6-Phosphate Dehydrogenase, NADPH Redox, and Stem Cells in Pulmonary Hypertension. *Adv. Exp. Med. Biol.* **2017**, *967*, 47–55. [CrossRef]
60. Packer, M. Uric Acid Is a Biomarker of Oxidative Stress in the Failing Heart: Lessons Learned from Trials With Allopurinol and SGLT2 Inhibitors. *J. Card. Fail.* **2020**, *26*, 977–984. [CrossRef] [PubMed]
61. Mervaala, E.; Cheng, Z.; Tikkanen, I.; Lapatto, R.; Nurminen, K.; Vapaatalo, H.; Müller, D.; Fiebeler, A.; Ganten, U.; Ganten, D.; et al. Endothelial Dysfunction and Xanthine Oxidoreductase Activity in Rats With Human Renin and Angiotensinogen Genes. *Hypertension* **2001**, *37*, 414–418. [CrossRef]
62. Battelli, M.G.; Polito, L.; Bolognesi, A. Xanthine oxidoreductase in atherosclerosis pathogenesis: Not only oxidative stress. *Atherosclerosis* **2014**, *237*, 562–567. [CrossRef]
63. Moi, P.; Chan, K.; Asunis, I.; Cao, A.; Kan, Y.W. Isolation of NF-E2-related factor 2 (Nrf2), a NF-E2-like basic leucine zipper transcriptional activator that binds to the tandem NF-E2/AP1 repeat of the beta-globin locus control region. *Proc. Natl. Acad. Sci. USA* **1994**, *91*, 9926–9930. [CrossRef]
64. Liou, S.F.; Nguyen, T.T.N.; Hsu, J.H.; Sulistyowati, E.; Huang, S.E.; Wu, B.N.; Lin, M.C.; Yeh, J.L. The preventive effects of xanthohumol on vascular calcification induced by vitamin D3 plus nicotine. *Antioxidants* **2020**, *9*, 956. [CrossRef] [PubMed]
65. Sarutipaiboon, I.; Settasatian, N.; Komanasin, N.; Kukongwiriyapan, U.; Sawanyawisuth, K.; Intharaphet, P.; Senthong, V.; Settasatian, C. Association of Genetic Variations in NRF2, NQO1, HMOX1, and MT with Severity of Coronary Artery Disease and Related Risk Factors. *Cardiovasc. Toxicol.* **2020**, *20*, 176–189. [CrossRef]
66. Yagishita, Y.; Gatbonton-schwager, T.N.; McCallum, M.L.; Kensler, T.W. Current landscape of NRF2 biomarkers in clinical trials. *Antioxidants* **2020**, *9*, 716. [CrossRef]
67. Zgorzynska, E.; Dziedzic, B.; Walczewska, A. An overview of the nrf2/are pathway and its role in neurodegenerative diseases. *Int. J. Mol. Sci.* **2021**, *22*, 9592. [CrossRef] [PubMed]
68. Mata, A.; Cadenas, S. The Antioxidant Transcription Factor Nrf2 in Cardiac Ischemia-Reperfusion Injury. *Int. J. Mol. Sci.* **2021**, *22*, 11939. [CrossRef]
69. Tan, X.; Jiao, P.L.; Sun, J.C.; Wang, W.; Ye, P.; Wang, Y.K.; Leng, Y.Q.; Wang, W.Z. β-Arrestin1 Reduces Oxidative Stress via Nrf2 Activation in the Rostral Ventrolateral Medulla in Hypertension. *Front. Neurosci.* **2021**, *15*, 1–12. [CrossRef] [PubMed]

70. Shin, J.M.; Lee, K.-M.; Lee, H.J.; Yun, J.H.; Nho, C.W. Physalin A regulates the Nrf2 pathway through ERK and p38 for induction of detoxifying enzymes. *BMC Complement. Altern. Med.* **2019**, *19*, 101. [CrossRef]
71. Koundouros, N.; Poulogiannis, G. Phosphoinositide 3-Kinase/Akt Signaling and Redox Metabolism in Cancer. *Front. Oncol.* **2018**, *8*, 160. [CrossRef]
72. Matzinger, M.; Fischhuber, K.; Pölöske, D.; Mechtler, K.; Heiss, E.H. AMPK leads to phosphorylation of the transcription factor Nrf2, tuning transactivation of selected target genes. *Redox Biol.* **2020**, *29*, 101393. [CrossRef]
73. Liu, H.; Johnston, L.J.; Wang, F.; Ma, X. Triggers for the nrf2/are signaling pathway and its nutritional regulation: Potential therapeutic applications of ulcerative colitis. *Int. J. Mol. Sci.* **2021**, *22*, 11411. [CrossRef]
74. Silva-Islas, C.A.; Maldonado, P.D. Canonical and non-canonical mechanisms of Nrf2 activation. *Pharmacol. Res.* **2018**, *134*, 92–99. [CrossRef] [PubMed]
75. Baird, L.; Yamamoto, M. The Molecular Mechanisms Regulating the KEAP1-NRF2 Pathway. *Mol. Cell. Biol.* **2020**, *40*, e00099-20. [CrossRef] [PubMed]
76. Liu, T.; Lv, Y.-F.; Zhao, J.-L.; You, Q.-D.; Jiang, Z.-Y. Regulation of Nrf2 by phosphorylation: Consequences for biological function and therapeutic implications. *Free Radic. Biol. Med.* **2021**, *168*, 129–141. [CrossRef] [PubMed]
77. Chen, B.; Lu, Y.; Chen, Y.; Cheng, J. The role of Nrf2 in oxidative stress-induced endothelial injuries. *J. Endocrinol.* **2015**, *225*, R83–R99. [CrossRef]
78. Zang, H.; Mathew, R.O.; Cui, T. The Dark Side of Nrf2 in the Heart. *Front. Physiol.* **2020**, *11*, 722. [CrossRef]
79. Kannan, S.; Muthusamy, V.R.; Whitehead, K.J.; Wang, L.; Gomes, A.V.; Litwin, S.E.; Kensler, T.W.; Abel, E.D.; Hoidal, J.R.; Rajasekaran, N.S. Nrf2 deficiency prevents reductive stress-induced hypertrophic cardiomyopathy. *Cardiovasc. Res.* **2013**, *100*, 63–73. [CrossRef]
80. Qin, Q.; Qu, C.; Niu, T.; Zang, H.; Qi, L.; Lyu, L.; Wang, X.; Nagarkatti, M.; Nagarkatti, P.; Janicki, J.S.; et al. Nrf2-Mediated Cardiac Maladaptive Remodeling and Dysfunction in a Setting of Autophagy Insufficiency. *Hypertension* **2016**, *67*, 107–117. [CrossRef]
81. Ooi, B.K.; Goh, B.H.; Yap, W.H. Oxidative stress in cardiovascular diseases: Involvement of Nrf2 antioxidant redox signaling in macrophage foam cells formation. *Int. J. Mol. Sci.* **2017**, *18*, 2336. [CrossRef]
82. Da Costa, R.M.; Rodrigues, D.; Pereira, C.A.; Silva, J.F.; Alves, J.V.; Lobato, N.S.; Tostes, R.C. Nrf2 as a potential mediator of cardiovascular risk in metabolic diseases. *Front. Pharmacol.* **2019**, *10*, 1–12. [CrossRef]
83. Karan, A.; Bhakkiyalakshmi, E.; Jayasuriya, R.; Sarada, D.V.L.; Ramkumar, K.M. The pivotal role of nuclear factor erythroid 2-related factor 2 in diabetes-induced endothelial dysfunction. *Pharmacol. Res.* **2020**, *153*, 104601. [CrossRef]
84. Behl, T.; Kaur, I.; Sehgal, A.; Sharma, E.; Kumar, A.; Grover, M.; Bungau, S. Unfolding Nrf2 in diabetes mellitus. *Mol. Biol. Rep.* **2021**, *48*, 927–939. [CrossRef] [PubMed]
85. Bayliak, M.M.; Abrat, O.B. Role of Nrf2 in Oxidative and Inflammatory Processes in Obesity and Metabolic Diseases BT—Nrf2 and its Modulation in Inflammation. In *Nrf2 and Its Modulation in Inflammation*; Deng, H., Ed.; Springer International Publishing: Cham, Switzerland, 2020; pp. 153–187. ISBN 978-3-030-44599-7. [CrossRef]
86. Li, S.; Eguchi, N.; Lau, H.; Ichii, H. The Role of the Nrf2 Signaling in Obesity and Insulin Resistance. *Int. J. Mol. Sci.* **2020**, *21*, 6973. [CrossRef] [PubMed]
87. Vasileva, L.V.; Savova, M.S.; Amirova, K.M.; Dinkova-Kostova, A.T.; Georgiev, M.I. Obesity and NRF2-mediated cytoprotection: Where is the missing link? *Pharmacol. Res.* **2020**, *156*, 104760. [CrossRef] [PubMed]
88. Cuadrado, A.; Manda, G.; Hassan, A.; Alcaraz, M.J.; Barbas, C.; Daiber, A.; Ghezzi, P.; León, R.; López, M.G.; Oliva, B.; et al. Transcription Factor NRF2 as a Therapeutic Target for Chronic Diseases: A Systems Medicine Approach. *Pharmacol. Rev.* **2018**, *70*, 348–383. [CrossRef]
89. McSweeney, S.R.; Warabi, E.; Siow, R.C.M. Nrf2 as an Endothelial Mechanosensitive Transcription Factor: Going With the Flow. *Hypertension* **2016**, *67*, 20–29. [CrossRef]
90. Polvani, S.; Tarocchi, M.; Galli, A. PPARγ and Oxidative Stress: Con(β) Catenating NRF2 and FOXO. *PPAR Res.* **2012**, *2012*, 641087. [CrossRef]
91. Kvandová, M.; Majzúnová, M.; Dovinová, I. The role of PPARγ in cardiovascular diseases. *Physiol. Res.* **2016**, *65*, S343–S363. [CrossRef]
92. Dovinova, I.; Kvandova, M.; Balis, P.; Gresova, L.; Majzunova, M.; Horakova, L.; Chan, J.Y.H.; Barancik, M. The Role of Nrf2 and PPARγ in the Improvement of Oxidative Stress in Hypertension and Cardiovascular Diseases. *Physiol. Res.* **2020**, *69*, S541–S553. [CrossRef]
93. Mussbacher, M.; Salzmann, M.; Brostjan, C.; Hoesel, B.; Schoergenhofer, C.; Datler, H.; Hohensinner, P.; Basílio, J.; Petzelbauer, P.; Assinger, A.; et al. Cell Type-Specific Roles of NF-κB Linking Inflammation and Thrombosis. *Front. Immunol.* **2019**, *10*, 85. [CrossRef]
94. Giridharan, S.; Srinivasan, M. Mechanisms of NF-κB p65 and strategies for therapeutic manipulation. *J. Inflamm. Res.* **2018**, *11*, 407–419. [CrossRef]
95. Bhandari, R.; Khanna, G.; Kaushik, D.; Kuhad, A. Divulging the Intricacies of Crosstalk Between NF-Kb and Nrf2-Keap1 Pathway in Neurological Complications of COVID-19. *Mol. Neurobiol.* **2021**, *58*, 3347–3361. [CrossRef] [PubMed]
96. Farooqui, Z.; Mohammad, R.S.; Lokhandwala, M.F.; Banday, A.A. Nrf2 inhibition induces oxidative stress, renal inflammation and hypertension in mice. *Clin. Exp. Hypertens.* **2021**, *43*, 175–180. [CrossRef] [PubMed]

97. Wang, C.; Luo, Z.; Carter, G.; Wellstein, A.; Jose, P.A.; Tomlinson, J.; Leiper, J.; Welch, W.J.; Wilcox, C.S.; Wang, D. NRF2 prevents hypertension, increased ADMA, microvascular oxidative stress, and dysfunction in mice with two weeks of ANG II infusion. *Am. J. Physiol. Regul. Integr. Comp. Physiol.* **2018**, *314*, R399–R406. [CrossRef]
98. Ahmed, S.M.U.; Luo, L.; Namani, A.; Wang, X.J.; Tang, X. Nrf2 signaling pathway: Pivotal roles in inflammation. *Biochim. Biophys. Acta-Mol. Basis Dis.* **2017**, *1863*, 585–597. [CrossRef] [PubMed]
99. Lopes, R.A.; Neves, K.B.; Tostes, R.C.; Montezano, A.C.; Touyz, R.M. Downregulation of Nuclear Factor Erythroid 2-Related Factor and Associated Antioxidant Genes Contributes to Redox-Sensitive Vascular Dysfunction in Hypertension. *Hypertension* **2015**, *66*, 1240–1250. [CrossRef] [PubMed]
100. Banday, A.A.; Lokhandwala, M.F. Transcription factor Nrf2 protects renal dopamine D1 receptor function during oxidative stress. *Hypertension* **2013**, *62*, 512–517. [CrossRef] [PubMed]
101. Kim, J.; Grotegut, C.A.; Wisler, J.W.; Li, T.; Mao, L.; Chen, M.; Chen, W.; Rosenberg, P.B.; Rockman, H.A.; Lefkowitz, R.J. β-arrestin 1 regulates β2-adrenergic receptor-mediated skeletal muscle hypertrophy and contractility. *Skelet. Muscle* **2018**, *8*, 39. [CrossRef] [PubMed]
102. Pugh, D.; Gallacher, P.J.; Dhaun, N. Management of Hypertension in Chronic Kidney Disease. *Drugs* **2019**, *79*, 365–379. [CrossRef]
103. Gray, Z.; Tu, W.; Chertow, G.M.; Bhalla, V. Aldosterone sensitivity: An opportunity to explore the pathogenesis of hypertension. *Am. J. Physiol. Physiol.* **2021**, *320*, F325–F335. [CrossRef]
104. Inoue, K.; Goldwater, D.; Allison, M.; Seeman, T.; Kestenbaum, B.R.; Watson, K.E. Serum Aldosterone Concentration, Blood Pressure, and Coronary Artery Calcium. *Hypertension* **2020**, *76*, 113–120. [CrossRef]
105. Ames, M.K.; Atkins, C.E.; Pitt, B. The renin-angiotensin-aldosterone system and its suppression. *J. Vet. Intern. Med.* **2019**, *33*, 363–382. [CrossRef] [PubMed]
106. Xiao, L.; Gao, L.; Lazartigues, E.; Zucker, I.H. Brain-selective overexpression of angiotensin-converting enzyme 2 attenuates sympathetic nerve activity and enhances baroreflex function in chronic heart failure. *Hypertension* **2011**, *58*, 1057–1065. [CrossRef] [PubMed]
107. Ma, A.; Gao, L.; Wafi, A.M.; Yu, L.; Rudebush, T.; Zhou, W.; Zucker, I.H. Overexpression of central ACE2 (angiotensin-converting enzyme 2) attenuates the pressor response to chronic central infusion of ang II (angiotensin II): A potential role for Nrf2 (nuclear factor [erythroid-derived 2]-like 2). *Hypertension* **2020**, *2*, 1514–1525. [CrossRef] [PubMed]
108. Satta, S.; Mahmoud, A.M.; Wilkinson, F.L.; Yvonne Alexander, M.; White, S.J. The Role of Nrf2 in Cardiovascular Function and Disease. *Oxid. Med. Cell. Longev.* **2017**, *2017*, 9237263. [CrossRef] [PubMed]
109. Robledinos-Antón, N.; Fernández-Ginés, R.; Manda, G.; Cuadrado, A. Activators and Inhibitors of NRF2: A Review of Their Potential for Clinical Development. *Oxid. Med. Cell. Longev.* **2019**, *2019*, 9372182. [CrossRef]
110. Kopacz, A.; Kloska, D.; Forman, H.J.; Jozkowicz, A.; Grochot-Przeczek, A. Beyond repression of Nrf2: An update on Keap1. *Free Radic. Biol. Med.* **2020**, *157*, 63–74. [CrossRef]
111. Tkachev, V.O.; Menshchikova, E.B.; Zenkov, N.K. Mechanism of the Nrf2/Keap1/ARE signaling system. *Biochemistry* **2011**, *76*, 407–422. [CrossRef]
112. Chin, M.P.; Bakris, G.L.; Block, G.A.; Chertow, G.M.; Goldsberry, A.; Inker, L.A.; Heerspink, H.J.L.; O'Grady, M.; Pergola, P.E.; Wanner, C.; et al. Bardoxolone Methyl Improves Kidney Function in Patients with Chronic Kidney Disease Stage 4 and Type 2 Diabetes: Post-Hoc Analyses from Bardoxolone Methyl Evaluation in Patients with Chronic Kidney Disease and Type 2 Diabetes Study. *Am. J. Nephrol.* **2018**, *47*, 40–47. [CrossRef]
113. Sun, Q.; Ye, F.; Liang, H.; Liu, H.; Li, C.; Lu, R.; Huang, B.; Zhao, L.; Tan, W.; Lai, L. Bardoxolone and bardoxolone methyl, two Nrf2 activators in clinical trials, inhibit SARS-CoV-2 replication and its 3C-like protease. *Signal Transduct. Target. Ther.* **2021**, *6*, 2020–2022. [CrossRef]
114. Nio, Y.; Sasai, M.; Akahori, Y.; Okamura, H.; Hasegawa, H.; Oshima, M.; Watashi, K.; Wakita, T.; Ryo, A.; Tanaka, Y.; et al. Bardoxolone methyl as a novel potent antiviral agent against hepatitis B and C viruses in human hepatocyte cell culture systems. *Antivir. Res.* **2019**, *169*, 104537. [CrossRef]
115. Cuadrado, A.; Pajares, M.; Benito, C.; Jiménez-Villegas, J.; Escoll, M.; Fernández-Ginés, R.; Garcia Yagüe, A.J.; Lastra, D.; Manda, G.; Rojo, A.I.; et al. Can Activation of NRF2 Be a Strategy against COVID-19? *Trends Pharmacol. Sci.* **2020**, *41*, 598–610. [CrossRef] [PubMed]
116. Yagishita, Y.; Fahey, J.W.; Dinkova-Kostova, A.T.; Kensler, T.W. Broccoli or sulforaphane: Is it the source or dose that matters? *Molecules* **2019**, *24*, 3593. [CrossRef] [PubMed]
117. Gwon, Y.; Oh, J.; Kim, J.S. Sulforaphane induces colorectal cancer cell proliferation through Nrf2 activation in a p53-dependent manner. *Appl. Biol. Chem.* **2020**, *63*, 86. [CrossRef]
118. Ruhee, R.T.; Suzuki, K. The integrative role of sulforaphane in preventing inflammation, oxidative stress and fatigue: A review of a potential protective phytochemical. *Antioxidants* **2020**, *9*, 521. [CrossRef]
119. Senanayake, G.V.K.; Banigesh, A.; Wu, L.; Lee, P.; Juurlink, B.H.J. The dietary phase 2 protein inducer sulforaphane can normalize the kidney epigenome and improve blood pressure in hypertensive rats. *Am. J. Hypertens.* **2012**, *25*, 229–235. [CrossRef] [PubMed]
120. Kim, S.; Chen, J.; Cheng, T.; Gindulyte, A.; He, J.; He, S.; Li, Q.; Shoemaker, B.A.; Thiessen, P.A.; Yu, B.; et al. PubChem in 2021: New data content and improved web interfaces. *Nucleic Acids Res.* **2021**, *49*, D1388–D1395. [CrossRef]
121. Blair, H.A. Dimethyl Fumarate: A Review in Moderate to Severe Plaque Psoriasis. *Drugs* **2018**, *78*, 123–130. [CrossRef]

122. Lipton, S.; Satoh, T. Recent advances in understanding NRF2 as a druggable target: Development of pro-electrophilic and non-covalent NRF2 activators to overcome systemic side effects of electrophilic drugs like dimethyl fumarate. *F1000Research* **2017**, *6*, 1–10. [CrossRef]
123. Grzegorzewska, A.P.; Seta, F.; Han, R.; Czajka, C.A.; Makino, K.; Stawski, L.; Isenberg, J.S.; Browning, J.L.; Trojanowska, M. Dimethyl Fumarate ameliorates pulmonary arterial hypertension and lung fibrosis by targeting multiple pathways. *Sci. Rep.* **2017**, *7*, 41605. [CrossRef]
124. Oh, C.J.; Park, S.; Kim, J.-Y.; Kim, H.-J.; Jeoung, N.H.; Choi, Y.-K.; Go, Y.; Park, K.-G.; Lee, I.-K. Dimethylfumarate attenuates restenosis after acute vascular injury by cell-specific and Nrf2-dependent mechanisms. *Redox Biol.* **2014**, *2*, 855–864. [CrossRef]
125. Hsu, C.N.; Lin, Y.J.; Yu, H.R.; Lin, I.C.; Sheen, J.M.; Huang, L.T.; Tain, Y.L. Protection of male rat offspring against hypertension programmed by prenatal dexamethasone administration and postnatal high-fat diet with the Nrf2 activator dimethyl fumarate during pregnancy. *Int. J. Mol. Sci.* **2019**, *20*, 3957. [CrossRef]
126. Kuang, Y.; Zhang, Y.; Xiao, Z.; Xu, L.; Wang, P.; Ma, Q. Protective effect of dimethyl fumarate on oxidative damage and signaling in cardiomyocytes. *Mol. Med. Rep.* **2020**, *22*, 2783–2790. [CrossRef] [PubMed]
127. Zhou, Y.; Zhang, F.; Jiang, H.; Xu, D.; Deng, D. Fumaric acid and succinic acid treat gestational hypertension by downregulating the expression of KCNMB1 and TET1. *Exp. Ther. Med.* **2021**, *22*, 1072. [CrossRef] [PubMed]
128. Kong, K.; Koontz, D.; Morse, C.; Roth, E.; Domsic, R.T.; Simon, M.A.; Stratton, E.; Buchholz, C.; Tobin-Finch, K.; Simms, R.; et al. A Pilot Study of Dimethyl Fumarate in Pulmonary Arterial Hypertension Associated with Systemic Sclerosis. *J. Scleroderma Relat. Disord.* **2021**, *6*, 242–246. [CrossRef] [PubMed]
129. Kourakis, S.; Timpani, C.A.; de Haan, J.B.; Gueven, N.; Fischer, D.; Rybalka, E. Dimethyl Fumarate and Its Esters: A Drug with Broad Clinical Utility? *Pharmaceuticals* **2020**, *13*, 306. [CrossRef]
130. Qader, M.; Xu, J.; Yang, Y.; Liu, Y.; Cao, S. Natural nrf2 activators from juices, wines, coffee, and cocoa. *Beverages* **2020**, *6*, 68. [CrossRef]
131. Sengupta, S.; Bhattacharyya, D.; Kasle, G.; Karmakar, S.; Sahu, O.; Ganguly, A.; Addya, S.; Das Sarma, J. Potential Immunomodulatory Properties of Biologically Active Components of Spices Against SARS-CoV-2 and Pan β-Coronaviruses. *Front. Cell. Infect. Microbiol.* **2021**, *11*, 1–12. [CrossRef]
132. Kim, D.W.; Kim, M.J.; Shin, Y.; Jung, S.K.; Kim, Y.J. Green pepper (Piper nigrum l.) extract suppresses oxidative stress and lps-induced inflammation via regulation of JNK signaling pathways. *Appl. Sci.* **2020**, *10*, 2519. [CrossRef]
133. Wafi, A.M.; Hong, J.; Rudebush, T.L.; Yu, L.; Hackfort, B.; Wang, H.; Schultz, H.D.; Zucker, I.H.; Gao, L. Curcumin improves exercise performance of mice with coronary artery ligation-induced HFrEF: Nrf2 and antioxidant mechanisms in skeletal muscle. *J. Appl. Physiol.* **2019**, *126*, 477–486. [CrossRef]
134. Ji, K.; Fang, L.; Zhao, H.; Li, Q.; Shi, Y.; Xu, C.; Wang, Y.; Du, L.; Wang, J.; Liu, Q. Ginger Oleoresin Alleviated γ-Ray Irradiation-Induced Reactive Oxygen Species via the Nrf2 Protective Response in Human Mesenchymal Stem Cells. *Oxid. Med. Cell. Longev.* **2017**, *2017*, 1480294. [CrossRef]
135. Mimura, J.; Inose-Maruyama, A.; Taniuchi, S.; Kosaka, K.; Yoshida, H.; Yamazaki, H.; Kasai, S.; Harada, N.; Kaufman, R.J.; Oyadomari, S.; et al. Concomitant Nrf2- and ATF4-Activation by Carnosic Acid Cooperatively Induces Expression of Cytoprotective Genes. *Int. J. Mol. Sci.* **2019**, *20*, 1706. [CrossRef]
136. Mohan Manu, T.; Anand, T.; Sharath Babu, G.R.; Patil, M.M.; Khanum, F. Bacopa monniera extract mitigates isoproterenol-induced cardiac stress via Nrf2/Keap1/NQO1 mediated pathway. *Arch. Physiol. Biochem.* **2019**, 1–11. [CrossRef]
137. He, T.; Li, X.; Wang, X.; Xu, X.; Yan, X.; Li, X.; Sun, S.; Dong, Y.; Ren, X.; Liu, X.; et al. Chemical composition and anti-oxidant potential on essential oils of Thymus quinquecostatus Celak. from Loess Plateau in China, regulating Nrf2/Keap1 signaling pathway in zebrafish. *Sci. Rep.* **2020**, *10*, 11280. [CrossRef]
138. Korenori, Y.; Tanigawa, S.; Kumamoto, T.; Qin, S.; Daikoku, Y.; Miyamori, K.; Nagai, M.; Hou, D.-X. Modulation of Nrf2/Keap1 system by Wasabi 6-methylthiohexyl isothiocyanate in ARE-mediated NQO1 expression. *Mol. Nutr. Food Res.* **2013**, *57*, 854–864. [CrossRef] [PubMed]
139. Kanlaya, R.; Khamchun, S.; Kapincharanon, C.; Thongboonkerd, V. Protective effect of epigallocatechin-3-gallate (EGCG) via Nrf2 pathway against oxalate-induced epithelial mesenchymal transition (EMT) of renal tubular cells. *Sci. Rep.* **2016**, *6*, 1–13. [CrossRef] [PubMed]
140. Paul, S.; Chakraborty, S.; Anand, U.; Dey, S.; Nandy, S.; Ghorai, M.; Saha, S.C.; Patil, M.T.; Kandimalla, R.; Próchów, J.; et al. Withania somnifera (L.) Dunal (Ashwagandha): A comprehensive review on ethnopharmacology, pharmacotherapeutics, biomedicinal and toxicological aspects. *Biomed. Pharmacother.* **2021**, *143*, 112175. [CrossRef] [PubMed]
141. Farkhondeh, T.; Folgado, S.L.; Pourbagher-Shahri, A.M.; Ashrafizadeh, M.; Samarghandian, S. The therapeutic effect of resveratrol: Focusing on the Nrf2 signaling pathway. *Biomed. Pharmacother.* **2020**, *127*, 110234. [CrossRef]
142. Yang, P.M.; Chen, H.Z.; Huang, Y.T.; Hsieh, C.W.; Wung, B.S. Lycopene inhibits NF-κB activation and adhesion molecule expression through Nrf2-mediated heme oxygenase-1 in endothelial cells. *Int. J. Mol. Med.* **2017**, *39*, 1533–1540. [CrossRef]
143. Ramyaa, P.; Padma, V.V. Ochratoxin-induced toxicity, oxidative stress and apoptosis ameliorated by quercetin—Modulation by Nrf2. *Food Chem. Toxicol.* **2013**, *62*, 205–216. [CrossRef]
144. Moussa, Z.; Judeh, Z.; Ahmed, S. Nonenzymatic Exogenous and Endogenous Antioxidants. In *Free Radical Medicine and Biology*; IntechOpen: London, UK, 2019; ISBN 978-1-78985-143-4. [CrossRef]

145. Dias, T.R.; Martin-Hidalgo, D.; Silva, B.M.; Oliveira, P.F.; Alves, M.G. Endogenous and Exogenous Antioxidants As a Tool to Ameliorate Male Infertility Induced by Reactive Oxygen Species. *Antioxid. Redox Signal.* **2020**, *33*, 767–785. [CrossRef] [PubMed]
146. Chang, X.; Zhao, Z.; Zhang, W.; Liu, D.; Ma, C.; Zhang, T.; Meng, Q.; Yan, P.; Zou, L.; Zhang, M. Natural Antioxidants Improve the Vulnerability of Cardiomyocytes and Vascular Endothelial Cells under Stress Conditions: A Focus on Mitochondrial Quality Control. *Oxid. Med. Cell. Longev.* **2021**, *2021*, 6620677. [CrossRef]
147. Seco-Cervera, M.; González-Cabo, P.; Pallardó, F.V.; Romá-Mateo, C.; García-Giménez, J.L. Thioredoxin and glutaredoxin systems as potential targets for the development of new treatments in Friedreich's ataxia. *Antioxidants* **2020**, *9*, 1257. [CrossRef] [PubMed]
148. Ahsan, M.K.; Lekli, I.; Ray, D.; Yodoi, J.; Das, D.K. Redox regulation of cell survival by the thioredoxin superfamily: An implication of redox gene therapy in the heart. *Antioxid. Redox Signal.* **2009**, *11*, 2741–2758. [CrossRef]
149. Suresh, S.C.; Selvaraju, V.; Thirunavukkarasu, M.; Goldman, J.W.; Husain, A.; Alexander Palesty, J.; Sanchez, J.A.; McFadden, D.W.; Maulik, N. Thioredoxin-1 (Trx1) engineered mesenchymal stem cell therapy increased pro-angiogenic factors, reduced fibrosis and improved heart function in the infarcted rat myocardium. *Int. J. Cardiol.* **2015**, *201*, 517–528. [CrossRef]
150. Cuadrado, A.; Rojo, A.I.; Wells, G.; Hayes, J.D.; Cousin, S.P.; Rumsey, W.L.; Attucks, O.C.; Franklin, S.; Levonen, A.-L.; Kensler, T.W.; et al. Therapeutic targeting of the NRF2 and KEAP1 partnership in chronic diseases. *Nat. Rev. Drug Discov.* **2019**, *18*, 295–317. [CrossRef]
151. Gupte, S.A.; Li, K.-X.; Okada, T.; Sato, K.; Oka, M. Inhibitors of pentose phosphate pathway cause vasodilation: Involvement of voltage-gated potassium channels. *J. Pharmacol. Exp. Ther.* **2002**, *301*, 299–305. [CrossRef]
152. Alzoubi, A.; Toba, M.; Abe, K.; O'Neill, K.D.; Rocic, P.; Fagan, K.A.; McMurtry, I.F.; Oka, M. Dehydroepiandrosterone restores right ventricular structure and function in rats with severe pulmonary arterial hypertension. *Am. J. Physiol. Heart Circ. Physiol.* **2013**, *304*, H1708–H1718. [CrossRef]
153. Ventetuolo, C.E.; Baird, G.L.; Barr, R.G.; Bluemke, D.A.; Fritz, J.S.; Hill, N.S.; Klinger, J.R.; Lima, J.A.C.; Ouyang, P.; Palevsky, H.I.; et al. Higher Estradiol and Lower Dehydroepiandrosterone-Sulfate Levels Are Associated with Pulmonary Arterial Hypertension in Men. *Am. J. Respir. Crit. Care Med.* **2016**, *193*, 1168–1175. [CrossRef]
154. Dumas de La Roque, E.; Savineau, J.-P.; Metivier, A.-C.; Billes, M.-A.; Kraemer, J.-P.; Doutreleau, S.; Jougon, J.; Marthan, R.; Moore, N.; Fayon, M.; et al. Dehydroepiandrosterone (DHEA) improves pulmonary hypertension in chronic obstructive pulmonary disease (COPD): A pilot study. *Ann. Endocrinol.* **2012**, *73*, 20–25. [CrossRef] [PubMed]
155. Sanghvi, V.R.; Leibold, J.; Mina, M.; Mohan, P.; Berishaj, M.; Li, Z.; Miele, M.M.; Lailler, N.; Zhao, C.; de Stanchina, E.; et al. The Oncogenic Action of NRF2 Depends on De-glycation by Fructosamine-3-Kinase. *Cell* **2019**, *178*, 807–819.e21. [CrossRef]
156. Beeraka, N.M.; Bovilla, V.R.; Doreswamy, S.H.; Puttalingaiah, S.; Srinivasan, A.; Madhunapantula, S. V The Taming of Nuclear Factor Erythroid-2-Related Factor-2 (Nrf2) Deglycation by Fructosamine-3-Kinase (FN3K)-Inhibitors-A Novel Strategy to Combat Cancers. *Cancers* **2021**, *13*, 281. [CrossRef]
157. Sartore, G.; Ragazzi, E.; Burlina, S.; Paleari, R.; Chilelli, N.C.; Mosca, A.; Avemaria, F.; Lapolla, A. Role of fructosamine-3-kinase in protecting against the onset of microvascular and macrovascular complications in patients with T2DM. *BMJ Open Diabetes Res. Care* **2020**, *8*, e001256. [CrossRef] [PubMed]
158. Daiber, A.; Chlopicki, S. Revisiting pharmacology of oxidative stress and endothelial dysfunction in cardiovascular disease: Evidence for redox-based therapies. *Free Radic. Biol. Med.* **2020**, *157*, 15–37. [CrossRef] [PubMed]
159. Berman, A.Y.; Motechin, R.A.; Wiesenfeld, M.Y.; Holz, M.K. The therapeutic potential of resveratrol: A review of clinical trials. *npj Precis. Oncol.* **2017**, *1*, 35. [CrossRef] [PubMed]

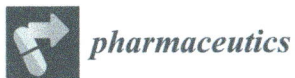 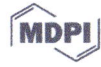

Article

Cardiac Sodium/Hydrogen Exchanger (NHE11) as a Novel Potential Target for SGLT2i in Heart Failure: A Preliminary Study

Lorena Pérez-Carrillo [1], Alana Aragón-Herrera [2,3], Isaac Giménez-Escamilla [1], Marta Delgado-Arija [1], María García-Manzanares [4], Laura Anido-Varela [2,3], Francisca Lago [2,3], Luis Martínez-Dolz [1,3], Manuel Portolés [1,3,†], Estefanía Tarazón [1,3,*,†] and Esther Roselló-Lletí [1,3,*,†]

1. Clinical and Translational Research in Cardiology Unit, Health Research Institute Hospital La Fe (IIS La Fe), 46026 Valencia, Spain
2. Cellular and Molecular Cardiology Research Unit, Department of Cardiology and Institute of Biomedical Research, University Clinical Hospital, 15706 Santiago de Compostela, Spain
3. Cardiovascular Biomedical Research Center Network (CIBERCV), 28029 Madrid, Spain
4. Department of Animal Medicine and Surgery, Veterinary Faculty, CEU Cardenal Herrera Unversity, 46115 Valencia, Spain
* Correspondence: tarazon_est@gva.es (E.T.); esther_rosello@iislafe.es (E.R.-L.); Tel.: +34-9-6124-6644 (E.T. & E.R.-L.)
† These authors contributed equally to this work.

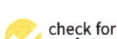

Citation: Pérez-Carrillo, L.; Aragón-Herrera, A.; Giménez-Escamilla, I.; Delgado-Arija, M.; García-Manzanares, M.; Anido-Varela, L.; Lago, F.; Martínez-Dolz, L.; Portolés, M.; Tarazón, E.; et al. Cardiac Sodium/Hydrogen Exchanger (NHE11) as a Novel Potential Target for SGLT2i in Heart Failure: A Preliminary Study. *Pharmaceutics* **2022**, *14*, 1996. https://doi.org/ 10.3390/pharmaceutics14101996

Academic Editors: Ionut Tudorancea and Radu Iliescu

Received: 29 July 2022
Accepted: 19 September 2022
Published: 21 September 2022

Publisher's Note: MDPI stays neutral with regard to jurisdictional claims in published maps and institutional affiliations.

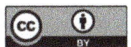

Copyright: © 2022 by the authors. Licensee MDPI, Basel, Switzerland. This article is an open access article distributed under the terms and conditions of the Creative Commons Attribution (CC BY) license (https:// creativecommons.org/licenses/by/ 4.0/).

Abstract: Despite the reduction of cardiovascular events, including the risk of death, associated with sodium/glucose cotransporter 2 inhibitors (SGLT2i), their basic action remains unclear. Sodium/hydrogen exchanger (NHE) has been proposed as the mechanism of action, but there are controversies related to its function and expression in heart failure (HF). We hypothesized that sodium transported-related molecules could be altered in HF and modulated through SGLT2i. Transcriptome alterations in genes involved in sodium transport in HF were investigated in human heart samples by RNA-sequencing. NHE11 and NHE1 protein levels were determined by ELISA; the effect of empagliflozin on NHE11 and NHE1 mRNA levels in rats' left ventricular tissues was studied through RT-qPCR. We highlighted the overexpression of *SLC9C2* and *SCL9A1* sodium transport genes and the increase of the proteins that encode them (NHE11 and NHE1). NHE11 levels were correlated with left ventricular diameters, so we studied the effect of SGLT2i on its expression, observing that NHE11 mRNA levels were reduced in treated rats. We showed alterations in several sodium transports and reinforced the importance of these channels in HF progression. We described upregulation in NHE11 and NHE1, but only NHE11 correlated with human cardiac dysfunction, and its levels were reduced after treatment with empagliflozin. These results propose NHE11 as a potential target of SGLT2i in cardiac tissue.

Keywords: SGLT2i; empagliflozin; heart failure; NHE1; NHE11; sodium channel

1. Introduction

Heart failure (HF) continues to be a public health problem in industrialized countries due to its high morbidity and mortality rate. There are currently no curative treatments, so many investigations are studying possible therapeutic targets [1,2]. Sodium/glucose cotransporter 2 inhibitors (SGLT2i), a novel anti-diabetic drug class, have been shown to reduce the incidence of cardiovascular events and have been found to have beneficial effects even in patients without type 2 diabetes [3,4]. At present, the study of the effects of SGLT2i HF is a hot topic since the underlying mechanisms involved in the cardiac protective actions of this pharmacological treatment remain unclear. Among the proposed mechanisms of action are the shifts in myocardial metabolism from glucose consumption to ketone body utilization, reduction of oxidative stress and inhibition of the sodium-hydrogen exchanger (NHE) [5].

It has been published that SGLT2i acts within the heart to directly inhibit sodium/hydrogen exchanger 1 (NHE1) [6]. Moreover, the inhibition of cardiac NHE1 reduces cytoplasmic Na^+ and Ca^{2+} concentrations, increasing mitochondrial Ca^{2+} levels and improving the viability of cardiomyocytes and mitochondrial function [7–9]. However, there are studies that question the direct inhibition of NHE1 in cardiac tissue and its effect on the regulation of intracellular Na^+ concentration [10]. Nevertheless, the NHE family consists of many molecules involved in pH homeostasis, including the unknown molecule NHE11. Published studies about NHE11 are currently scarce. *SLC9C2* (NHE11 protein) belongs to the mammalian sperm-NHE-like subfamily (*SLC9C*). *SLC9Cs* encode an NHE-like N-terminal domain and a long non-conserved C-terminal part with similarity to the Na-transporting carboxylic acid decarboxylase transporter family [11]. Previously Wang D et al. [12] described that sperm NHE could perform as functional NHE. However, the specific activity of NHE11 is unknown. Furthermore, other sodium transporters expressed in the heart are proposed as possible targets of SGLT2i, such as the role of glucose/sodium transporters in the action mechanism of these drugs [13].

Therefore, due to the existing controversy in relation to the effect of SGLT2i on NHE and the lack of evidence on the expression and alterations in the levels of other sodium transporters in pathological and healthy human hearts, we analyzed the status of the main sodium transporters in HF. In addition, we delved into the study of the sodium/hydrogen exchangers deregulated by analyzing their protein levels and their relationship with cardiac function parameters. Furthermore, we studied the effect of empagliflozin (EMPA) on NHE11 expression in vivo, using an animal model, for the first time.

2. Materials and Methods

2.1. Human Sample Collection

In this study, we used a total of 84 human left ventricular tissue samples from patients with end-stage HF undergoing heart transplantation (mean age of 54 ± 10 years, 85% were men). Patients had previously been diagnosed with significant comorbidities, including hypertension (38%) and type 2 diabetes (34%). Patients were classified according to the functional criteria of the New York Heart Association (NYHA) and received medical treatment according to the guidelines of the European Society of Cardiology [14]. The clinical characteristics of the patients used in each study are summarized in Table 1.

Table 1. Clinical characteristics of patients with heart failure (HF).

	RNA-Seq Analysis	Protein Analysis
	HF (n = 26)	HF (n = 70)
Age (years)	53 ± 10	54 ± 10
Gender male (%)	96	84
NYHA class	III–IV	III–IV
BMI (kg/m^2)	27 ± 5	26 ± 5
Hypercholesterolemia (%)	13	21
Prior hypertension (%)	25	38
Prior type 2 diabetes (%)	29	35
Hemoglobin (mg/mL)	14 ± 3	13 ± 2
Hematocrit (%)	40 ± 7	39 ± 6
LVEF (%)	21 ± 8	23 ± 8
LVESD (mm)	66 ± 12	60 ± 11
LVEDD (mm)	74 ± 11	68 ± 10

Data are shown as the mean value $\pm$ SD; NYHA, New York Heart Association; BMI, body mass index; LVEF, left ventricle ejection fraction; LVESD, left ventricular end-systolic diameter; LVEDD, left ventricular end-diastolic diameter.

A total of 16 control donors (CNT) were used (mean age 54 ± 18 years, 80% were men). The CNT samples were obtained from non-diseased hearts that could not be transplanted owing to surgical reasons or blood type incompatibility. The cause of death of these donors was a cerebrovascular event or a motor vehicle accident. All control donors had normal left ventricular function (ejection fraction > 50%) and no history of cardiac disease. Comorbidities and other echocardiographic data were not available for the CNT group in accordance with the Spanish Organic Law on Data Protection 15/1999.

The left ventricle is an integral part of the cardiovascular system; it pumps blood at a higher pressure compared with the other heart chambers, as it faces a much higher workload and mechanical afterload, so it is essential for normal function [15]. Specifically, fresh transmural samples were obtained from near the apex of the left ventricle at the time of transplantation and preserved in 0.9% NaCl at 4 °C for a maximum of 6 h from the time of removal from coronary circulation. The tissue samples were stored at −80 °C until use. A reduced time between sample receipt and storage yielded higher-quality samples, as evidenced by the RNA integrity numbers of ≥ 9.

This study was approved by the Ethics Committee (Biomedical Investigation Ethics Committee of La Fe University Hospital of Valencia, Valencia, Spain). Prior to tissue collection, signed informed consent was obtained from each patient. The study was conducted in accordance with the guidelines of the Declaration of Helsinki [16].

2.2. Transcriptomic Analysis

Transcriptome-level differences between the HF and CNT samples were investigated by means of large-scale screening of 36 heart samples (HF, n = 26; CNT, n = 10). The RNA isolation and RNA-seq procedures and analyses have been extensively described previously by Roselló-Lletí et al. [17]. Briefly, RNA extractions were performed using a PureLink™ Kit (Ambion Life Technologies, Waltham, MA, USA), and cDNA libraries were obtained following Illumina's recommendations. Transcriptome libraries were sequenced on the SOLiD 5500 XL (Applied Biosystems, Waltham, MA, USA) platform. The data used in this publication have been deposited in the NCBI Gene Expression Omnibus (GEO) and can be retrieved using the GEO Series accession number GSE55296 (http://www.ncbi.nlm.nih.gov/geo/query/acc.cgi?acc=GSE55296, accessed on 28 April 2014).

2.3. NHE11 and NHE1 Protein Concentration

NHE11 and NHE1 protein levels were determined on 80 heart samples (HF, n = 70; CNT, n = 10). Protein extraction has been extensively described previously by Roselló-Lletí et al. [18]. Briefly, twenty-five milligrams of the frozen left ventricle were homogenized in an extraction buffer (2% SDS, 10 mM EDTA, 6 mM Tris–HCl, pH 7.4) in a FastPrep-24 homogenizer (MP Biomedicals) with specifically designed Lysing Matrix D tubes. The homogenates were centrifuged, and the supernatant was aliquoted. Protein concentrations of NHE11 and NHE1 were determined using a specific sandwich enzyme-linked immunosorbent assay (NHE11 ELISA Kit MBS9323174 from MyBioSource, and NHE1 ELISA Kit SEG374Hu from Cloud-Clone Corp.) following the manufacturer's specifications. The test had a limit of detection of 0.1 and 0.052 ng/mL for NHE11 and NHE1, respectively. The intra- and inter-assay coefficients of variation were <15% for NHE11 and <12% and <10% for NHE1. No significant cross-reactivity or interference between NHE11, NHE1, and analogs was observed. The tests were quantified at 450 nm in a dual-wavelength microplate reader (Sunrise; TECAN, Tecan Ibérica Instrumentación S.L., Barcelona, Spain) using Magellan version 2.5 software (TECAN).

2.4. In Vivo Study

Adult male ZDF (Zucker diabetic fatty) rats (ZDF-Lepr$^{fa/fa}$), purchased from Charles River Laboratories at 7 weeks of age with a body weight range of 200–250 g, were used in this study. The information related to their housing, feeding and treatment was extensively explained by Aragón-Herrera et al. [19]. The animals were fed ad libitum with the special rodent chow Formulab 5008 (LabDiet). The rats were accommodated in individual cages under controlled conditions. The rats were randomly divided into two groups: CNT (n = 10) with mineral drink treatment and treated (n = 12) with EMPA 30 mg/kg/d for 6 weeks.

EMPA was provided by Boehringer Ingelheim Pharma GmbH&Co and administered p. o. via drinking water (dissolved by sonication) and initiated when the rats achieved fasting glucose levels of 350.75 ± 18.59 mg/dL (12 weeks old). After 6 weeks from the start of treatment, the animals were killed by decapitation. At the time of sacrifice, the rats were 19 weeks old, and the mean weight was 425 g in the EMPA-treated rats and 399 g in the untreated rats. The tissues were collected and quickly frozen on liquid nitrogen and stored at −80 °C until subsequent analysis.

SLC9C2 (NHE11) and *SLC9A1* (NHE1) mRNA levels were determined in the left ventricle of CNT and EMPA-treated rats through RT-qPCR. RNA was extracted using a NucleoSpin kit (Macherey-Nagel GmbH & Co., Allentown, PA, USA), according to the manufacturer's instructions. One microgram of total RNA was reverse transcribed into cDNA using the Transcriptor First Stand cDNA Synthesis Kit (F. Hoffman-La Roche Ltd., Basel, Switzerland). Perfect Master Mix SYBER®Green kit (with LOW ROX) and specific primers provided by Anygenes® for rat *Slc9c2* (GenBank accession no. XM_008769700.2), rat *Slc9a1* (GenBank accession no. NM_012652.2), and rat *Rn18S* (GenBank accession no. NR_046237.1) were used to normalize the expression data. RT-qPCR was performed on the Stratagene MX3000p according to the manufacturer's instructions (Agilent Technologies, Santa Clara, CA, USA). The relative expression of the *SLC9C2* and *SLC9A1* genes was calculated according to the Livak method of $2^{-\Delta\Delta Ct}$ [20].

The study was performed in accordance with the ARRIVE guidelines (Animals in Research: Reporting In Vivo Experiments) and the European Union Directive 2010/63. All animals were maintained and killed using protocols approved by the Animal Care Committee of the University of Santiago de Compostela in accordance with European Union Directive 2010/63. The application approval number for these experimental procedures was 15005/2015/003. The number of animals employed in the experimental procedures was the minimum necessary to develop our objectives and to ensure a pertinent statistical power.

2.5. Statistical Analysis

Clinical characteristics were expressed as mean ± standard deviation for continuous variables and percentages for discrete variables. Results for each variable were tested for normality using the Kolmogorov-Smirnov method. Continuous variables not following normal distribution were compared using the Mann-Whitney test, and categorical clinical variables were compared using the chi-square test. Variables with a normal distribution were compared using Student's *t*-test for continuous variables and Fisher's exact test for discrete variables. The Pearson and Spearman correlation coefficient was calculated to analyze the association between variables. A $p < 0.05$ was considered statistically significant. All statistical analyses were performed using SPSS software (version 20.0; IBM SPSS Inc., Armonk, NY, USA).

3. Results

3.1. Human Left Ventricle mRNA Expression of the Main Sodium Channels

Differences in transcriptome-level between HF and CNT samples were investigated with a large-scale screening of 36 heart samples (HF, n = 26 and CNT, n = 10) using RNA-seq technology. We analyzed the main sodium transporters expressed in cardiac tissue (Supplementary Table S1), which were classified in relation to the type of transport used for the exchange of molecules in the cell. Among analyzed uniporter (Figure 1A), we observed *SCN1A* under-expression (FC = −1.802, $p = 0.013$), a voltage-dependent ion channel, *ASIC1* over-expression (FC = 1.588, $p = 0.026$), and a voltage-independent ion channel. Moreover, we observed differential expressions in several cotransporters (Figure 1B,C), specifically, alterations in the symporter *SLC5A7* (FC = −1.495, $p = 0.049$) and the antiporters *SLC8A1* (FC = −1.210, $p = 0.041$), *SCL9A1* (FC = 1.170, $p = 0.020$) and *SLC9C2* (FC = 4.459, $p = 0.005$). *SLC9A1* and *SLC9C2* are sodium/hydrogen exchangers which encode the NHE1 and NHE11 proteins, respectively. Regulatory molecules of the different sodium transporters analyzed were also altered (Figure 1D), such as *GPD1L* (FC = −1.373, *p* = 0.014), *SLC9A3R2* (FC = 1.147, *p* = 0.036), *SCN2B* (FC = 1.806, *p* = 0.001), and *SCN3B* (FC = 1.564, *p* = 0.031).

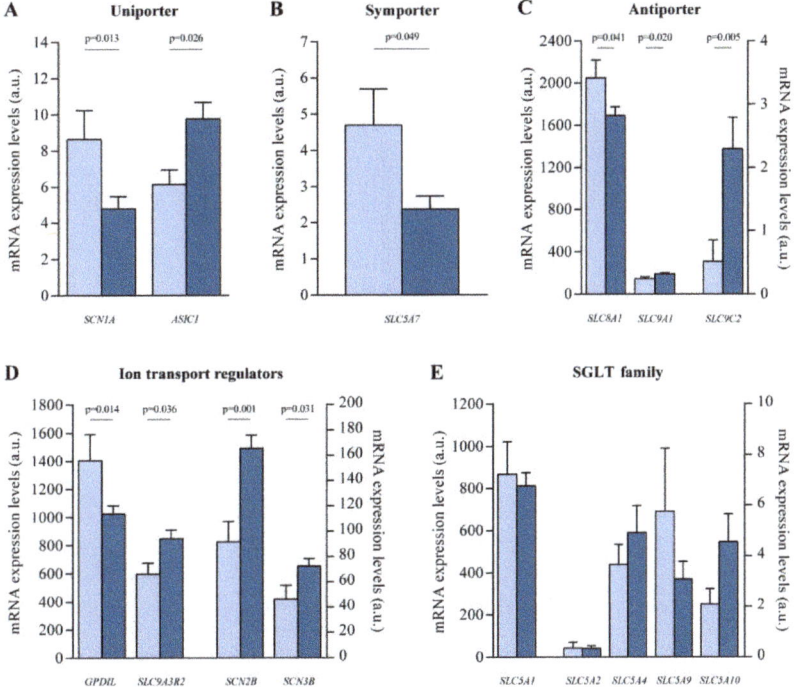

Figure 1. mRNA expression levels of altered genes involved in sodium transport in human heart failure (HF) hearts. (**A**) Uniporter (*SCN1A* and *ASIC1*). (**B**) Symporter (*SLC5A7*). (**C**) Antiporter (*SLC8A1*, *SCL9A1* and *SLC9C2*). (**D**) Regulators of sodium transporters (*GPD1L*, *SLC9A3R2*, *SCN2B* and *SCN3B*). (**E**) Sodium/glucose cotransporter (SGLT family). Bars represent mean ± SEM values. a.u., arbitrary units. Controls subjects (n = 10; light blue) and heart failure patients (n = 26; dark blue).

Moreover, the analyzed genes that code for the different sodium/glucose transporters, potential targets of the SGLT2i, including *SLC5A1* (SGLT1 protein) and *SLC5A2* (SGLT2 protein), were detected in the human hearts of patients with HF and CNT individuals, but we did not observe statistically significant differences in the expression between both groups (Figure 1E).

3.2. Human Protein Expression of NHE11 and NHE1

In addition, using a specific enzyme-linked immunosorbent assay, with total heart samples increased to 80 (HF, n = 70 and CNT, n = 10), we found significant upregulation in the protein levels of NHE11 (FC = 1.614, *p* = 0.042) and NHE1 (FC = 1.518, *p* = 0.018) in the HF hearts (Figure 2A). Moreover, we did not find significant differences in NHE11 and NHE1 cardiac protein levels between the HF group with type 2 diabetes and those without (Figure 2B).

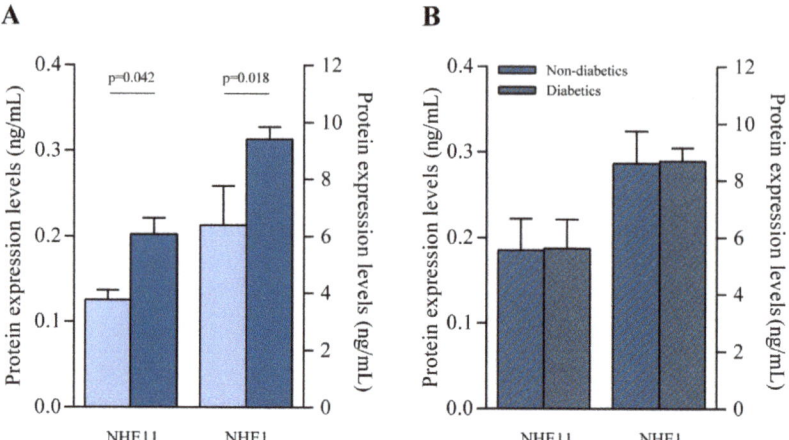

Figure 2. NHE11 and NHE1 protein concentration in human heart failure (HF) hearts. (**A**) NHE11 and NHE1 protein levels in control versus HF samples. (**B**) NHE11 and NHE1 protein levels in HF without type 2 diabetes versus HF with type 2 diabetes. Bars represent mean ± SEM values. Controls subjects (n = 10; light blue) and heart failure patients (n = 70; dark blue). HF without type 2 diabetes (dark blue and grey stripes), HF with type 2 diabetes (dark blue and grey squares).

Furthermore, NHE11 protein expression levels showed a positive correlation with established echocardiographic parameters (Table 2), specifically left ventricular end-systolic (r = 0.334, p = 0.011) and left ventricular end-diastolic (r = 0.290, p = 0.029) diameters.

Table 2. Relationships between NHEs protein levels and ventricular parameters.

	LVESD	LVEDD
NHE11	r = 0.334 p = 0.011	r = 0.290 p = 0.029
NHE1	ns	ns

LVESD, left ventricular end-systolic diameter; LVEDD, left ventricular end-diastolic diameter; ns, not significant.

3.3. SLC9C2 (NHE11) and SLC9A1 (NHE1) mRNA Levels in Empagliflozin-Treated Rats

The effects of SGLT2i treatment on *SLC9C2* (NHE11 protein) and *SLC9A1* (NHE1 protein) mRNA levels were analyzed in the rat models' left ventricular tissues by RT-qPCR. For this, untreated rats (n = 10) and rats treated with EMPA (n = 12) were used. Our results showed a reduction in the expression of both *SLC9C2* (FC = −2.047, p = 0.010; Figure 3A) and *SLC9A1* (FC = −1.504, p = 0.034; Figure 3B) in the rats treated with EMPA.

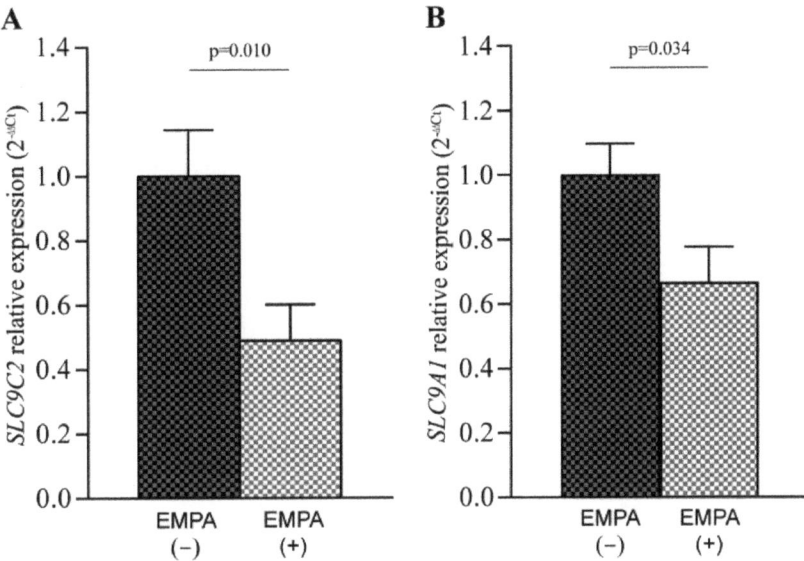

Figure 3. *SLC9C2* (NHE11 protein) (**A**) and *SLC9A1* (NHE1 protein) (**B**) mRNA levels in rat left ventricular tissue after treatment with empagliflozin (EMPA). Bars represent mean ± SEM values. Control rats (n = 10; black and grey squares) and rats treated with EMPA (n = 12; white and grey squares).

4. Discussion

Our findings showed alterations in several sodium transporters, highlighting the upregulation in two sodium/hydrogen exchangers (NHE1 and NHE11) in the left ventricular tissue of HF patients with and without diabetes. Furthermore, NHE11 protein levels were positively correlated with ventricular diameters, supporting the importance of this sodium transporter in cardiac pathology. For this reason, we analyzed, for the first time, the effect of empagliflozin, an SGLT2i, on NHE11 levels. Our results showed a relevant reduction of NHE11 mRNA levels in empagliflozin-treated rats.

Many studies have attempted to identify the pathophysiological mechanisms on which SGLT2i acts in the context of HF. One of the main proposed mechanisms is the inhibition of the sodium/hydrogen exchanger [6,7]. In this study, we demonstrated the upregulation of unknown sodium/hydrogen exchanger 11 in human heart tissue. The most relevant finding was the reduction of NHE11 mRNA expression levels in the left ventricular tissue of rats treated with empagliflozin. Currently, there is a lack of knowledge about the function of this molecule [11]; however, in the context of periodontitis, a chronic inflammatory disease, the association between the *SLC9C2* gene and systolic and diastolic blood pressure has been described [21].

NHE1 is the most studied sodium transporter in the context of cardiac pathology. In addition, it has been published that SGLT2i acts within the heart to directly inhibit NHE1 [6,7]. Controversially, Chung et al. [10] have shown that SGLT2i did not act as direct inhibitors of NHE1 activity under physiological pH conditions in an animal model. On the other hand, it has been described that SGLT2i reduces NHE1 mRNA expression in mouse cardiofibroblasts and in the left ventricle of infarcted rats, acting as an indirect inhibitor of its function [22,23]. Additionally, we confirmed the reduction of NHE1 mRNA levels in empagliflozin-treated rats. Still, little is known regarding NHE1 expression in human myocardium. In a previous study, the abundance of NHE1 protein was similar in ventricular tissue from hearts with end-stage HF and in patients with low ejection fraction [24]. We described, for the first time, the upregulation of NHE1 mRNA and protein levels in the left ventricular tissue from HF patients when compared with healthy donor hearts.

In recent years, a hypothesis that has gained strength describes that beneficial action of SGLT2i on HF is due to a systemic effect [5]. SGLT2i could act as modulators of metabolic fuel used by the myocardium, specifically reducing glucose consumption and increasing the use of ketone bodies, which ameliorate adverse left ventricle remodeling [25,26]. Previously, we observed alterations in lipids metabolism in HF patients [27], as well as in animal models treated with empagliflozin [19]. In addition, sodium/hydrogen exchangers are related to different functions in the cell. NHE1 has been related to the regulation of cellular pH, the cellular response to insulin stimuli and the process of apoptosis [28,29]. These are some of the described mechanisms on which SGLT2i acts [30,31], so it is interesting to know the modulation of NHE1 in relation to these processes. Furthermore, the structure of the isoform NHE11 is similar to NHE1 [11], but further studies are necessary to know the function of NHE11 in heart tissue.

Furthermore, the expression of sodium/glucose receptors (SGLTs) was analyzed. There is controversy regarding the presence of SGLT2 in the heart [32–35], but we have shown that SGLT2 is expressed in the human left ventricle, although at a low level. This sodium/glucose cotransporter did not seem to have a relevant role in HF since we did not find alterations in its mRNA expression. In fact, it should be noted that none of the sodium/glucose cotransporters expressed in the heart were altered in HF. However, over-expression of SGLT1 (*SLC5A1* gene) has been described in patients with ischemic cardiomyopathy and diabetic cardiomyopathy [36]. In addition, Sayour et al. [13] showed an over-expression of SGLT1 in HF patients of different etiology and the control group was composed of patients with a preserved systolic function who went through mitral valve replacement.

Our study was limited on several points, and the results must be interpreted in this context. This study does not distinguish cell types and we have determined the gene expression profiles in an animal model treated with SGLT2i, but we do not know its effect in HF patients. However, we believe that the current analyses provide substantial evidence and our findings represent a necessary first step for future research.

5. Conclusions

Our findings showed alterations in several sodium transports and reinforced the importance of these channels in HF progression. We described upregulation in NHE11 and NHE1 in HF patients, but only NHE11 correlated with cardiac dysfunction. In addition, the most relevant finding was the change observed in the expression of the unknown NHE11 after treatment with empagliflozin. These results propose NHE11 as a potential target of SGLT2i in cardiac tissue.

Supplementary Materials: The following supporting information can be downloaded at: https://www.mdpi.com/article/10.3390/pharmaceutics14101996/s1, Table S1: Genes related to sodium channels in heart failure patients.

Author Contributions: Conceptualization, M.P., E.T. and E.R.-L.; methodology, L.P.-C. and A.A.-H.; validation, M.G.-M., I.G.-E., M.D.-A.; formal analysis, M.P.; investigation, E.T.; resources, L.M.-D.; writing—original draft preparation, L.P.-C., M.P., E.T. and E.R.-L.; writing—review and editing, A.A.-H., I.G.-E., M.D.-A., M.G.-M., L.A.-V., F.L. and L.M.-D.; supervision, E.R.-L.; funding acquisition, E.T., L.M.-D. and E.R.-L. All authors have read and agreed to the published version of the manuscript.

Funding: This research was funded by the National Institute of Health Fondo de Investigaciones Sanitarias del Instituto de Salud Carlos III [PI20/01469, PI20/00071, CP18/00145, CP21/00041, FI21/00034, FI21/00186], Consorcio Centro de Investigación Biomédica en Red, M.P. [CIBERCV, under Grant CB16/11/00261], and co-funded by European Union.

Institutional Review Board Statement: The study was conducted in accordance with the Declaration of Helsinki and approved by the Ethics Committee (Biomedical Investigation Ethics Committee of La Fe University Hospital of Valencia, Spain). The study was performed in accordance with the ARRIVE guidelines (Animals in Research: Reporting In Vivo Experiments) and the European Union Directive 2010/63. The protocol used was approved by the Galician Clinical Research Ethics Committee (2007/304) (protocol number 15005/2015/003).

Informed Consent Statement: Prior to tissue collection, signed informed consent was obtained from each patient.

Data Availability Statement: The data used in this publication has been deposited in the NCBI Gene Expression Omnibus (GEO) and can be retrieved using the GEO Series accession number GSE55296 (http://www.ncbi.nlm.nih.gov/geo/query/acc.cgi?acc=GSE55296, accessed on 28 April 2014).

Acknowledgments: We thank the Transplant Coordination Unit (Hospital Universitario La Fe, Valencia, Spain) for their help in obtaining the heart tissue samples.

Conflicts of Interest: The authors declare no conflict of interest.

References

1. Rosello-Lleti, E.; Tarazon, E.; Ortega, A.; Gil-Cayuela, C.; Carnicer, R.; Lago, F.; Gonzalez-Juanatey, J.R.; Portoles, M.; Rivera, M. Protein Inhibitor of NOS1 Plays a Central Role in the Regulation of NOS1 Activity in Human Dilated Hearts. *Sci. Rep.* **2016**, *6*, 30902. [CrossRef] [PubMed]
2. Nabeebaccus, A.; Zheng, S.; Shah, A.M. Heart failure-potential new targets for therapy. *Br. Med. Bull.* **2016**, *119*, 99–110. [CrossRef] [PubMed]
3. Zelniker, T.A.; Wiviott, S.D.; Raz, I.; Im, K.; Goodrich, E.L.; Bonaca, M.P.; Mosenzon, O.; Kato, E.T.; Cahn, A.; Furtado, R.H.M.; et al. SGLT2 inhibitors for primary and secondary prevention of cardiovascular and renal outcomes in type 2 diabetes: A systematic review and meta-analysis of cardiovascular outcome trials. *Lancet* **2019**, *393*, 31–39. [CrossRef]
4. Brito, D.; Bettencourt, P.; Carvalho, D.; Ferreira, J.; Fontes-Carvalho, R.; Franco, F.; Moura, B.; Silva-Cardoso, J.C.; de Melo, R.T.; Fonseca, C. Sodium-Glucose Co-transporter 2 Inhibitors in the Failing Heart: A Growing Potential. *Cardiovasc. Drugs Ther.* **2020**, *34*, 419–436. [CrossRef]
5. Santos-Gallego, C.G.; Garcia-Ropero, A.; Mancini, D.; Pinney, S.P.; Contreras, J.P.; Fergus, I.; Abascal, V.; Moreno, P.; Atallah-Lajam, F.; Tamler, R.; et al. Rationale and Design of the EMPA-TROPISM Trial (ATRU-4): Are the "Cardiac Benefits" of Empagliflozin Independent of its Hypoglycemic Activity? *Cardiovasc. Drugs Ther.* **2019**, *33*, 87–95. [CrossRef]
6. Baartscheer, A.; Schumacher, C.A.; Wust, R.C.; Fiolet, J.W.; Stienen, G.J.; Coronel, R.; Zuurbier, C.J. Empagliflozin decreases myocardial cytoplasmic Na$^{(+)}$ through inhibition of the cardiac Na$^{(+)}$/H$^{(+)}$ exchanger in rats and rabbits. *Diabetologia* **2017**, *60*, 568–573. [CrossRef]
7. Uthman, L.; Baartscheer, A.; Bleijlevens, B.; Schumacher, C.A.; Fiolet, J.W.T.; Koeman, A.; Jancev, M.; Hollmann, M.W.; Weber, N.C.; Coronel, R.; et al. Class effects of SGLT2 inhibitors in mouse cardiomyocytes and hearts: Inhibition of Na$^{(+)}$/H$^{(+)}$ exchanger, lowering of cytosolic Na$^{(+)}$ and vasodilation. *Diabetologia* **2018**, *61*, 722–726. [CrossRef]
8. Packer, M. Reconceptualization of the Molecular Mechanism by Which Sodium-Glucose Cotransporter 2 Inhibitors Reduce the Risk of Heart Failure Events. *Circulation* **2019**, *140*, 443–445. [CrossRef]
9. Zuurbier, C.J.; Baartscheer, A.; Schumacher, C.A.; Fiolet, J.W.T.; Coronel, R. Sodium-glucose co-transporter 2 inhibitor empagliflozin inhibits the cardiac Na+/H+ exchanger 1: Persistent inhibition under various experimental conditions. *Cardiovasc. Res.* **2021**, *117*, 2699–2701. [CrossRef]
10. Chung, Y.J.; Park, K.C.; Tokar, S.; Eykyn, T.R.; Fuller, W.; Pavlovic, D.; Swietach, P.; Shattock, M.J. Off-target effects of sodium-glucose co-transporter 2 blockers: Empagliflozin does not inhibit Na$^+$/H$^+$ exchanger-1 or lower [Na$^+$]i in the heart. *Cardiovasc. Res.* **2021**, *117*, 2794–2806. [CrossRef]
11. Donowitz, M.; Ming Tse, C.; Fuster, D. SLC9/NHE gene family, a plasma membrane and organellar family of Na$^{(+)}$/H$^{(+)}$ exchangers. *Mol. Aspects Med.* **2013**, *34*, 236–251. [CrossRef] [PubMed]
12. Wang, D.; King, S.M.; Quill, T.A.; Doolittle, L.K.; Garbers, D.L. A new sperm-specific Na$^+$/H$^+$ exchanger required for sperm motility and fertility. *Nat. Cell Biol.* **2003**, *5*, 1117–1122. [CrossRef] [PubMed]
13. Sayour, A.A.; Olah, A.; Ruppert, M.; Barta, B.A.; Horvath, E.M.; Benke, K.; Polos, M.; Hartyanszky, I.; Merkely, B.; Radovits, T. Characterization of left ventricular myocardial sodium-glucose cotransporter 1 expression in patients with end-stage heart failure. *Cardiovasc. Diabetol.* **2020**, *19*, 159. [CrossRef] [PubMed]
14. Ponikowski, P.; Voors, A.A.; Anker, S.D.; Bueno, H.; Cleland, J.G.; Coats, A.J.; Falk, V.; Gonzalez-Juanatey, J.R.; Harjola, V.P.; Jankowska, E.A.; et al. 2016 ESC Guidelines for the diagnosis and treatment of acute and chronic heart failure: The Task Force for the diagnosis and treatment of acute and chronic heart failure of the European Society of Cardiology (ESC). Developed with the special contribution of the Heart Failure Association (HFA) of the ESC. *Eur. J. Heart Fail.* **2016**, *18*, 891–975.
15. Harbo, M.B.; Norden, E.S.; Narula, J.; Sjaastad, I.; Espe, E.K.S. Quantifying left ventricular function in heart failure: What makes a clinically valuable parameter? *Prog. Cardiovasc. Dis.* **2020**, *63*, 552–560. [CrossRef]

16. Macrae, D.J. The Council for International Organizations and Medical Sciences (CIOMS) guidelines on ethics of clinical trials. *Proc. Am. Thorac. Soc.* **2007**, *4*, 176–179. [CrossRef]
17. Rosello-Lleti, E.; Tarazon, E.; Barderas, M.G.; Ortega, A.; Molina-Navarro, M.M.; Martinez, A.; Lago, F.; Martinez-Dolz, L.; Gonzalez-Juanatey, J.R.; Salvador, A.; et al. ATP synthase subunit alpha and LV mass in ischaemic human hearts. *J. Cell Mol. Med.* **2015**, *19*, 442–451. [CrossRef]
18. Rosello-Lleti, E.; Carnicer, R.; Tarazon, E.; Ortega, A.; Gil-Cayuela, C.; Lago, F.; Gonzalez-Juanatey, J.R.; Portoles, M.; Rivera, M. Human Ischemic Cardiomyopathy Shows Cardiac Nos1 Translocation and its Increased Levels are Related to Left Ventricular Performance. *Sci. Rep.* **2016**, *6*, 24060. [CrossRef]
19. Aragon-Herrera, A.; Feijoo-Bandin, S.; Otero Santiago, M.; Barral, L.; Campos-Toimil, M.; Gil-Longo, J.; Costa Pereira, T.M.; Garcia-Caballero, T.; Rodriguez-Segade, S.; Rodriguez, J.; et al. Empagliflozin reduces the levels of CD36 and cardiotoxic lipids while improving autophagy in the hearts of Zucker diabetic fatty rats. *Biochem. Pharmacol.* **2019**, *170*, 113677. [CrossRef]
20. Livak, K.J.; Schmittgen, T.D. Analysis of relative gene expression data using real-time quantitative PCR and the 2(-Delta Delta C(T)) Method. *Methods* **2001**, *25*, 402–408. [CrossRef]
21. Moon, K.H. Screening of Genetic Factor in the Interaction Between Periodontitis and Metabolic Traits Using Candidate Gene Association Study (CGAS). *Biochem. Genet.* **2019**, *57*, 466–474. [CrossRef] [PubMed]
22. Ye, Y.; Jia, X.; Bajaj, M.; Birnbaum, Y. Dapagliflozin Attenuates $Na^{(+)}/H^{(+)}$ Exchanger-1 in Cardiofibroblasts via AMPK Activation. *Cardiovasc. Drugs Ther.* **2018**, *32*, 553–558. [CrossRef] [PubMed]
23. Goerg, J.; Sommerfeld, M.; Greiner, B.; Lauer, D.; Seckin, Y.; Kulikov, A.; Ivkin, D.; Kintscher, U.; Okovityi, S.; Kaschina, E. Low-Dose Empagliflozin Improves Systolic Heart Function after Myocardial Infarction in Rats: Regulation of MMP9, NHE1, and SERCA2a. *Int. J. Mol. Sci.* **2021**, *22*, 5437. [CrossRef] [PubMed]
24. Yokoyama, H.; Gunasegaram, S.; Harding, S.E.; Avkiran, M. Sarcolemmal Na^+/H^+ exchanger activity and expression in human ventricular myocardium. *J. Am. Coll. Cardiol.* **2000**, *36*, 534–540. [CrossRef]
25. Santos-Gallego, C.G.; Requena-Ibanez, J.A.; San Antonio, R.; Ishikawa, K.; Watanabe, S.; Picatoste, B.; Flores, E.; Garcia-Ropero, A.; Sanz, J.; Hajjar, R.J.; et al. Empagliflozin Ameliorates Adverse Left Ventricular Remodeling in Nondiabetic Heart Failure by Enhancing Myocardial Energetics. *J. Am. Coll. Cardiol.* **2019**, *73*, 1931–1944. [CrossRef] [PubMed]
26. Feijóo-Bandín, S.; Aragón-Herrera, A.; Otero-Santiago, M.; Anido-Varela, L.; Moraña-Fernández, S.; Tarazón, E.; Roselló-Lletí, E.; Portolés, M.; Gualillo, O.; González-Juanatey, J.R.; et al. Role of Sodium-Glucose Co-Transporter 2 Inhibitors in the Regulation of Inflammatory Processes in Animal Models. *Int. J. Mol. Sci.* **2022**, *23*, 5634. [CrossRef] [PubMed]
27. Pérez-Carrillo, L.; Giménez-Escamilla, I.; Martínez-Dolz, L.; Sánchez-Lázaro, I.J.; Portolés, M.; Roselló-Lletí, E.; Tarazón, E. Implication of Sphingolipid Metabolism Gene Dysregulation and Cardiac Sphingosine-1-Phosphate Accumulation in Heart Failure. *Biomedicines* **2022**, *10*, 135. [CrossRef]
28. Sauvage, M.; Maziere, P.; Fathallah, H.; Giraud, F. Insulin stimulates NHE1 activity by sequential activation of phosphatidylinositol 3-kinase and protein kinase C zeta in human erythrocytes. *Eur. J. Biochem.* **2000**, *267*, 955–962. [CrossRef]
29. Prasad, V.; Lorenz, J.N.; Miller, M.L.; Vairamani, K.; Nieman, M.L.; Wang, Y.; Shull, G.E. Loss of NHE1 activity leads to reduced oxidative stress in heart and mitigates high-fat diet-induced myocardial stress. *J. Mol. Cell Cardiol.* **2013**, *65*, 33–42. [CrossRef]
30. Vaduganathan, M.; Inzucchi, S.E.; Sattar, N.; Fitchett, D.H.; Ofstad, A.P.; Brueckmann, M.; George, J.T.; Verma, S.; Mattheus, M.; Wanner, C.; et al. Effects of empagliflozin on insulin initiation or intensification in patients with type 2 diabetes and cardiovascular disease: Findings from the EMPA-REG OUTCOME trial. *Diabetes Obes. Metab.* **2021**, *23*, 2775–2784. [CrossRef]
31. Uthman, L.; Li, X.; Baartscheer, A.; Schumacher, C.A.; Baumgart, P.; Hermanides, J.; Preckel, B.; Hollmann, M.W.; Coronel, R.; Zuurbier, C.J.; et al. Empagliflozin reduces oxidative stress through inhibition of the novel inflammation/NHE/$[Na^{(+)}]c$/ROS-pathway in human endothelial cells. *Biomed. Pharmacother.* **2022**, *146*, 112515. [CrossRef] [PubMed]
32. Xue, M.; Li, T.; Wang, Y.; Chang, Y.; Cheng, Y.; Lu, Y.; Liu, X.; Xu, L.; Li, X.; Yu, X.; et al. Empagliflozin prevents cardiomyopathy via sGC-cGMP-PKG pathway in type 2 diabetes mice. *Clin. Sci.* **2019**, *133*, 1705–1720. [CrossRef] [PubMed]
33. Zhou, L.; Cryan, E.V.; D'Andrea, M.R.; Belkowski, S.; Conway, B.R.; Demarest, K.T. Human cardiomyocytes express high level of Na+/glucose cotransporter 1 (SGLT1). *J. Cell Biochem.* **2003**, *90*, 339–346. [CrossRef] [PubMed]
34. Chen, J.; Williams, S.; Ho, S.; Loraine, H.; Hagan, D.; Whaley, J.M.; Feder, J.N. Quantitative PCR tissue expression profiling of the human SGLT2 gene and related family members. *Diabetes Ther.* **2010**, *1*, 57–92. [CrossRef]
35. Von Lewinski, D.; Rainer, P.P.; Gasser, R.; Huber, M.S.; Khafaga, M.; Wilhelm, B.; Haas, T.; Machler, H.; Rossl, U.; Pieske, B. Glucose-transporter-mediated positive inotropic effects in human myocardium of diabetic and nondiabetic patients. *Metabolism* **2010**, *59*, 1020–1028. [CrossRef]
36. Banerjee, S.K.; McGaffin, K.R.; Pastor-Soler, N.M.; Ahmad, F. SGLT1 is a novel cardiac glucose transporter that is perturbed in disease states. *Cardiovasc. Res.* **2009**, *84*, 111–118. [CrossRef]

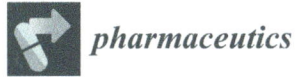

Article

Paracrine Factors of Stressed Peripheral Blood Mononuclear Cells Activate Proangiogenic and Anti-Proteolytic Processes in Whole Blood Cells and Protect the Endothelial Barrier

Dragan Copic [1,2], Martin Direder [1,2], Klaudia Schossleitner [3], Maria Laggner [1,2], Katharina Klas [1,2], Daniel Bormann [1,2], Hendrik Jan Ankersmit [1,2,*,†] and Michael Mildner [4,*,†]

1. Department of Thoracic Surgery, Medical University of Vienna, 1090 Vienna, Austria; dragan.copic@meduniwien.ac.at (D.C.); martin.direder@meduniwien.ac.at (M.D.); laggner.maria@gmail.com (M.L.); katharina.klas@meduniwien.ac.at (K.K.); daniel.bormann@meduniwien.ac.at (D.B.)
2. Laboratory for Cardiac and Thoracic Diagnosis and Regeneration, Department of Thoracic Surgery, Medical University of Vienna, 1090 Vienna, Austria
3. Skin and Endothelium Research Division, Department of Dermatology, Medical University of Vienna, 1090 Vienna, Austria; klaudia.schossleitner@meduniwien.ac.at
4. Department of Dermatology, Medical University of Vienna, 1090 Vienna, Austria
* Correspondence: hendrik.ankersmit@meduniwien.ac.at (H.J.A.); michael.mildner@meduniwien.ac.at (M.M.)
† These authors contributed equally to this work.

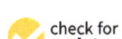

Citation: Copic, D.; Direder, M.; Schossleitner, K.; Laggner, M.; Klas, K.; Bormann, D.; Ankersmit, H.J.; Mildner, M. Paracrine Factors of Stressed Peripheral Blood Mononuclear Cells Activate Proangiogenic and Anti-Proteolytic Processes in Whole Blood Cells and Protect the Endothelial Barrier. *Pharmaceutics* 2022, 14, 1600. https://doi.org/10.3390/pharmaceutics14081600

Academic Editors: Ionut Tudorancea and Radu Iliescu

Received: 7 June 2022
Accepted: 28 July 2022
Published: 30 July 2022

Publisher's Note: MDPI stays neutral with regard to jurisdictional claims in published maps and institutional affiliations.

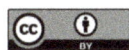

Copyright: © 2022 by the authors. Licensee MDPI, Basel, Switzerland. This article is an open access article distributed under the terms and conditions of the Creative Commons Attribution (CC BY) license (https://creativecommons.org/licenses/by/4.0/).

Abstract: Tissue-regenerative properties have been attributed to secreted paracrine factors derived from stem cells and other cell types. In particular, the secretome of γ-irradiated peripheral blood mononuclear cells (PBMCsec) has been shown to possess high tissue-regenerative and proangiogenic capacities in a variety of preclinical studies. In light of future therapeutic intravenous applications of PBMCsec, we investigated the possible effects of PBMCsec on white blood cells and endothelial cells lining the vasculature. To identify changes in the transcriptional profile, whole blood was drawn from healthy individuals and stimulated with PBMCsec for 8 h ex vivo before further processing for single-cell RNA sequencing. PBMCsec significantly altered the gene signature of granulocytes (17 genes), T-cells (45 genes), B-cells (72 genes), and, most prominently, monocytes (322 genes). We detected a strong upregulation of several tissue-regenerative and proangiogenic cyto- and chemokines in monocytes, including *VEGFA*, *CXCL1*, and *CXCL5*. Intriguingly, inhibitors of endopeptidase activity, such as *SERPINB2*, were also strongly induced. Measurement of the trans-endothelial electrical resistance of primary human microvascular endothelial cells revealed a strong barrier-protective effect of PBMCsec after barrier disruption. Together, we show that PBMCsec induces angiogenic and proteolytic processes in the blood and is able to attenuate endothelial barrier damage. These regenerative properties suggest that systemic application of PBMCsec might be a promising novel strategy to restore damaged organs.

Keywords: regenerative medicine; cell-free secretomes; paracrine factors; single-cell RNA sequencing; serine protease inhibitor; endothelial barrier

1. Introduction

Central goals in modern regenerative medicine are the repair of injured tissues and organs along with restoration of their innate functions [1]. Cell-based therapies have made tangible progress in this field over the past decades [2]. Mesenchymal stem cells (MSC) possess high capacities for self-renewal and differentiation, which makes them a highly attractive option to promote tissue regeneration. However, in spite of encouraging preclinical data, most of the first-in-men clinical trials failed to show effectivity in patients [3,4]. Beyond that, it became increasingly apparent that released paracrine factors, rather than engraftment and differentiation of applied stem cells, are crucial for most of the beneficial biological effects and, thus, predominantly contribute to the observed tissue-regenerative effects [5–8]. In addition, stem-cell secretome-based therapies bear considerable limitations, including the need for invasive procedures for isolation, low abundance, and high costs for expansion and preservation. This highlights the need for alternative sources [9].

Recently, several studies suggested peripheral blood mononuclear cells (PBMCs) as a valuable alternative source to MSCs [10,11]. In addition, γ-irradiation of PBMCs has been shown to promote the production and release of soluble factors and to exert tissue protection [10]. In-depth functional analyses of the secretome of γ-irradiated PBMCs (PBMCsec) revealed a vast array of proteins, lipids, and extracellular vesicles as the main biological constituents and confirmed that the presence of all fractions is required in order for PBMCsec to exert its biological effects to full capacity [12,13]. The modes of action via which PBMCsec exerts its beneficial effects range from promotion of angiogenesis [12], antimicrobial activity [14], cytoprotection [15], immunomodulation [16], improvement of re-epithelization [17] to vasodilation and the inhibition of platelet aggregation [18]. More recently, Laggner and colleagues were able to demonstrate a decrease of dendritic cell-mediated skin inflammation in a murine model of contact hypersensitivity, as well as inhibition of basophil and mast cell degranulation after treatment with PBMCsec, further expanding the broad spectrum of possible clinical implications of this investigational medicinal product [19,20]. Beneficial effects of PBMCsec have thus far been examined in numerous preclinical setups of experimental tissue damage, including acute myocardial infarction, autoimmune myocarditis, stroke, and spinal cord injury (for a review, see [21]). Topical administration of PBMCsec enhanced wound healing in a murine full-thickness skin model [17] and improved tissue survival in a rodent epigastric flap model [22]. Similar results were observed in a porcine model of burn injury, where the application of PBMCsec markedly improved epidermal thickness after injury [23]. In addition, beneficial effects of PBMCsec were also observed after intraperitoneal or intravenous administration. PBMCsec decreased the affected area and improved neurological outcome in rodent models of cerebral ischemia and acute spinal cord injury after systemic application [24,25]. Furthermore, PBMCsec ameliorated myocardial damage, improved overall cardiac performance, and promoted cytoprotection of cardiomyocytes in rodent and porcine models of acute myocardial infarction (AMI) [10,15]. Interestingly, transcriptional changes were not restricted to the infarcted myocardium and the circumjacent heart tissue but also detected in the liver and the spleen, suggesting a systemic effect of PBMCsec beyond the site of injury [26].

For the treatment of cardiovascular pathologies caused by thromboembolic occlusion of arterial blood flow such as acute myocardial infarction and ischemic stroke, the rapid interventional re-establishment of vessel perfusion still remains the first-line therapy as it maximizes the rescue of ischemic tissue and, thus, decisively determines the primary outcome in affected patients [27]. However, increasing emphasis is attributed to the attenuation of damages secondary to reperfusion injury, as it represents a considerable risk factor for long-term tissue functions [28]. During extended periods of oxygen deprivation, cells suffer from intracellular calcium overload [29] and disturbed mitochondrial energy production [30], which ultimately lead to cell death and the release of inflammatory mediators and reactive oxygen species [31]. In turn, inflammatory cells infiltrate the damaged area and release proinflammatory cyto- and chemokines. In addition, neutrophils release serine proteases [32,33], which contribute to endothelial barrier dysfunction, further enhancing vascular injury in small arterial blood vessels and downstream capillaries [34]. As a result, large amounts of intravascular fluids along with the damaging mediators diffuse into the interstitial space to cause further damage [34].

Since PBMCsec has shown tissue-regenerative properties in several animal models and there is an urgent need for novel systemic tissue-regenerative therapeutic interventions, we investigated the effects of PBMCsec on white blood cells and on the endothelial barrier function.

2. Materials and Methods

2.1. Ethics Statement

This study was conducted in accordance with the Declaration of Helsinki and local regulations. Blood samples were obtained from healthy volunteers who had given their consent to donate. Use of primary HUVECs, primary DMECs, and blood samples was approved by the Institutional Review Board of the Medical University of Vienna (Ethics committee votes: 1280/2015, 1539/2017, and 1621/2020). All donors provided written informed consent.

2.2. Generation of PBMCsec

Isolation of PBMCs and generation of PBMCsec have previously been described in detail [35], and a graphical overview is given in Figure 1A. In brief, PBMCs of volunteer blood donors aged 18–45 years were enriched by Ficoll-Paque PLUS (GE Healthcare, Chicago, IL, USA) density centrifugation, diluted to a concentration of 2.5×10^7 cells/mL in CellGenix granulocyte–monocyte progenitor dendritic cell medium (CellGenix, Freiburg, Germany) and exposed to 60 Gy cesium-137 γ-irradiation (IBL 437C, Isotopen Diagnostik CIS GmbH, Dreieich, Germany). Following 24 h of incubation, cells and cellular debris were removed by centrifugation at $800 \times g$ for 15 min, and supernatants were passed through a 0.2 mm filter. The cell-free secretome generated by 2.5×10^7 cells/mL corresponds to 25 units/mL PBMCsec. Next, methylene blue treatment was performed for viral clearance [35]. Secretomes were lyophilized, terminally sterilized by high-dosage-irradiation (Gammatron 1500, UKEM60Co irradiator with a maximum capacity of 1.5 MCi), and cryopreserved. Lyophilized compounds were reconstituted in 0.9% NaCl (B. Braun Melsungen AG, Melsungen, Germany) to the desired concentrations.

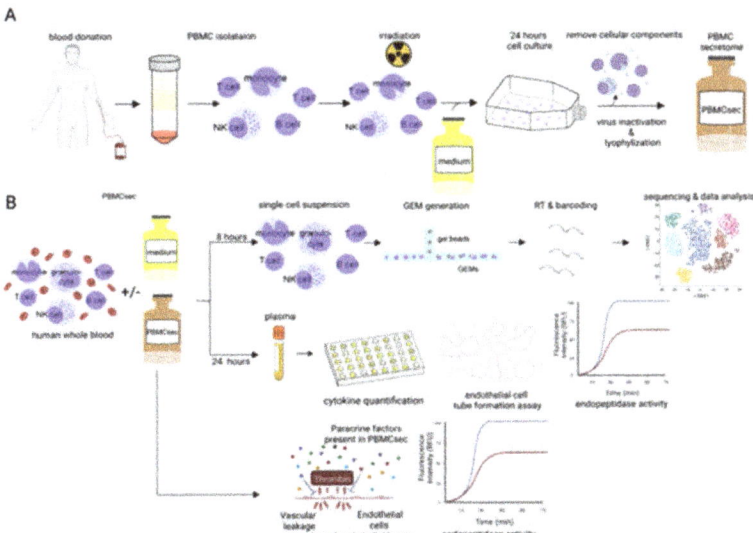

Figure 1. Experimental overview (**A**) Isolation of PBMCs from healthy donors and subsequent procedures necessary for the generation of PBMCsec. (**B**) The experimental setup involved two branches. In order to investigate pharmacodynamics effects of PBMCsec, human whole blood cells were treated with PBMCsec or left untreated for 8 h prior to further processing them for single-cell RNA sequencing. Plasma was collected from PBMCsec-treated whole blood and controls after 24 h of incubation and analyzed in a series of functional assays. In addition, we evaluated effects mediated directly by PBMCsec on endopeptidase activity and endothelial barrier protection. This figure was generated using Biorender.com (accessed on 6 June 2022).

2.3. Preparation of Single-Cell Suspension of Human Whole Blood

For scRNA-seq, heparinized human whole blood was drawn from two age-matched male donors (age donor 1: 29 years; age donor 2: 29 years). A total of 3 mL of whole blood was either treated with PBMCsec (GMP APOSEC lot number: A00918399135; diluted in 0.9% NaCl; final concentration: 12.5 units/mL) or left untreated. Samples were incubated at 37 °C for 8 h. Red blood cells were removed by Red Blood Cell Lysis Buffer (Abcam, Cambridge, MA, USA). Cells were then washed twice with PBS containing 0.04% bovine serum albumin (BSA) and sequentially passed through 100 and 40 µm cell strainers. Using the LUNA-FL Dual Fluorescence Cell Counter (BioCat, Heidelberg, Germany) and the Acridine Orange/Propidium Iodide Cell Viability Kit (Logos Biosystems, Gyeonggi-do, South Korea), samples were set at a concentration of 1×10^6 cells/mL and displayed a viability above 90%.

2.4. Dermal Microvascular Endothelial Cell Culture

Dermal microvascular endothelial cells (DMECs) were isolated from human foreskin. Foreskin was digested with dispase (Corning). The epidermis was removed, and the foreskin was scraped to dislodge endothelial cells. Cells were sorted for CD31 with magnetic beads (Thermo Fisher Scientific). Endothelial cells were cultured in endothelial growth medium (EGM-2; Lonza) containing 15% fetal bovine serum (FCS; Thermo Fisher Scientific, Waltham, MA, USA) and supplements for microvascular cells (Lonza). Cells were maintained in a humidified atmosphere containing 5% CO_2 at 37 °C and passaged at 90% confluence. Prior to experiments, cells were authenticated and confirmed to be free of contamination by mycoplasma. Endothelial cells were used at passages 2–8.

2.5. Tube Formation Assay

Proangiogenic properties of PBMCsec and plasma of PBMCsec-treated whole blood were compared in a tube formation assay with human umbilical vein endothelial cells (HUVECs, passage 8) as described previously [36]. HUVECs (Lonza, Basel, Switzerland) were thawed and routinely cultured in polystyrene culture flasks (Merck Millipore, Burlington, MA, USA) containing endothelial cell basal medium-2 (EBM-2; Lonza) supplemented with endothelial cell growth medium-2 (EGM-2, Lonza) until fully confluent. The medium was changed every other day for a total of two passages. Prior to the tube formation assay, cells were maintained in EBM-2 containing 3% (v/v) heat-inactivated fetal bovine serum (Lonza) overnight and starved in basal EBM-2 without supplements for 3 h. Cells were seeded on growth factor-reduced Matrigel Matrix (Corning Inc. Life Sciences, Tewksbury, MA, USA) in µ-slides Angiogenesis (ibidi GmbH, Graefelfing, Germany) at a density of 10×10^4 cells per well and stimulated with the supernatant obtained from 3 mL of whole blood cells for 4 h. Micrographs were acquired by an inverted phase contrast microscope (CKX41 Olympus Corporation; Tokyo, Japan) equipped with a 10× objective (CAch N, 10×/0.25 PhP; Olympus) using a SC30 camera (Olympus) and cellSens Entry software (version 1.8; Olympus). Tubule formation was quantified by the Angiogenesis Analyzer plugin [37] of ImageJ (version 1.53, java 1.8.0_172) using default settings.

2.6. Protein Quantification by Enzyme-Linked Immunosorbent Assay (ELISA)

For in vitro experiments, heparinized human whole blood was drawn from male donors (age donor 1:29 years; age donor 2:29 years; age donor 3:30 years). A total of 3 mL of whole blood was centrifuged ($1000 \times g$ for 10 min at room temperature) freshly after venipuncture or after 24 h long cultivation of whole blood in absence or presence of 12.5 units/mL PBMCsec. Plasma samples were then stored at −20 °C until further use. Protein levels of Human CXCL1, human CXCL5, human SERPINB2, human VEGF-A, and human urokinase (R&D Systems, Biotechne, Minneapolis, MN, USA) were quantified by ELISA as recommended by the manufacturer. Absorbance was measured at 450 nm by a Spark multimode microplate reader (Tecan, Männedorf, Switzerland), and analyte quantifications were determined using external standard curves.

2.7. Protease Activity Assays

To test the inhibitory effects of PBMCsec on protease activity, we performed a fluorometric enzyme activity assay (Enzcheck) using the unselective serine protease trypsin (ThermoFisher Scientific, Waltham, MA, USA) at a concentration of 0.05%. Enzyme substrate was diluted in provided assay buffer according to manufacturer's instruction. Equal amounts of trypsin were 1:2 diluted in assay buffer, control medium, or PBMCsec concentrated at 12.5 units/mL for 5 min before adding 10 µL to the prepared substrate mixture adding up to a total volume of 100 µL per well. The Urokinase Inhibitor Screening Kit (Sigma-Aldrich, St. Louis, MO, USA) was used to test the effect of the investigated plasma samples and PBMCsec on urokinase activity. In brief, 45 µL plasma sample were diluted in an equal volume of provided assay buffer. Human urokinase and substrate were added as suggested by the protocol, adding up to a total reaction volume of 100 µL per well. Samples from three donors were analyzed. For both tests, samples were then incubated at room temperature for a total of 60 min. Absorbance at 450 nm was measured by FluoStar Optima microplate reader (BMG Labtech, Ortenberg, Germany) in 15 min intervals.

2.8. Electrical Cell-Substrate Impedance Sensing (ECIS)

Electrical cell-substrate impedance sensing (ECIS, Applied Biophysics, Troy, NY, USA) was used to measure the electrical resistance of endothelial monolayers. A total of 12,000 endothelial cells were seeded on array plates (Ibidi) coated with gelatin (Sigma). After the resistance at 4000 Hz reached a stable plateau of >1000 Ω, endothelial cells were treated with indicated substances. Electrical resistance of cell monolayers was continuously monitored at 250 Hz [38].

2.9. Gel Bead-In Emulsion (GEMs) and Library Preparation

Single-cell RNA-seq was performed using the 10X Genomics Chromium Single-Cell Controller (10X Genomics, Pleasanton, CA, USA) with the Chromium Single-Cell 3' V3 Kit following the manufacturer's instructions. After quality control, RNA sequencing was performed by the Biomedical Sequencing Core Facility of the Center for Molecular Medicine (Center for Molecular Medicine, Vienna, Austria) on an Illumina HiSeq 3000/4000 (Illumina, San Diego, CA, USA). For donor 1, we detected 2003 cells in the untreated sample and 1281 cells in the PBMCsec-treated sample, while donor 2 had 12,356 cells in the untreated sample and 10,865 cells in the PBMCsec-treated sample. Raw sequencing data were then processed with the Cell Ranger v3.0.2 software (10X Genomics, Pleasanton, CA, USA) for demultiplexing and alignment to a reference genome (GRCh38).

2.10. Data Analysis

Secondary data analysis was performed using R Studio in R (Version 4.0.4; The R Foundation, Vienna, Austria) using the R software package "Seurat" (Seurat v.4.0.0, Satija Lab, New York, NY, USA). Cells were first analyzed for their unique molecular identifiers (UMI) and mitochondrial gene counts to remove unwanted variations in the scRNA-seq data. Cells with UMI counts below 200 or above 2500 and more than 10% of mitochondrial genes were excluded from the dataset. Next, we followed the recommended standard workflow for integration of scRNA-seq datasets [39]. Data were scaled, and principal component analysis (PCA) was performed. Statistically significant principal components (PCs) were identified by visual inspection. Using the Louvain algorithm at a resolution of 0.025, we identified a total of four communities. The preselected PCs and identified clusters served for Uniform Manifold Approximation and Projection for Dimension Reduction (UMAP). After bioinformatics integration of datasets of untreated and PBMCsec-treated samples, erythrocytes were removed by excluding all cells with expression of hemoglobin subunit beta (HBB) >0.5. Clusters were then annotated on the basis of the expression of well-established cell-type-defining marker genes. We used UMAP-plots, feature plots, heat maps, volcano plots, and violin plots to visualize differences between the investigated conditions. To determine DEGs, normalized count numbers were used. We applied the FindMarkers argument using default settings to calculate DEGs for clusters of interest between conditions with a log-foldchange threshold of 0.25 and an adjusted p-value <0.05. A $\log_2$ fold-change increase in gene expression above 1 was considered as upregulation, while a decrease below -1 was considered as downregulation. Only genes with an avgLog$_2$FC above 1 and below -1 were forwarded to the Metascape [40] online software package to identify significantly enriched pathways ($-\log_{10}(p$-value) >2). Additionally, the same gene sets were processed by Cytoscape plug-in ClueGO [41] to visualize significantly (p-value <0.05, kappa score: 0.4) enriched molecular functions for the investigated conditions.

2.11. Statistical Analysis

For single-cell RNA-seq, two donors were analyzed. Negative binomial regression was performed to normalize data and achieve variance stabilization. The Wilcoxon rank sum test was applied, followed by the Bonferroni post hoc test, to calculate differentially expressed genes. For in vitro experiments, at least three different donors were used. For data analysis of the tube formation assay, investigators were blinded to treatments. Data were statistically evaluated using GraphPad Prism v8.0.1 software (GraphPad Software, San Diego, CA, USA). When analyzing three or more groups, ordinary one-way ANOVA and multiple comparison post hoc tests with Dunnett's correction were calculated, and p-values <0.05 were considered statistically significant. Data are presented as the mean ± standard error of the mean (SEM).

3. Results

3.1. PBMCsec Modulates the Gene Signature of T Cells, B Cells, Granulocytes, and Monocytes

To investigate the degree to which PBMCsec alters the transcriptional landscape of immune cells in human whole blood, we conducted single-cell RNA sequencing (scRNA-seq) of whole-blood samples treated ex vivo with PBMCsec for 8 h. A methodological overview of the experimental approach employed in this study is provided in Figure 1. Bioinformatics analysis and UMAP clustering revealed four main cell populations consisting of monocytes, T-cells, B-cells, and granulocytes in all investigated conditions (Figure 2A). Identification was based on the expression of cluster marker genes including the CD14 molecule (*CD14*), CD3D molecule (*CD3D*), membrane spanning four domains A1 (*MS4A1*), and peptidase inhibitor 3 (*PI3*) for the respective cell types (Figure S1). Although significantly fewer cells were analyzed from donor 1, all cell types were found in both donors (Figure S2A). Treatment with PBMCsec did not result in a significant change in relative cell numbers (percentage of cells in untreated vs PBMCsec for T-cells: 75.73% vs. 74.86%; monocytes: 14.31% vs. 14.97%; B-cells: 8.89% vs. 8.09%; granulocytes 1.03% vs. 1.90%) (Figure 2B). The transcriptional heterogeneity between cell types was confirmed in a heatmap showing the average expression of cluster-defining genes of each cell type (Figure 2C). Next, we assessed changes in gene expression for all cell populations after treatment with PBMCsec. We calculated the number and distribution of significantly up- (Figure 2D) and downregulated genes (Figure 2E) for each cell type compared to the untreated control. A total number of 45 differentially expressed genes (DEG) (16 upregulated; 29 downregulated) were detected in T-cells, along with 72 in B-cells (28 upregulated, 44 downregulated) and 17 in granulocytes (two upregulated; 15 downregulated) (Figure S3A–C). Monocytes displayed the highest number of differentially expresses genes (173 upregulated; 148 downregulated), including upregulation of serpin family B member 2 (SERPINB2), epiregulin (EREG), interleukin 1 beta (IL1B), C–X–C motif chemokine ligand 1 (CXCL1), C–X–C motif chemokine ligand 3 (CXCL3), (CXCL5), and vascular endothelial growth factor A (VEGFA), and downregulation of S100 calcium-binding protein A8 (S100A8), S100 calcium-binding protein A9 (S100A9), allograft inflammatory factor 1 (AIF1), CD36 molecule (CD36), and CD163 molecule (CD163), amongst others (Figure 2F). From this, we can conclude that ex vivo stimulation of human whole blood with PBMCsec significantly changed gene expression in blood immune cells, most prominently in monocytes.

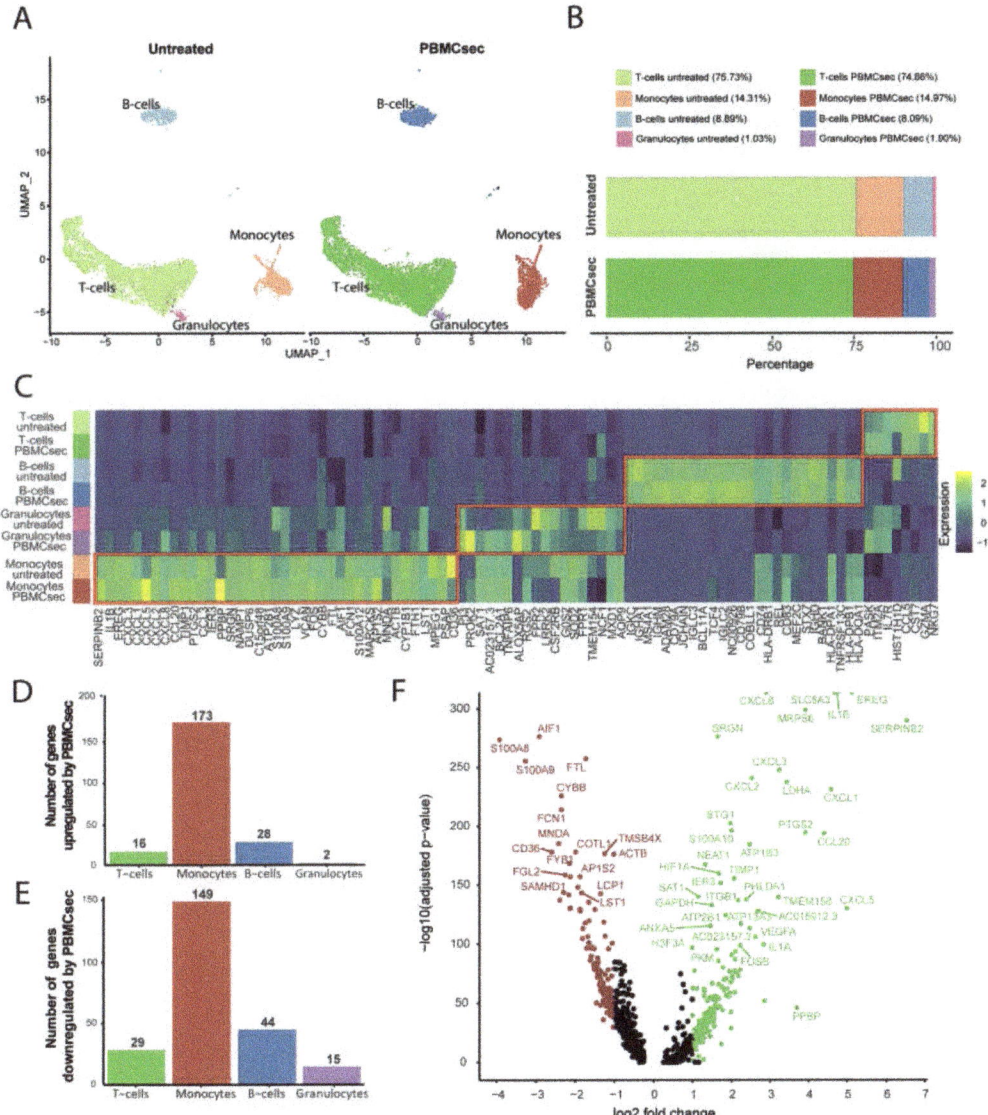

Figure 2. Ex vivo treatment of human whole blood cells alters the transcriptional profile in the monocyte subset and upregulates pathways associated with tissue regeneration. (**A**) UMAP clustering identified T-cells, monocytes, B-cells, and granulocytes in untreated and PBMCsec-treated samples with (**B**) similar cell frequency for each cluster between the investigated conditions. (**C**) Heatmap of cluster-defining marker genes of normalized gene expression showing distinct gene patterns between T-cells, monocytes, B-cells, and granulocytes. Bar plots represent the number of (**D**) up- and (**E**) downregulated genes in PBMCsec-treated samples compared to untreated control. Genes with an adjusted p-value < 0.05 and an average $\log_2$ fold change ≥ 1 or ≤ -1 were considered as DEGs. (**F**) Volcano plot showing the regulated genes in monocytes treated with PBMCsec when compared to untreated monocytes. Upregulated genes are marked in green, while downregulated genes are shown in red.

3.2. PBMCsec Induces Tissue-Regenerative Pathways in Monocytes from Human Whole Blood

Next, we identified biological pathways associated with the differentially regulated genes across the identified cell types. Biological functions such as angiogenesis and cytokine production were enriched in T- and B-cells treated with PBMCsec (Figure S3D,F), while activation of myeloid cells and responses to oxidative stress were associated with the downregulated gene sets (Figure S3E,G). No significantly regulated pathways were identified in granulocytes. The top Gene Ontology pathways associated with upregulated genes in monocytes after treatment with PBMCsec included response to lipid and to interleukin 1, along with terms strongly associated with wound healing, angiogenesis, regulation and production of cytokines, and regulation of endopeptidase activity (Figure 3A). Upregulated gene sets in monocytes treated with PBMCsec were highly comparable between the two donors (Figure S2B,C), and expression of *SERPINB2*, *VEGFA*, *CXCL1*, and *CXCL5* was significantly upregulated by PBMCsec in monocytes from both donors (Figure S2D,E), indicating a low donor variability. Major pathways associated with biological processes resulting from the downregulated gene set in monocytes treated with PBMCsec involved activation and differentiation of leukocytes, generation of reactive oxide species, and processing and presentation of antigens (Figure 3B). The complete lists of all up- and downregulated pathways (Figure S4A,B) and genes (Supplementary Files S1 and S2, respectively) are provided as Supplementary Materials. A closer look at the genes involved in the degranulation and cell activation of leukocytes revealed different members of the S100 and leukocyte immunoglobulin-like receptor (LILR) families to be downregulated in monocytes treated with PBMCsec (Figure S5A). Furthermore, we observed a downregulation of genes associated with the generation of reactive oxygen species, including the scavenger receptor CD36, the pattern recognition receptor CLEC7A, and a subunit of the NADPH oxidase complex in NCF1 (Figure S5B). We further sought to confirm our findings using ClueGO to investigate molecular functions related to these gene sets. In line with the initial analysis, we again identified strong associations with molecular functions related to cyto- and chemokine activity, signaling, and negative regulation of cysteine-type endopeptidase activity for the upregulated genes (Figure 3C), while functions related to immune receptor signaling, oxidoreductase activity, and antigen presentation were significantly associated with the set of downregulated genes (Figure 3D). From this analysis, we can conclude that monocytes were mostly affected by PBMCsec, resulting in the induction of tissue-regenerative processes, while processes associated with leukocyte activation and reactive oxygen species generation were downregulated.

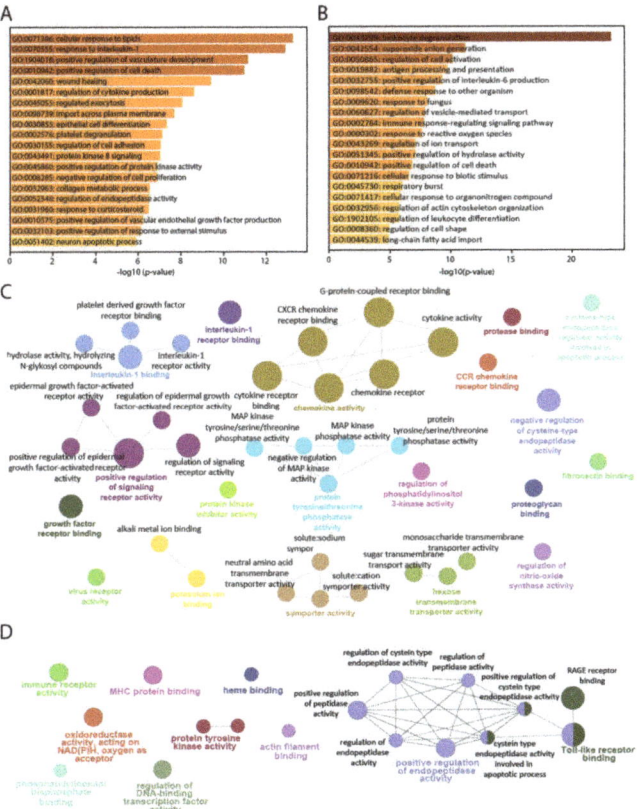

Figure 3. Tissue-regenerative pathways are upregulated in monocytes treated with PBMCsec Gene ontology pathway analysis was performed in Metascape. The top 20 biological processes affected by the upregulated (**A**) and downregulated (**B**) DEG in monocytes treated with PBMCsec are listed and hierarchically sorted by $-\log_{10}(p\text{-value})$ and enrichment factor (>2). (**C**) ClueGO visualization of molecular functions associated with upregulated and (**D**) downregulated genes in monocytes treated with PBMCsec.

3.3. Paracrine Factors in the Plasma of PBMCsec-Treated Whole Blood Exert Proangiogenetic Effects In Vitro

Since several cytokines and growth factors were upregulated in monocytes treated with PBMCsec (Figure 2F), we next assessed the protein levels of selected factors in plasma derived from PBMCsec-treated whole blood. PBMCsec, fresh plasma collected immediately after venipuncture, and untreated plasma after ex vivo incubation for 24 h served as controls. Gene expression of CXCL1, CXCL5, and VEGFA showed strong upregulation in monocytes after stimulation with PBMCsec (Figure 4A). This was confirmed on a protein level, when CXCL1 (2873 ± 2093 pg/mL), CXCL5 (6413 ± 1911 pg/mL), and VEGF-A (117.2 ± 13.04 pg/mL) were strongly elevated in plasma PBMCsec, while being undetectable in controls (Figure 4B). In contrast, several proinflammatory factors, such as IL-1β, TNF-α, and IFN-γ were not detectable in the plasma of PBMCsec-treated whole blood (data not shown). We next aimed to assess the proangiogenic capacity of fresh plasma, plasma of untreated whole blood, and plasma of PBMCsec-treated whole blood in an in vitro endothelial cell tube formation assay (Figure 4C). While controls showed little ability to induce tube formation, plasma of PBMCsec-treated whole blood displayed the highest proangiogenic properties as indicated by a significant increase in total segment length, as well as in numbers of nodes and junctions (Figure 4D). In summary, we could demonstrate that the expression and secretion of proangiogenic paracrine factors were strongly increased in whole blood cells following treatment with PBMCsec.

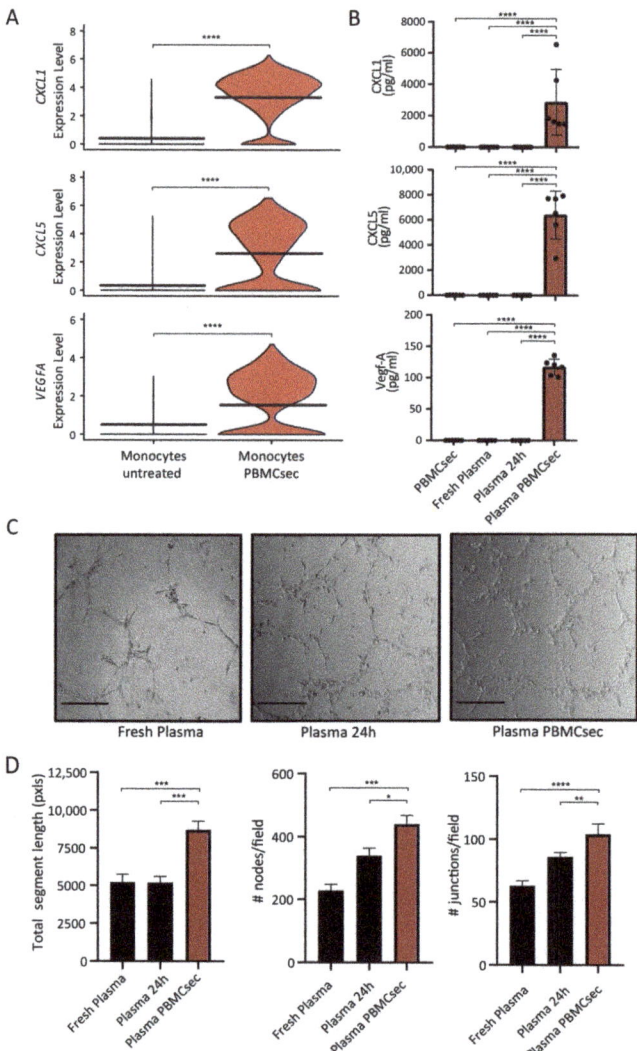

Figure 4. Paracrine factors are induced by PBMCsec in human plasma and enhance endothelial cell tube formation in vitro. (**A**) Gene expression of the proangiogenic chemokines *CXCL1* and *CXCL5*, as well as growth factor *VEGFA*, is strongly induced in monocytes treated with PBMCsec when compared to untreated monocytes (**B**) Assessment of protein levels for CXCL1, CXCL5, and VEGF-A by ELISA in plasma from PBMCsec-treated whole blood and controls (n = 3 biological replicates measured in duplicates). (**C**) Representative images of HUVEC tube formation assay in presence of fresh plasma, plasma from untreated whole blood, and plasma obtained from PBMCsec-treated whole blood after 24 h of ex vivo cultivation (scale bar 250 µm) with (**D**) analysis of number of nodes and junctions per field and total segment length (n = 3). Ordinary one-way ANOVA was performed. Dunnett's multiple comparison test was carried out to compare groups; * $p < 0.05$, ** $p < 0.01$, *** $p < 0.001$, **** $p < 0.0001$.

3.4. PBMCsec Inhibits Protease Activity In Vitro and Induces the Selective Serine Protease SERPINB2 in Human Whole Blood Ex Vivo

Increased protease activity, as seen in acute cardiovascular or inflammatory diseases, has been shown to significantly contribute to tissue destruction, thus representing an attractive target for tissue regeneration [42,43]. Evidence from previous studies identified monocytes as a source of protease inhibitors [44]. As our pathway analysis also revealed an association of upregulated genes in monocytes with the regulation of endopeptidase activity, we next aimed to confirm this finding in functional assays in vitro. Therefore, we performed a protease activity assay to test a potential anti-proteolytic effect of PBMCsec on the nonselective serine protease trypsin. While the medium control showed a negligible inhibitory effect on protease activity (3.72 ± 0.55%), PBMCsec led to a significant inhibition of the enzymatic activity (40.51 ± 4.728%) (Figure 5A). Furthermore, SERPINB2 displayed the highest positive $\log_2$ fold-change induction (Figure 5B) of all DEGs in monocytes treated with PBMCsec in our sequencing analysis. SERPINB2 is a member of the serpin superfamily of serine proteases and encodes plasminogen activator inhibitor type II (PAI-2), which is involved in the irreversible inhibition of urokinase [45]. First, we determined the protein levels of SERPINB2 in PBMCsec, fresh plasma, plasma of untreated whole blood, and then compared them to plasma of PBMCsec-treated whole blood. In accordance with the present literature, only very low levels of SERPINB2 were detectable in the control samples. In contrast, plasma obtained from PBMCsec-treated whole blood showed significantly elevated levels of SERPINB2 (11908 ± 3530 pg/mL) (Figure 5C). As SERPINB2 mainly acts as an inhibitor for urokinase [45], we next evaluated the plasma levels of urokinase, as well as the inhibitory effect of plasma PBMCsec on its activity in vitro. Whereas high levels of urokinase were still detected (Figure 5D), urokinase activity was strongly reduced by PBMCsec-treated plasma (Figure 5E), indicating that the observed urokinase inhibitory action was a result of the presence of a urokinase inhibitor rather than a quantitative decrease in available urokinase. While in vitro urokinase activity was not affected by PBMCsec alone, addition of fresh plasma (38.45% ± 5.94%) and plasma of untreated whole blood (40.78% ± 17.07%) resulted in a considerable inhibition of urokinase activity. Interestingly, this effect was even more pronounced in the presence of plasma obtained from PBMCsec-treated whole blood (79.48 ± 2.15%) (Figure 5E). Together, these data show that soluble factors with anti-proteolytic activities were present in PBMCsec or strongly induced in white blood cells after treatment with PBMCsec.

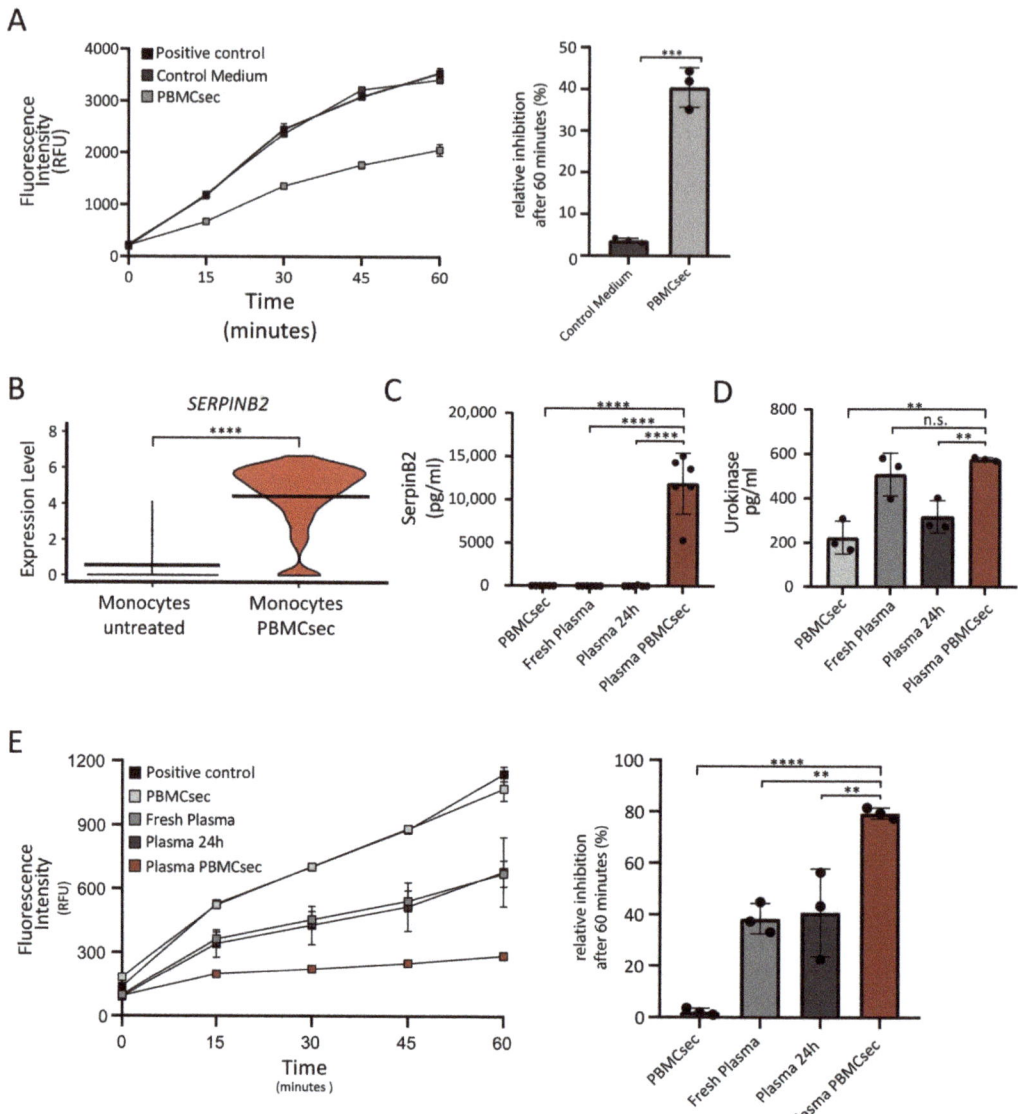

Figure 5. PBMCsec inhibits serine protease activity in vitro and increases levels of SERPINB2 in plasma of PBMCsec-treated whole blood. (**A**) Trypsin activity measured by increase in fluorescence intensity of cleaved substrate over time in the presence and absence of PBMCsec ($n = 3$ biological replicates). (**B**) Gene expression of the urokinase inhibitor *SERPINB2* in monocytes treated with PBMCsec (p-value < 0.0001) compared to untreated monocytes. (**C**) SerpinB2 ($n = 3$ biological replicates measured in duplicates) and (**D**) urokinase ($n = 3$ biological replicates) protein levels of fresh plasma, untreated plasma, and plasma of PBMCsec-treated whole blood. (**E**) In vitro assessment of urokinase activity of fresh plasma, plasma from untreated whole blood, and plasma obtained from PBMCsec-treated whole blood. ** $p < 0.01$, *** $p < 0.001$, **** $p < 0.0001$.

3.5. PBMCsec Ameliorates Thrombin-Induced Decrease in Endothelial Barrier Function

The activity of inflammatory mediators and serine proteases has been shown to support angiogenesis, as well as increase vascular leakage, by decreasing the endothelial barrier function [38,46]. Electrical cell-substrate impedance sensing enables the continuous assessment of changes in quality and function of a cellular barrier in response to different stimuli over time [47]. Loss of barrier function in endothelial cells can result in increased extravasation of immune cells and harmful mediators into the extravasal space, further increasing tissue damage [48]. Hence, we examined whether PBMCsec affected the thrombin-induced drop in endothelial barrier function by utilizing electrical cell-substrate impedance sensing. Addition of thrombin resulted in a transient decrease in trans-endothelial resistance, reaching the lowest point 5 min after stimulation (29% ± 12% barrier function relative to untreated basal medium control) (Figure 6). While the simultaneous addition of thrombin and control medium resulted in a similar change in barrier resistance (38% ± 2%) compared to basal medium, PBMCsec inhibited the thrombin-induced decrease in endothelial resistance (84% ± 14%) (Figure 6). Therefore, PBMCsec positively influenced endothelial barrier function in vitro by attenuating thrombin-mediated changes in endothelial cells.

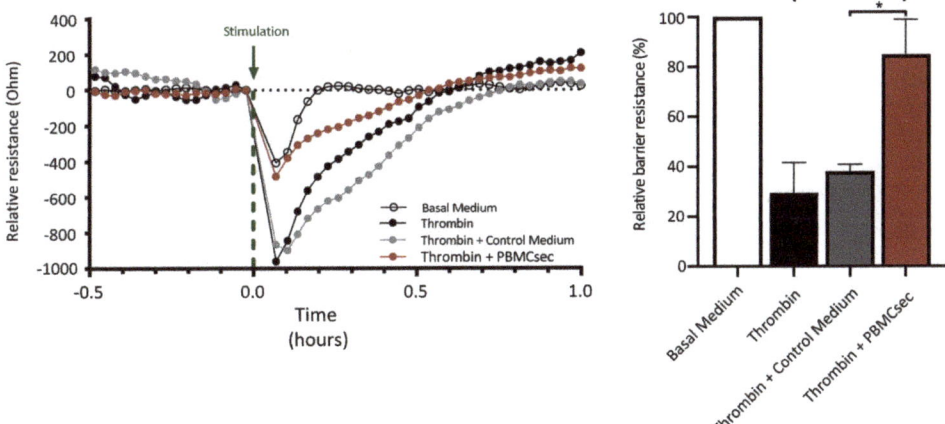

Figure 6. PBMCsec ameliorated the thrombin-induced decrease in endothelial cell barrier function. Representative evaluation of one of three independently conducted experiments. Paracellular resistance at 250 Hz was measured in DMECs challenged with 2 units/mL thrombin alone or in combination with control medium (CellGenix) or PBMCsec at 12.5 units/mL over time. The green arrow marks the time point of stimulation with the respective treatments. The bar plot shows the changes in endothelial barrier function for the investigated conditions relative to the basal medium (EBM-2) control. One-way ANOVA was performed with post hoc Dunnett's multiple comparison test to compare groups to basal medium; * $p < 0.05$, ** $p < 0.01$.

4. Discussion

The beneficial effects of PBMC-derived cell secretomes in the regeneration of damaged tissues and organs have already been well described [10,15,21,24,25]. In order to transit from these promising preclinical studies to the treatment of patients, the safety and tolerability of topical administration of autologous PBMCsec in dermal wounds was successfully assessed in a clinical phase I trial (MARSYAS I, NCT02284360) [49]. On the basis of these results, an ongoing clinical phase I/II trial has been initiated to evaluate the safety and efficacy of topically administered allogeneic PBMCsec for the treatment of diabetic foot ulcers (MARSYAS II, NCT04277598) [50]. In light of future therapeutic approaches using systemic administration of PBMCsec to regenerate inner organs, we analyzed in the present study the effects of PBMCsec on whole blood and the endothelium in more detail.

Using scRNA-seq, we identified a strong induction of tissue-regenerative pathways after treatment of human whole blood with PBMCsec ex vivo. In particular, biological processes associated with the regulation of vasculature development, wound healing, and regulation of endopeptidase activity, as well as decreased superoxide anion generation and leukocyte degranulation, all of which contribute to tissue regeneration, were significantly overrepresented in our analysis. The observed changes of the transcriptional profile of white blood cells treated with PBMCsec were most pronounced in monocytes, while all other cell types showed comparably low alterations in gene expression. Our finding is in line with previous publications where functional changes were mainly reported in monocytes after stimulation with conditioned medium from MSCs [51,52]. As monocytes are an important part of the innate immune system, a rapid response to extracellular stimuli, such as PBMCsec, was expected. Interestingly, only few granulocytes, which also represent a main constituent of innate immunity, were detected in our single-cell analysis. A low detectability of the different granulocyte populations in scRNA-seq has been reported before and might be due to their overall low RNA content and presence of RNAses [53]. This assumption is further supported by the extremely low mRNA counts in the few granulocytes detected in our analysis. Interestingly, T- and B-cells also showed only minor gene regulation after exposure to the secretome. As both cell types belong to the adaptive branch of the immune system, it is tempting to speculate that repeated exposure of lymphoid cellular subsets to PBMCsec might result in a more pronounced adaptive immune response. Furthermore, the natural process of aging may lead to various changes in immune cells from whole blood, which manifest as decreased immunological activity in older individuals. Indeed, previous studies in animal models have reported on positive age-associated effects of blood from young donors [54]. However, in light of our ongoing and future clinical studies, we here used PBMCsec produced under GMP conditions, which represents a pool of donors in the age range of 18–45 years. As pooling averages all active factors in PBMCsec, further studies will be necessary to fully address age-related effects.

Examination of the altered gene sets in monocytes revealed upregulation of several members of the chemokine (C–X–C motif) ligand (CXCL) family (*CXCL1*, *CXCL2*, *CXCL3*, *CXCL5*, and *CXCL8*), as well as different growth factors after stimulation with PBMCsec. In addition, high protein levels of CXCL1, CXCL5, and VEGF-A were detected in the plasma of PBMCsec-treated whole blood. These factors have previously been described as important constituents of PBMCsec, contributing to its tissue-regenerative actions [13,15]. Yet, we were not able to detect these proteins in PBMCsec in our assays. This discrepancy could be explained by the lower concentration of PBMCsec that we used in our ex vivo study. The lower concentration of PBMCsec had to be used for the stimulation of PBMCs, and endothelial cells as 1:2 dilutions with fresh medium were necessary for cell viability. Nevertheless, all these factors were strongly induced in whole blood and abundantly present in the plasma derived from PBMCsec-treated whole blood, indicating a significant amplification of the production of tissue regenerative factors. In addition, our transcriptional analysis revealed a downregulation of genes involved in the generation of superoxide anion species with an inhibitory effect on the formation of reactive oxygen species in PBMCsec-treated monocytes. Expression of the scavenger receptor CD36 on monocytes treated with PBMCsec was amongst the most strongly downregulated genes. In monocytes and macrophages, activation of this receptor promotes increased production of reactive oxygen species, which in turn reinforced damage to the vasculature [55]. Furthermore, CD36 is known to modulate the uptake of oxidized lipid species by macrophages, leading to functional changes in these cells. As they accumulate lipids, these so-called foam cells then promote proliferation and inflammation of endothelial and smooth muscle cells, which contributes to the formation of atherosclerotic plaques [56]. Given that reactive oxygen species increase after re-establishment of perfusion and aggravate tissue damage in a series of cardiovascular pathologies, our data offer a potential mechanism via which PBMCsec might directly and/or indirectly reduce tissue damage after ischemic conditions.

Future studies will elucidate the influence of PBMCsec on the generation and amelioration of reactive oxygen species.

Various biological active components have already been identified, contributing to the diverse effects of PBMCsec, including cytokines, growth factors, lipids, and exosomes. In particular, lipids present in PBMCsec have been shown to strongly impact immune cell functions. Laggner et al., recently demonstrated that PBMCsec-derived lipids interfere with dendritic cell differentiation and mast cell and basophil granulocyte degranulation, thereby improving skin inflammation and allergic symptoms, respectively [19,20]. This special composition of biologically active cytokines, growth factors, lipids, and exosomes, amongst other yet unidentified substances, makes PBMCsec a highly effective compound against tissue damage and inflammation. Previous work from our group demonstrated that paracrine factors released from γ-irradiated PBMCs positively influence tissue regeneration by affecting endothelial cell survival and sprouting [12]. In addition, we here showed that PBMCsec was also able to inhibit thrombin-induced disruption of the endothelial barrier in dermal microvascular endothelial cells. This effect might counteract increased leakage of blood vessels, thereby preventing insufficient perfusion of the vital part of the injured organ and amplification of the damage. We also observed an inhibitory effect of the plasma of PBMCsec-treated whole blood on the serine protease urokinase, which was not detected in PBMCsec alone. Thus, de novo synthesis of the urokinase inhibitor SERPINB2 could mediate this effect. Serine protease inhibitors are widely discussed as promising therapeutic approaches for several disease entities. Recently, Vorstandlechner et al. identified dipeptidyl-peptidase 4 (DPP4) and urokinase (PLAU) as important drivers of skin fibrosis, and targeted inhibition of both molecules was shown to reduce myo-fibroblast formation and improve scar quality [57]. Implications for therapeutic targeting of serine proteases are also evident for myocardial infarction [58,59]. While early re-vascularization of occluded blood vessels still remains the gold-standard intervention to maximize rescue of functional tissue, increasing emphasis is being put on the reduction of late onset events caused by accumulation of proinflammatory stimuli, proteases, and other detrimental factors, secondary to reperfusion injury [32]. Mauro and colleagues reported reduced infarction sizes following treatment with alpha-1-antitrypsin, in addition to revascularization, in a murine model of myocardial infarction [60]. This was further reinforced by a report by Hooshdaran et al., where inhibition of the serine proteases cathepsin G and chymase was shown to reduce adverse cardiac remodeling, myocyte apoptosis, and fibrosis in a murine model of myocardial ischemia reperfusion injury [61]. In addition, a recent publication by Sen and colleagues reported a central role for SerpinB2 in the coordinated resolution and repair of damaged tissue after ischemia/reperfusion in a murine kidney injury model [62]. These data suggest that, in addition to the protective action of serine protease inhibitors investigated in our study, they might also show valuable tissue-regenerative and antifibrotic properties. Further studies are needed to fully decipher the contribution of protease inhibitors already present in PBMCsec, as well as de novo induced inhibitors such as SerpinB2, and their respective roles in the inhibition of tissue-damage or the restoration of damaged tissue and organs.

Paracrine signaling for the prevention of a proinflammatory response and cell death, as well as induction of angiogenesis, is essential to restore damaged tissues and organs [52,63]. We previously showed that PBMCsec was able to positively modulate all of these events [12,15,64], and administration of a single dose of PBMCsec was sufficient to almost completely inhibit heart damage in a porcine model of experimental myocardial infarction [15]. However, given that pharmacodynamic investigations revealed that several main components of PBMCsec were only traceable for minutes to a maximum of 5 h in the blood of rats and dogs after intravenous application of human PBMCsec, this finding was rather unexpected [65]. Whether human PBMCsec induces a comparable release of pro-regenerative factors in these animal models has not been investigated so far. Our new data provide a reasonable explanation for this observation and suggest that PBMCsec induces the production of a new secretome in human white blood cells with additional regenerative properties. This is in line with our findings of increased endothelial cell sprouting after treatment of HUVECs with plasma of PBMCsec-treated whole blood. Cell types other than PBMCs, which could also contribute to the regenerative effects, can be found in whole blood. Thrombocytes are known for their proangiogenic properties, which are mainly due to the release of VEGF upon thrombocyte activation [66]. Interestingly, previous work from our group identified an inhibitory effect of PBMCsec on platelet activation and aggregation [18], suggesting that PBMCsec does not promote the release of proangiogenic mediators from thrombocytes. In contrast, an increased activity was observed in untreated plasma after cultivating whole blood for 24 h, as compared to fresh plasma, which might be a result of thrombocyte activation in the absence of PBMCsec. Importantly, our results indicate that the pharmacodynamic effect of a single application of PBMCsec can be significantly prolonged by continuous stimulation, comparable to the behavior of a damped wave. Therefore, this induced secretome, produced over an extended period of time, might multiply the pro-regenerative properties of PBMCsec by combining them with those of the newly induced factors. However, further studies in a human setting will be necessary to fully explore the tissue-regenerative potential of the newly formed secretome and to examine for how long this effect can be maintained.

In summary, our scRNA-seq analysis identified key mechanisms, potentially contributing to tissue regeneration, which might occur after systemic application of a cell secretome derived from irradiated PBMCs. PBMCsec displays a broad spectrum of mechanistic modes of actions that greatly complement each other and, therefore, positively contribute to tissue regeneration in a wide range of pathological settings. In addition, our data suggest that the effects in vivo are not restricted to direct actions of PBMCsec but also arise from further stimulation of circulating monocytes in the blood. Further human clinical studies in the future will clarify the underlying mechanisms and the therapeutic benefit of systemic treatment of damaged organs with PBMC-derived secretomes.

5. Patents

The Medical University of Vienna has claimed financial interest. H.J.A. holds patents related to this work (WO 2010/079086 A1; WO 2010/070105 A1; EP 3502692; European Patent Office application #19165340.1).

Supplementary Materials: The following supporting information can be downloaded at https://www.mdpi.com/article/10.3390/pharmaceutics14081600/s1: Figure S1. Identification of cell clusters based on expression of cluster-defining marker genes for T-cells, B- cells, monocytes, and granulocytes; Figure S2. Donor comparability of detected cell types and identification of pathways associated with upregulated genes in monocytes treated with PBMCsec; Figure S3. Transcriptional changes in T-cells, B-cells, and granulocytes and their predicted regulation of biological processes; Figure S4. Biological processes affected by up- and downregulated genes in monocytes treated with PBMCsec; Figure S5. Downregulated genes in monocytes treated with PBMCsec associated with leukocyte degranulation and generation of reactive oxygen species; Supplementary sheet 1. Pathways associated with significantly upregulated genes in monocytes treated with PBMCsec; Supplementary sheet 2. Pathways associated with significantly downregulated genes in monocytes treated with PBMCsec.

Author Contributions: M.M., H.J.A. and D.C. conceptualized and planned the experiments; H.J.A. and M.M. acquired funding; D.C., M.D. and K.S. performed the experiments; D.C., M.D., K.S., M.L., K.K., D.B., H.J.A. and M.M. participated in data interpretation; D.C., M.L. and M.M. drafted the manuscript. All authors have read and agreed to the published version of the manuscript.

Funding: This research project was financed by the Austrian Research Promotion Agency FFG Grant "APOSEC" (852748 and 862068; 2015–2019), by the Vienna Business Agency "APOSEC to clinic" (2343727, 2018–2020), and by the Aposcience AG under group leader H.J.A.

Institutional Review Board Statement: This study was conducted in accordance with the Declaration of Helsinki and local regulations. Use of primary HUVECs, primary DMECs, and blood samples was approved by the Institutional Review Board of the Medical University of Vienna (Ethics committee votes: 1280/2015, 1539/2017, and 1621/2020). All donors provided written informed consent.

Informed Consent Statement: Informed consent was obtained from all subjects involved in the study.

Data Availability Statement: ScRNA-seq data are available upon request.

Acknowledgments: We are thankful to HP Haselsteiner and the CRISCAR Familienstiftung for their belief in this private–public partnership to augment basic and translational clinical research. The authors acknowledge the core facilities of the Medical University of Vienna, a member of Vienna Life Science.

Conflicts of Interest: The Medical University of Vienna has claimed financial interest. H.J.A. holds patents related to this work (WO 2010/079086 A1; WO 2010/070105 A1; EP 3502692; European Patent Office application #19165340.1). All other authors declare no conflicts of interest.

References

1. Kumar, P.; Kandoi, S.; Misra, R.; Vijayalakshmi, S.; Rajagopal, K.; Verma, R.S. The mesenchymal stem cell secretome: A new paradigm towards cell-free therapeutic mode in regenerative medicine. *Cytokine Growth Factor Rev.* **2019**, *46*, 1–9.
2. Vizoso, F.J.; Eiro, N.; Cid, S.; Schneider, J.; Perez-Fernandez, R. Mesenchymal Stem Cell Secretome: Toward Cell-Free Therapeutic Strategies in Regenerative Medicine. *Int. J. Mol. Sci.* **2017**, *18*, 1852. [CrossRef]
3. Zheng, H.; Zhang, B.; Chhatbar, P.Y.; Dong, Y.; Alawieh, A.; Lowe, F.; Hu, X.; Feng, W. Mesenchymal Stem Cell Therapy in Stroke: A Systematic Review of Literature in Pre-Clinical and Clinical Research. *Cell Transpl.* **2018**, *27*, 1723–1730. [CrossRef]
4. Gyöngyösi, M.; Haller, P.M.; Blake, D.J.; Rendon, E.M. Meta-Analysis of Cell Therapy Studies in Heart Failure and Acute Myocardial Infarction. *Circ. Res.* **2018**, *123*, 301–308. [CrossRef]
5. Eggenhofer, E.; Benseler, V.; Kroemer, A.; Popp, F.C.; Geissler, E.; Schlitt, H.J.; Baan, C.C.; Dahlke, M.H.; Hoogduijn, M.J. Mesenchymal stem cells are short-lived and do not migrate beyond the lungs after intravenous infusion. *Front. Immunol.* **2012**, *3*, 297. [CrossRef]
6. Thum, T.; Bauersachs, J.; Poole-Wilson, P.A.; Volk, H.D.; Anker, S.D. The dying stem cell hypothesis: Immune modulation as a novel mechanism for progenitor cell therapy in cardiac muscle. *J. Am. Coll. Cardiol.* **2005**, *46*, 1799–1802. [CrossRef]
7. Takahashi, M.; Li, T.-S.; Suzuki, R.; Kobayashi, T.; Ito, H.; Ikeda, Y.; Matsuzaki, M.; Hamano, K. Cytokines produced by bone marrow cells can contribute to functional improvement of the infarcted heart by protecting cardiomyocytes from ischemic injury. *Am. J. Physiol. Heart Circ. Physiol.* **2006**, *291*, H886–H893. [CrossRef]
8. Gnecchi, M.; He, H.; Noiseux, N.; Liang, O.D.; Zhang, L.; Morello, F.; Mu, H.; Melo, L.G.; Pratt, R.E.; Ingwall, J.S.; et al. Evidence supporting paracrine hypothesis for Akt-modified mesenchymal stem cell-mediated cardiac protection and functional improvement. *FASEB J.* **2006**, *20*, 661–669. [CrossRef] [PubMed]
9. Chu, D.-T.; Phuong, T.N.T.; Tien, N.L.B.; Tran, D.K.; Van Thanh, V.; Quang, T.L.; Truong, D.T.; Pham, V.H.; Ngoc, V.T.N.; Chu-Dinh, T.; et al. An Update on the Progress of Isolation, Culture, Storage, and Clinical Application of Human Bone Marrow Mesenchymal Stem/Stromal Cells. *Int. J. Mol. Sci.* **2020**, *21*, 708. [CrossRef] [PubMed]
10. Ankersmit, H.J.; Hoetzenecker, K.; Dietl, W.; Soleiman, A.; Horvat, R.; Wolfsberger, M.; Gerner, C.; Hacker, S.; Mildner, M.; Moser, B.; et al. Irradiated cultured apoptotic peripheral blood mononuclear cells regenerate infarcted myocardium. *Eur. J. Clin. Investig.* **2009**, *39*, 445–456. [CrossRef] [PubMed]
11. Korf-Klingebiel, M.; Kempf, T.; Sauer, T.; Brinkmann, E.; Fischer, P.; Meyer, G.P.; Ganser, A.; Drexler, H.; Wollert, K.C. Bone marrow cells are a rich source of growth factors and cytokines: Implications for cell therapy trials after myocardial infarction. *Eur. Heart J.* **2008**, *29*, 2851–2858. [CrossRef]
12. Wagner, T.; Traxler, D.; Simader, E.; Beer, L.; Narzt, M.-S.; Gruber, F.; Madlener, S.; Laggner, M.; Erb, M.; Vorstandlechner, V.; et al. Different pro-angiogenic potential of γ-irradiated PBMC-derived secretome and its subfractions. *Sci. Rep.* **2018**, *8*, 18016. [CrossRef]
13. Beer, L.; Zimmermann, M.; Mitterbauer, A.; Ellinger, A.; Gruber, F.; Narzt, M.-S.; Zellner, M.; Gyöngyösi, M.; Madlener, S.; Simader, E.; et al. Analysis of the Secretome of Apoptotic Peripheral Blood Mononuclear Cells: Impact of Released Proteins and Exosomes for Tissue Regeneration. *Sci. Rep.* **2015**, *5*, 16662. [CrossRef]
14. Kasiri, M.M.; Beer, L.; Nemec, L.; Gruber, F.; Pietkiewicz, S.; Haider, T.; Simader, E.M.; Traxler-Weidenauer, D.; Schweiger, T.; Janik, S.; et al. Dying blood mononuclear cell secretome exerts antimicrobial activity. *Eur. J. Clin. Investig.* **2016**, *46*, 853–863. [CrossRef]
15. Lichtenauer, M.; Mildner, M.; Hoetzenecker, K.; Zimmermann, M.; Podesser, B.K.; Sipos, W.; Berényi, E.; Dworschak, M.; Tschachler, E.; Gyöngyösi, M.; et al. Secretome of apoptotic peripheral blood cells (APOSEC) confers cytoprotection to cardiomyocytes and inhibits tissue remodelling after acute myocardial infarction: A preclinical study. *Basic Res. Cardiol.* **2011**, *106*, 1283–1297. [CrossRef]
16. Hoetzenecker, K.; Zimmermann, M.; Hoetzenecker, W.; Schweiger, T.; Kollmann, D.; Mildner, M.; Hegedus, B.; Mitterbauer, A.; Hacker, S.; Birner, P.; et al. Mononuclear cell secretome protects from experimental autoimmune myocarditis. *Eur. Heart J.* **2015**, *36*, 676–685. [CrossRef]

17. Mildner, M.; Hacker, S.; Haider, T.; Gschwandtner, M.; Werba, G.; Barresi, C.; Zimmermann, M.; Golabi, B.; Tschachler, E.; Ankersmit, H.J. Secretome of peripheral blood mononuclear cells enhances wound healing. *PLoS ONE* **2013**, *8*, e60103. [CrossRef]
18. Hoetzenecker, K.; Assinger, A.; Lichtenauer, M.; Mildner, M.; Schweiger, T.; Starlinger, P.; Jakab, A.; Berényi, E.; Pavo, N.; Zimmermann, M.; et al. Secretome of apoptotic peripheral blood cells (APOSEC) attenuates microvascular obstruction in a porcine closed chest reperfused acute myocardial infarction model: Role of platelet aggregation and vasodilation. *Basic Res. Cardiol.* **2012**, *107*, 292. [CrossRef]
19. Laggner, M.; Copic, D.; Nemec, L.; Vorstandlechner, V.; Gugerell, A.; Gruber, F.; Peterbauer, A.; Ankersmit, H.J.; Mildner, M. Therapeutic potential of lipids obtained from γ-irradiated PBMCs in dendritic cell-mediated skin inflammation. *EBioMedicine* **2020**, *55*, 102774. [CrossRef]
20. Laggner, M.; Acosta, G.S.; Kitzmüller, C.; Copic, D.; Gruber, F.; Altenburger, L.M.; Vorstandlechner, V.; Gugerell, A.; Direder, M.; Klas, K.; et al. The secretome of irradiated peripheral blood mononuclear cells attenuates activation of mast cells and basophils. *eBioMedicine* **2022**, *81*, 104093. [CrossRef]
21. Beer, L.; Mildner, M.; Gyöngyösi, M.; Ankersmit, H.J. Peripheral blood mononuclear cell secretome for tissue repair. *Apoptosis* **2016**, *21*, 1336–1353. [CrossRef]
22. Hacker, S.; Mittermayr, R.; Traxler, D.; Keibl, C.; Resch, A.; Salminger, S.; Leiss, H.; Hacker, P.; Gabriel, C.; Golabi, B.; et al. The secretome of stressed peripheral blood mononuclear cells increases tissue survival in a rodent epigastric flap model. *Bioeng. Transl. Med.* **2021**, *6*, e10186. [CrossRef]
23. Hacker, S.; Mittermayr, R.; Nickl, S.; Haider, T.; Lebherz-Eichinger, D.; Beer, L.; Mitterbauer, A.; Leiss, H.; Zimmermann, M.; Schweiger, T.; et al. Paracrine Factors from Irradiated Peripheral Blood Mononuclear Cells Improve Skin Regeneration and Angiogenesis in a Porcine Burn Model. *Sci. Rep.* **2016**, *6*, 25168. [CrossRef]
24. Altmann, P.; Mildner, M.; Haider, T.; Traxler, D.; Beer, L.; Ristl, R.; Golabi, B.; Gabriel, C.; Leutmezer, F.; Ankersmit, H.J. Secretomes of apoptotic mononuclear cells ameliorate neurological damage in rats with focal ischemia. *F1000Research* **2014**, *3*, 131. [CrossRef]
25. Haider, T.; Höftberger, R.; Rüger, B.; Mildner, M.; Blumer, R.; Mitterbauer, A.; Buchacher, T.; Sherif, C.; Altmann, P.; Redl, H.; et al. The secretome of apoptotic human peripheral blood mononuclear cells attenuates secondary damage following spinal cord injury in rats. *Exp. Neurol.* **2015**, *267*, 230–242. [CrossRef]
26. Mildner, C.S.; Copic, D.; Zimmermann, M.; Lichtenauer, M.; Direder, M.; Klas, K.; Bormann, D.; Gugerell, A.; Moser, B.; Hoetzenecker, K.; et al. Secretome of Stressed Peripheral Blood Mononuclear Cells Alters Transcriptome Signature in Heart, Liver, and Spleen after an Experimental Acute Myocardial Infarction: An In Silico Analysis. *Biology* **2022**, *11*, 116. [CrossRef]
27. Neumann, F.J.; Sousa-Uva, M.; Ahlsson, A.; Alfonso, F.; Banning, A.P.; Benedetto, U.; Byrne, R.A.; Collet, J.P.; Falk, V.; Head, S.J.; et al. 2018 ESC/EACTS Guidelines on myocardial revascularization. *Eur. Heart J.* **2019**, *40*, 87–165. [CrossRef]
28. Neri, M.; Riezzo, I.; Pascale, N.; Pomara, C.; Turillazzi, E. Ischemia/Reperfusion Injury following Acute Myocardial Infarction: A Critical Issue for Clinicians and Forensic Pathologists. *Mediat. Inflamm.* **2017**, *2017*, 7018393. [CrossRef]
29. Garcia-Dorado, D.; Ruiz-Meana, M.; Inserte, J.; Rodriguez-Sinovas, A.; Piper, H.M. Calcium-mediated cell death during myocardial reperfusion. *Cardiovasc. Res.* **2012**, *94*, 168–180. [CrossRef]
30. Javadov, S.; Karmazyn, M. Mitochondrial permeability transition pore opening as an endpoint to initiate cell death and as a putative target for cardioprotection. *Cell Physiol. Biochem.* **2007**, *20*, 1–22. [CrossRef]
31. He, P.; Talukder, M.A.H.; Gao, F. Oxidative Stress and Microvessel Barrier Dysfunction. *Front. Physiol.* **2020**, *11*, 472. [CrossRef] [PubMed]
32. Toldo, S.; Mauro, A.G.; Cutter, Z.; Abbate, A. Inflammasome, pyroptosis, and cytokines in myocardial ischemia-reperfusion injury. *Am. J. Physiol. Heart Circ. Physiol.* **2018**, *315*, H1553–H1568. [CrossRef] [PubMed]
33. Sharony, R.; Yu, P.-J.; Park, J.; Galloway, A.C.; Mignatti, P.; Pintucci, G. Protein targets of inflammatory serine proteases and cardiovascular disease. *J. Inflamm.* **2010**, *7*, 45. [CrossRef] [PubMed]
34. Carden, D.L.; Granger, D.N. Pathophysiology of ischaemia-reperfusion injury. *J. Pathol.* **2000**, *190*, 255–266. [CrossRef]
35. Laggner, M.; Gugerell, A.; Bachmann, C.; Hofbauer, H.; Vorstandlechner, V.; Seibold, M.; Gouya Lechner, G.; Peterbauer, A.; Madlener, S.; Demyanets, S.; et al. Reproducibility of GMP-compliant production of therapeutic stressed peripheral blood mononuclear cell-derived secretomes, a novel class of biological medicinal products. *Stem Cell Res. Ther.* **2020**, *11*, 9. [CrossRef]
36. DeCicco-Skinner, K.L.; Henry, G.H.; Cataisson, C.; Tabib, T.; Gwilliam, J.C.; Watson, N.J.; Bullwinkle, E.M.; Falkenburg, L.; O'Neill, R.C.; Morin, A.; et al. Endothelial cell tube formation assay for the in vitro study of angiogenesis. *J. Vis. Exp.* **2014**, *91*, e51312. [CrossRef]
37. Carpentier, G.; Berndt, S.; Ferratge, S.; Rasband, W.; Cuendet, M.; Uzan, G.; Albanese, P. Angiogenesis Analyzer for ImageJ—A comparative morphometric analysis of "Endothelial Tube Formation Assay" and "Fibrin Bead Assay". *Sci. Rep.* **2020**, *10*, 11568. [CrossRef]
38. Holzner, S.; Bromberger, S.; Wenzina, J.; Neumüller, K.; Holper, T.-M.; Petzelbauer, P.; Bauer, W.; Weber, B.; Schossleitner, K. Phosphorylated cingulin localises GEF-H1 at tight junctions to protect vascular barriers in blood endothelial cells. *J. Cell Sci.* **2021**, *134*, jcs258557. [CrossRef]
39. Stuart, T.; Butler, A.; Hoffman, P.; Hafemeister, C.; Papalexi, E.; Mauck, W.M., III; Hao, Y.; Stoeckius, M.; Smibert, P.; Satija, R. Comprehensive Integration of Single-Cell Data. *Cell* **2019**, *177*, 1888–1902.e21. [CrossRef]
40. Zhou, Y.; Zhou, B.; Pache, L.; Chang, M.; Khodabakhshi, A.H.; Tanaseichuk, O.; Benner, C.; Chanda, S.K. Metascape provides a biologist-oriented resource for the analysis of systems-level datasets. *Nat. Commun.* **2019**, *10*, 1523. [CrossRef]

41. Bindea, G.; Mlecnik, B.; Hackl, H.; Charoentong, P.; Tosolini, M.; Kirilovsky, A.; Fridman, W.-H.; Pagès, F.; Trajanoski, Z.; Galon, J. ClueGO: A Cytoscape plug-in to decipher functionally grouped gene ontology and pathway annotation networks. *Bioinformatics* **2009**, *25*, 1091–1093. [CrossRef]
42. Julier, Z.; Park, A.J.; Briquez, P.S.; Martino, M.M. Promoting tissue regeneration by modulating the immune system. *Acta Biomater.* **2017**, *53*, 13–28. [CrossRef]
43. Urso, A.; Prince, A. Anti-Inflammatory Metabolites in the Pathogenesis of Bacterial Infection. *Front. Cell Infect. Microbiol.* **2022**, *12*, 925746. [CrossRef]
44. Kłoczko, J.; Bielawiec, M.; Giedrojć, J.; Radziwon, P.; Galar, M. Human monocytes release plasma serine protease inhibitors in vitro. *Haemostasis* **1990**, *20*, 229–232. [CrossRef]
45. Ritchie, H.; Robbie, L.A.; Kinghorn, S.; Exley, R.; Booth, N.A. Monocyte plasminogen activator inhibitor 2 (PAI-2) inhibits u-PA-mediated fibrin clot lysis and is cross-linked to fibrin. *Thromb. Haemost.* **1999**, *81*, 96–103.
46. Slack, M.A.; Gordon, S.M. Protease Activity in Vascular Disease. *Arterioscler. Thromb. Vasc. Biol.* **2019**, *39*, e210–e218. [CrossRef]
47. Szulcek, R.; Bogaard, H.J.; van Nieuw Amerongen, G.P. Electric cell-substrate impedance sensing for the quantification of endothelial proliferation, barrier function, and motility. *J. Vis. Exp.* **2014**, *3*, e51300. [CrossRef]
48. Park-Windhol, C.; D'Amore, P.A. Disorders of Vascular Permeability. *Annu. Rev. Pathol. Mech. Dis.* **2016**, *11*, 251–281. [CrossRef]
49. Simader, E.; Traxler, D.; Kasiri, M.M.; Hofbauer, H.; Wolzt, M.; Glogner, C.; Storka, A.; Mildner, M.; Gouya, G.; Geusau, A.; et al. Safety and tolerability of topically administered autologous, apoptotic PBMC secretome (APOSEC) in dermal wounds: A randomized Phase 1 trial (MARSYAS I). *Sci. Rep.* **2017**, *7*, 6216. [CrossRef]
50. Gugerell, A.; Gouya-Lechner, G.; Hofbauer, H.; Laggner, M.; Trautinger, F.; Almer, G.; Peterbauer-Scherb, A.; Seibold, M.; Hoetzenecker, W.; Dreschl, C.; et al. Safety and clinical efficacy of the secretome of stressed peripheral blood mononuclear cells in patients with diabetic foot ulcer-study protocol of the randomized, placebo-controlled, double-blind, multicenter, international phase II clinical trial MARSYAS II. *Trials* **2021**, *22*, 10.
51. Beez, C.M.; Haag, M.; Klein, O.; Van Linthout, S.; Sittinger, M.; Seifert, M. Extracellular vesicles from regenerative human cardiac cells act as potent immune modulators by priming monocytes. *J. Nanobiotechnol.* **2019**, *17*, 72. [CrossRef]
52. Guillén, M.I.; Platas, J.; del Caz, M.D.P.; Mirabet, V.; Alcaraz, M.J. Paracrine Anti-inflammatory Effects of Adipose Tissue-Derived Mesenchymal Stem Cells in Human Monocytes. *Front. Physiol.* **2018**, *9*, 661. [CrossRef]
53. Monaco, G.; Lee, B.; Xu, W.; Mustafah, S.; Hwang, Y.Y.; Carré, C.; Burdin, N.; Visan, L.; Ceccarelli, M.; Poidinger, M.; et al. RNA-Seq Signatures Normalized by mRNA Abundance Allow Absolute Deconvolution of Human Immune Cell Types. *Cell Rep.* **2019**, *26*, 1627–1640.e7. [CrossRef]
54. Lee, K.A.; Flores, R.R.; Jang, I.H.; Saathoff, A.; Robbins, P.D. Immune Senescence, Immunosenescence and Aging. *Front. Aging* **2022**, *3*, 900028. [CrossRef]
55. Chen, Y.; Yang, M.; Huang, W.; Chen, W.; Zhao, Y.; Schulte, M.L.; Volberding, P.; Gerbec, Z.; Zimmermann, M.T.; Zeighami, A.; et al. Mitochondrial Metabolic Reprogramming by CD36 Signaling Drives Macrophage Inflammatory Responses. *Circ. Res.* **2019**, *125*, 1087–1102. [CrossRef]
56. Bekkering, S.; Quintin, J.; Joosten, L.A.; van der Meer, J.W.; Netea, M.G.; Riksen, N.P. Oxidized low-density lipoprotein induces long-term proinflammatory cytokine production and foam cell formation via epigenetic reprogramming of monocytes. *Arterioscler. Thromb. Vasc. Biol.* **2014**, *34*, 1731–1738. [CrossRef]
57. Vorstandlechner, V.; Laggner, M.; Copic, D.; Klas, K.; Direder, M.; Chen, Y.; Golabi, B.; Haslik, W.; Radtke, C.; Tschachler, E.; et al. The serine proteases dipeptidyl-peptidase 4 and urokinase are key molecules in human and mouse scar formation. *Nat. Commun.* **2021**, *12*, 6242. [CrossRef]
58. Petrera, A.; Gassenhuber, J.; Ruf, S.; Gunasekaran, D.; Esser, J.; Shahinian, J.H.; Hübschle, T.; Rütten, H.; Sadowski, T.; Schilling, O. Cathepsin A inhibition attenuates myocardial infarction-induced heart failure on the functional and proteomic levels. *J. Transl. Med.* **2016**, *14*, 153. [CrossRef]
59. Ogura, Y.; Tajiri, K.; Murakoshi, N.; Xu, D.; Yonebayashi, S.; Li, S.; Okabe, Y.; Feng, D.; Shimoda, Y.; Song, Z.; et al. Neutrophil Elastase Deficiency Ameliorates Myocardial Injury Post Myocardial Infarction in Mice. *Int. J. Mol. Sci.* **2021**, *22*, 722. [CrossRef]
60. Mauro, A.G.; Mezzaroma, E.; Marchetti, C.; Narayan, P.; Del Buono, M.G.; Capuano, M.; Prestamburgo, D.; Catapano, S.; Salloum, F.N.; Abbate, A.; et al. A Preclinical Translational Study of the Cardioprotective Effects of Plasma-Derived Alpha-1 Anti-trypsin in Acute Myocardial Infarction. *J. Cardiovasc. Pharmacol.* **2017**, *69*, 273–278. [CrossRef] [PubMed]
61. Hooshdaran, B.; Kolpakov, M.A.; Guo, X.; Miller, S.A.; Wang, T.; Tilley, D.; Rafiq, K.; Sabri, A. Dual inhibition of cathepsin G and chymase reduces myocyte death and improves cardiac remodeling after myocardial ischemia reperfusion injury. *Basic Res. Cardiol.* **2017**, *112*, 62. [CrossRef] [PubMed]
62. Sen, P.; Helmke, A.; Liao, C.M.; Sörensen-Zender, I.; Rong, S.; Bräsen, J.-H.; Melk, A.; Haller, H.; Von Vietinghoff, S.; Schmitt, R. SerpinB2 Regulates Immune Response in Kidney Injury and Aging. *J. Am. Soc. Nephrol.* **2020**, *31*, 983–995. [CrossRef] [PubMed]
63. BBouchentouf, M.; Paradis, P.; Forner, K.A.; Cuerquis, J.; Boivin, M.N.; Zheng, J.; Boulassel, M.R.; Routy, J.P.; Schiffrin, E.; Galipeau, J. Monocyte derivatives promote angiogenesis and myocyte survival in a model of myocardial infarction. *Cell Transpl.* **2010**, *19*, 369–386. [CrossRef] [PubMed]
64. Simader, E.; Beer, L.; Laggner, M.; Vorstandlechner, V.; Gugerell, A.; Erb, M.; Kalinina, P.; Copic, D.; Moser, D.; Spittler, A.; et al. Tissue-regenerative potential of the secretome of γ-irradiated peripheral blood mononuclear cells is mediated via TNFRSF1B-induced necroptosis. *Cell Death Dis.* **2019**, *10*, 729. [CrossRef]

65. Wuschko, S.; Gugerell, A.; Chabicovsky, M.; Hofbauer, H.; Laggner, M.; Erb, M.; Ostler, T.; Peterbauer, A.; Suessner, S.; Demyanets, S.; et al. Toxicological testing of allogeneic secretome derived from peripheral mononuclear cells (APOSEC): A novel cell-free therapeutic agent in skin disease. *Sci. Rep.* **2019**, *9*, 5598. [CrossRef]
66. Webb, N.J.; Bottomley, M.J.; Watson, C.J.; Brenchley, P.E. Vascular endothelial growth factor (VEGF) is released from platelets during blood clotting: Implications for measurement of circulating VEGF levels in clinical disease. *Clin. Sci.* **1998**, *94*, 395–404. [CrossRef]

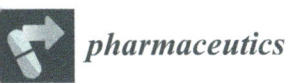

Article

HDAC Inhibition Regulates Cardiac Function by Increasing Myofilament Calcium Sensitivity and Decreasing Diastolic Tension

Deborah M. Eaton [1,2,†], Thomas G. Martin [3,†], Michael Kasa [4], Natasa Djalinac [4], Senka Ljubojevic-Holzer [4], Dirk Von Lewinski [4], Maria Pöttler [4], Theerachat Kampaengsri [3], Andreas Krumphuber [4], Katharina Scharer [4], Heinrich Maechler [5], Andreas Zirlik [4], Timothy A. McKinsey [6,7], Jonathan A. Kirk [3], Steven R. Houser [1], Peter P. Rainer [4,8] and Markus Wallner [1,4,*]

1. Cardiovascular Research Center, Lewis Katz School of Medicine, Temple University, Philadelphia, PA 19140, USA; deborah.eaton@pennmedicine.upenn.edu (D.M.E.); srhouser@temple.edu (S.R.H.)
2. Penn Cardiovascular Institute, University of Pennsylvania Perelman School of Medicine, Philadelphia, PA 19104, USA
3. Department of Cell and Molecular Physiology, Loyola University Chicago Stritch School of Medicine, Chicago, IL 60153, USA; thomas.martin-2@colorado.edu (T.G.M.); june.thk39@gmail.com (T.K.); jkirk2@luc.edu (J.A.K.)
4. Division of Cardiology, Medical University of Graz, 8036 Graz, Austria; michael.kasa@gmx.at (M.K.); natasa.djalinac@medunigraz.at (N.D.); senka.ljubojevic@medunigraz.at (S.L.-H.); dirk.von-lewinski@medunigraz.at (D.V.L.); maria.poettler@medunigraz.at (M.P.); andreas.krumphuber@stud.medunigraz.at (A.K.); katharina.scharer@stud.medunigraz.at (K.S.); andreas.zirlik@medunigraz.at (A.Z.); peter.rainer@medunigraz.at (P.P.R.)
5. Department of Cardiothoracic Surgery, Medical University of Graz, 8036 Graz, Austria; heinrich.maechler@medunigraz.at
6. Division of Cardiology, Department of Medicine, University of Colorado Anschutz Medical Campus, Aurora, CO 80045, USA; timothy.mckinsey@cuanschutz.edu
7. Consortium for Fibrosis Research & Translation, University of Colorado Anschutz Medical Campus, Aurora, CO 80045, USA
8. BioTechMed Graz, 8010 Graz, Austria
* Correspondence: markus.wallner@medunigraz.at
† These authors contributed equally to this work.

Abstract: We recently established a large animal model that recapitulates key clinical features of heart failure with preserved ejection fraction (HFpEF) and tested the effects of the pan-HDAC inhibitor suberoylanilide hydroxamic acid (SAHA). SAHA reversed and prevented the development of cardiopulmonary impairment. This study evaluated the effects of SAHA at the level of cardiomyocyte and contractile protein function to understand how it modulates cardiac function. Both isolated adult feline ventricular cardiomyocytes (AFVM) and left ventricle (LV) trabeculae isolated from non-failing donors were treated with SAHA or vehicle before recording functional data. Skinned myocytes were isolated from AFVM and human trabeculae to assess myofilament function. SAHA-treated AFVM had increased contractility and improved relaxation kinetics but no difference in peak calcium transients, with increased calcium sensitivity and decreased passive stiffness of myofilaments. Mass spectrometry analysis revealed increased acetylation of the myosin regulatory light chain with SAHA treatment. SAHA-treated human trabeculae had decreased diastolic tension and increased developed force. Myofilaments isolated from human trabeculae had increased calcium sensitivity and decreased passive stiffness. These findings suggest that SAHA has an important role in the direct control of cardiac function at the level of the cardiomyocyte and myofilament by increasing myofilament calcium sensitivity and reducing diastolic tension.

Keywords: heart failure; contractility; calcium; cardiomyocyte; myofilament; HDAC inhibitor

1. Introduction

Heart failure (HF) represents a major global health crisis. There are currently an estimated 26 million adults living with heart failure worldwide and this number is predicted to rise in the future [1]. About half of all heart failure patients are diagnosed with heart failure with preserved ejection fraction (HFpEF) and the other half with heart failure with (mildly) reduced ejection fraction (HFmrEF, HFrEF) [2]. There is a stark contrast in the etiology of the syndrome and treatment options available for patients with HFrEF and HFpEF. While there are several drug classes that have proven to effectively improve mortality in HFrEF, until recently no therapeutics have improved the outcome in patients with HFpEF. EMPEROR-Preserved, a randomized clinical trial comparing empagliflozin vs. placebo in HF patients with an EF greater or equal to 40%, produced a positive outcome [3]. To address this lack of treatments, we must bridge the gap from basic science where novel therapeutic targets are identified to pre-clinical and translational medicine. Part of the solution involves developing representative animal models that capture multiple aspects of the complex human syndrome of HFpEF [4]. Our lab previously published an in-depth characterization of the feline model of slow progressive pressure overload, which recapitulates several key clinical features of HFpEF [5,6]. While these animals have preserved ejection fraction, they develop systolic and diastolic dysfunction when assessed using speckle-tracking-based strain analysis and invasive hemodynamics. Aortic banded animals also develop pulmonary hypertension secondary to elevated LV filling pressures, which is accompanied by structural remodeling, reduced lung compliance, increased intrapulmonary shunting, and impaired oxygenation. This robust and extensively characterized cardiopulmonary phenotype is a useful platform for testing potential therapies for heart failure [6].

While developing new treatments is important, repurposing Federal Drug Administration (FDA)/European Medicine Agency (EMA)-approved therapies for HF has gained attention in recent years as these drugs have already been clinically evaluated for other diseases [7]. In line with this idea, we decided to focus on epigenetic/post-translational modifications as a therapeutic target by testing suberoylanilide hydroxamic acid (SAHA, vorinostat), which is a pan-histone deacetylase (HDAC) inhibitor, and was the first in class therapy to earn FDA approval in 2006 as a treatment for cutaneous T-cell lymphoma [8]. HDACs are enzymes that have genomic and non-genomic effects. Deacetylation of histones by HDACs leads to chromatin compaction, acting as an off switch for mRNA synthesis and regulating gene expression. HDACs can also facilitate post-translational protein modifications by catalyzing the removal of lysine acetyl groups from ε-amino groups of lysine residues [9,10]. HDACs are activated in cardiomyocytes subjected to pressure overload [11]. Using HDAC inhibitors to harness this integral catalytic activity is a promising therapeutic strategy. We previously showed that SAHA treatment improved systolic and diastolic cardiac, pulmonary, and mitochondrial function in an animal model of HFpEF [5]. More in-depth analyses provided a potential mechanism for the improvement in diastolic function. Using isolated myofibrils, we found a significant improvement in the linear relaxation duration with SAHA. Linear relaxation duration represents inactivation of thin filament regulatory proteins after Ca^{2+} unbinds [12]. This finding indicates that SAHA may have a direct role in modulating diastolic function via direct control of relaxation properties of myofibrils.

However, mechanisms and substrates for acetylation/deacetylation responsible for the improvements in systolic and diastolic cardiac function are poorly understood. Several studies have assessed the effect of SAHA in cardiomyocytes isolated from rodents and provided valuable insight [13,14], but there were still many unanswered questions. Furthermore, no study has assessed the functional effects of SAHA on human cardiac tissue. To address this gap in knowledge, we performed an in-depth analysis using tissue and cellular components from both non-failing human hearts and a large mammalian model with comparable physiological properties (action potential duration) and myosin heavy chain composition [15,16]. Our aim was to develop a better understanding of how SAHA treatment modulates systolic and diastolic function at a cellular and molecular level and its contractile components and identify potential substrates for acetylation/deacetylation.

2. Materials and Methods

Figure S1 details the experimental design.

2.1. AFVM Isolation

AFVMs were isolated from the left ventricle of domestic short hair kittens (n = 4, 6 months old) (Marshall Laboratories) as previously described [5,17–19]. Animals were sedated with 50 mg/kg of ketamine and 0.1 mg/kg of acepromazine (intramuscular), then 50 mg/kg of sodium pentobarbital (intraperitoneal). The heart was excised via cardiectomy, washed in ice cold Krebs-Henseleit Buffer (KHB) (12.5 mmol/L glucose, 5.4 mmol/L KCl, 1 mmol/L lactic acid, 1.2 mmol/L $MgSO_4$, 130 mmol/L NaCl, 1.2 mmol/L NaH_2PO_4, 25 mmol/L $NaHCO_3$, and 2 mmol/L Na-pyruvate, pH 7.4) and then the aorta was cannulated. The coronary arteries were then flushed with KHB to clear out any remaining blood. The heart was retrograde perfused with KHB using a modified Langendorff apparatus, then switched to digestion buffer (KHB, 180 units/mL collagenase type II (Worthington Biochemical Corporation, NJ, USA) and 50 µmol/L $CaCl_2$). All solutions were heated to 37 °C prior to perfusion through the heart and aerated with 95% oxygen and 5% CO_2 to maintain pH at 7.4. The heart was continuously checked to monitor digestion and then the left ventricle was separated from the rest of the heart and minced. The cardiomyocytes were then filtered, resuspended, and equilibrated in room temperature KHB with 200 µmol/L $CaCl_2$, and 1% bovine serum albumin (BSA) added.

2.2. AFVM Acute SAHA Treatment and Contractility/Calcium Recordings

Once AFVM had settled via gravity, they were washed with Normal Tyrode's solution (NT) (10 mM glucose, 5 mM HEPES, 5.4 mM KCl, 1.2 mM ($MgCl_2$) ($6H_2O$), 150 mM NaCl, and 2 mM NA-pyruvate, pH 7.4) with 1mM $CaCl_2$ (NT + 1 mM $CaCl_2$) added. A stock solution of 5 mM SAHA was prepared and then serially diluted to 2.5 µM of SAHA using NT + 1 mM $CaCl_2$. Corresponding dilutions of DMSO were prepared in NT + 1 mM $CaCl_2$ to use as the vehicle treatment. Cells were treated with SAHA or vehicle and incubated for 90 min. After 90 min, cells were incubated with Fluo-4am (ThermoFisher Scientific, Waltham, MA, USA) and Pluronic™ F-127 (ThermoFisher Scientific) for 12–15 min. Cells were then loaded onto a heated chamber of an inverted microscope and perfused with NT + 1 mM $CaCl_2$ with 2.5 µM SAHA or corresponding DMSO dilution added. Cells were first paced at 0.5 Hz to check for any not following stimulation. Once the steady state was reached, a minimum of 15 contractions was recorded using the IonOptix Calcium and Contractility platform. Background fluorescence was recorded for all cells. Analysis was performed offline using the IonOptix IonWizard software. Background fluorescence was subtracted from the calcium recording prior to performing calculations during analysis. Peak calcium transient was calculated as F/F_0, where F is peak calcium and F_0 is baseline calcium. Fractional shortening was calculated as ((baseline sarcomere length—peak sarcomere length/baseline sarcomere length) × 100).

2.3. Trabeculae Harvest

Trabeculae were isolated from the ventricles of human non-failing donor hearts that were not suitable for transplantation (n = 7 patients) or right atrial appendages (n = 30) as previously described [20]. A small piece of myocardium (5–8 mm × 5–8 mm) was excised and immediately stored in ice-cold cardioplegic solution for transportation to the lab. Using a stereomicroscope, small endocardial trabeculae (cross-sectional area < 0.8 mm^2) (LV: n = 18, RA: n = 28) were dissected off the larger piece of tissue.

2.4. Trabeculae Developed Force Experiments

The individual trabeculae were then moved to an organ bath where it was mounted on miniature hooks attached to a force-transducer and superfused with modified Tyrode's solution at 37 °C (127 mM NaCl, 2.3 mM KCl, 25 mM NaHCO$_3$, 0.6 mM MgSO$_4$, 1.3 mM KH$_2$PO$_4$, 2.5 mM CaCl$_2$, 11.2 mM glucose, 5IE/L insulin). The trabeculae were then electrically stimulated (STM1 Scientific Instruments) at 1 Hz (voltage 25% over threshold) and gradually stretched to reach the optimum preload, which is considered baseline. Developed force (systolic force—diastolic force) was recorded using a force transducer (Scientific instruments) and stored digitally (Labview) as well as with a thermorecorder (Graphtec Linearcorder WR 3320) for offline analysis. Baseline measurements were recorded and then trabeculae were treated with 10 μM SAHA or vehicle (DMSO) for 120 min. For selective HDAC inhibitor studies, data was collected using both low (Rodin-A: 2 μM; IRBM-D: 100 nM) and high (Rodin-A: 10 μM; IRBM-D: 250 nM) concentrations, in addition to a control group (DMSO 10 μM). Measurements were recorded at 15 min intervals for the entire 120 min treatment period for all trabeculae experiments. In profiling against isolated recombinant HDAC isoforms for inhibition of enzymatic activity, Rodin-A selectively inhibited the HDAC1 and HDAC2 isoforms. The half maximum inhibitory concentration (IC50) for HDAC1 and HDAC2 was 0.15 μM and 0.43 μM, respectively. IRBM-D selectively inhibited the HDAC1, HDAC2, and HDAC3 isoforms. The IC50 for HDAC1, HDAC2, and HDAC3 was 13 nM, 18 nM, and 11 nM, respectively. Detailed pharmacokinetic data has been previously reported [21,22].

2.5. Skinned Myocyte Functional Experiments

Skinned cardiomyocytes from human trabeculae were prepared as described previously [23]. Briefly, tissue was suspended in Isolation solution (108 mM KCl, 10 mM Imidazole, 8.9 mM KOH, 7.1 mM MgCl$_2$, 5.8 mM ATP, 2 mM EGTA) containing 0.5% Triton and 1:100 protease/phosphatase inhibitors (Halt, Thermo Fisher Scientific) and mechanically homogenized at 7000 RPM. The homogenate was then passed through a 70 μm filter and left on ice for 20 min. The filtered myocytes were pelleted by centrifugation at 120 RCF for 2 min and then resuspended in isolation solution without Triton. For the isolated adult feline ventricular myocytes (AFVMs), this same procedure was adopted except for mechanical homogenization and filtering.

To perform the active tension experiments, single cardiomyocytes were attached to two pins (one attached to a calibrated force transducer and the other to a piezo length controller) with UV-curing glue (Thor Labs, Newton, NJ, USA). The myocyte was then perfused with solutions of varying calcium concentration and the force exhibited by the cell in response to each was recorded and normalized to the myocyte cross-sectional area. The data were fit to a Hill equation to determine the F_{max} and EC_{50}. All experiments were performed at a sarcomere length of 2.1 μm and at room temperature. For the AFVM, n = 3 felines. For non-failing human, n = 7 patients.

To determine the myocyte passive tension, the cell was moved to a bath free of calcium. Using the length controller pin, the cell was next stretched in 0.2 μm increments from resting sarcomere length of 1.6–2.8 μm. The passive force at each sarcomere length was measured with the force transducer and normalized to the myocyte cross-sectional area. The data were fit to an exponential growth equation. These experiments were performed at room temperature. For the AFVM, n = 3 felines. For non-failing human, n = 7 patients.

2.6. Myofilament Protein Enrichment

Tissue was homogenized at 7000 RPM in a standard rigor buffer (SRB) containing 0.5% Triton and 1:100 protease/phosphatase inhibitors and left on ice for 20 min. The homogenate was then centrifuged at 1800 RCF to pellet the myofilament proteins. The pellet was washed twice in triton-free SRB by resuspension and centrifugation at 1800 RCF. The myofilament protein pellet was next solubilized in 9M urea, sonicated, and centrifuged at 10,000 RCF. The now solubilized myofilament proteins were collected as the supernatant and stored in aliquots at −80 °C. Protein concentration was determined by Pierce BCA Assay (Thermo Fisher Scientific).

2.7. Myofilament Immunoblots

Samples of 20 µg myofilament protein were combined in a 1:1 (v/v) ratio with SDS-Tris Glycine gel loading buffer (Novex) supplemented 1:5 with Bolt reducing buffer (Novex) and heated at 95 °C for 10 min. The samples were then loaded on 4–12% Bis Tris Plus gradient gels and proteins were separated by electrophoresis at 200 volts and then transferred onto a nitrocellulose membrane. The membrane was incubated in Revert Total Protein Stain (LICOR) to verify equal loading and serve as a loading control and then blocked for 1 h at room temperature in 1:1 0.1% Tween-TBS/Intercept TBS blocking buffer (LICOR). The Anti-Lysine Acetylation antibody (Cytoskeleton, 19C4B2.1) was added at 1:500 dilution in blocking buffer and incubated overnight at 4 °C. The blot was washed in TBS-T and then IR-dye donkey anti-mouse 680RD secondary antibody (LICOR) was added at 1:10,000 dilution for 1 hour at room temperature. The results were visualized using the Azure c600 imaging system and analyzed using LICOR Image Studio. For analysis, the lysine-acetylation signal was normalized to the total protein signal.

2.8. Mass Spectrometry

Myofilament protein lysates were separated by SDS-PAGE as above. The gel was then fixed in 50% methanol/10% acetic acid for 15 min and incubated in Coomassie Brilliant Blue for 30 min with gentle agitation, followed by destaining overnight (10% methanol, 7.5% acetic acid). Approximately 24 h after adding the destain solution, the gel was washed with HPLC-grade water twice for 1 h each.

The bands of interest (20 kDa) were cut from the gel and added to 1.5 mL Eppendorf tubes containing 100 mM ammonium bicarbonate. The tubes were incubated at 37 °C for 15 min and 600 RPM in a shaking incubator. The solution was discarded, replaced with a 1:1 (v/v) ammonium bicarbonate/acetonitrile solution, and then incubated again in the same fashion. After 15 min, a 100% acetonitrile solution was added, and the shaking incubation repeated. These three incubations constitute the "wash" step, which is repeated later. The gel pieces were next suspended in 250 mM DTT in 100 mM ammonium bicarbonate and incubated at 56 °C for 1 h and 600 RPM to reduce disulfide bonds. Alkylation was performed with 50 mM iodoacetamide in 100 mM ammonium bicarbonate at room temperature for 45 min in a dark room. Following this incubation, the iodoacetamide was removed and the wash step detailed above was repeated.

To digest the protein, 5 µg of Trypsin/LysC protease was added to the gel pieces in 200 µL 100 mM ammonium bicarbonate and incubated at 37 °C for 18 h and 600 RPM. The peptide-containing solution was then collected, and the gel pieces were washed twice in 50% acetonitrile/5% formic acid to collect the remaining peptides. The peptide solutions were dried by vacuum centrifugation, reconstituted in 3% acetonitrile/0.1% formic acid, and ~100 ng was subjected to high pressure liquid chromatography in a 25 cm PepMap RSLC C18 column coupled to tandem mass spectrometry on a LTQ Orbitrap XL mass spectrometer. Three technical replicates were run for each of the three samples in the vehicle and SAHA treatment groups. The acquired raw data files were analyzed using the Peaks Bioinformatics software and matched to the *Felis catus* proteome FASTA database downloaded from Uniprot. The fixed modification was cysteine carbamidomethylation (+57.02) and the variable modification was lysine acetylation (+42.01). For analysis, acetylated RLC peptides were normalized to total RLC peptides identified for each sample. Outliers greater than two standard deviations from the mean were removed.

2.9. Western Blot for Calcium Handling Proteins

Right atrium samples (n = 8 patients) were homogenized in homogenization buffer and protein concentration was determined using Pierce BCA assay (Thermo Fisher Scientific). A total amount of 10 µg of protein per sample was loaded on a 4–12%—Bis-TRIS Gradient

Gel (BioRad, Hercules, CA, USA) or in case of PLB a 16.5% TRIS-TRICINE-Gel (BioRad). Samples were transferred to nitrocellulose membranes (Amersham Protram) of 0.45 µm or 0.1 µm for PLB and probed with the following antibodies: GAPDH (Cell Signaling Technology #5174, Danvers MA, USA), RyR_2808_Ser (Badrilla #A010-30, Leeds, UK), ph-CaMKII Thr286 (Abcam #32678, Cambridge, UK), Serca2a (Badrilla #A010-20), Acetylated Lysine (Cell Signaling Technology # Ac-K-103), RyR-total (Abcam #2827), CamKII-total (Santa Cruz #sc-9035, Dallas, TX, USA), NCX (Abcam #177952), and Cav1.2 (Alomone Labs #ACC-003, Jerusalem, Israel). For secondary antibodies, HRP-conjugated ECL-Anti mouse IgG (GE Healthcare #NA931, Marlborough, MA, USA) and ECL-Anti Rabbit IgG (GE Healthcare #NA934) were used. Blots were imaged with the ChemiDoc Touch (BioRad) and band intensity was quantified using Image Lab Software 6.0.1 (BioRad).

2.10. Statistical Analysis

Data management and statistical analyses were performed using Graph Pad PRISM 7.05 (La Jolla, CA, USA). All data are expressed as the mean ± the standard error. Comparisons of two independent groups were performed using a two-sided Student's t-test for unpaired samples or Mann–Whitney test in the case where data were not normally distributed. Normality distribution was assessed by using Shapiro–Wilk normality test. When three or more groups were included, one-way ANOVA was performed. For the functional measurements in human trabeculae, a repeated measure two-way ANOVA was performed. If a significant interaction was identified, the Tukey post-hoc test for multiple comparisons was used. Two-sided testing was used for all statistical tests. A p-value of ≤ 0.05 was used to determine significance for all statistical tests. The data that supports the images and plots within this paper, as well as other findings from this study, are available from the corresponding author upon reasonable request.

3. Results

3.1. SAHA Improves Cardiomyocyte Contractility and Calcium Handling

We assessed the acute effects of SAHA treatment on cardiomyocyte function using adult feline ventricular myocytes (AFVM) isolated from healthy males. Freshly isolated cells were treated with 2.5 µM SAHA or vehicle (Dimethyl sulfoxide (DMSO)) for 90 min and then paced using field stimulation (0.5 Hz). Once cells reached a steady state, contractions and calcium transients were recorded. Representative traces for the contraction and calcium transient are shown in Figure 1A,E. There was a significant increase in contraction magnitude assessed by fractional shortening in SAHA vs. vehicle cells (veh: 6.36 ± 0.71 vs. SAHA: 4.00 ± 0.36; p = 0.0099), in addition to faster relaxation kinetics (time to 50% baseline) (0.67 s ± 0.05 vs. 0.55 s ± 0.04; p = 0.0142) and return velocity (0.34 µm/s ± 0.05 vs. 0.87 µm/s ± 0.15; p = 0.0250) (Figure 1B–D). While there was no difference in peak calcium transients between groups (Figure 1F), there was a significant shortening of the recovery phase of calcium transients, reflected by the time to 30% of fluorescence signal decay (Time to BL 30%) in SAHA vs. veh-treated cells (0.37 s ± 0.02 vs. 0.30 s ± 0.01; p = 0.0044) (Figure 1G). The time to 30% return to BL was selected because mammals with long action potential duration have two phases of calcium reuptake with the first phase being primarily mediated by sarcoendoplasmic reticulum calcium transport ATPase (SERCA), while the second phase includes a contribution of the sodium–calcium exchanger (NCX), which is activated with repolarization [24]. Choosing 30% to BL is a conservative approach to capture primarily the first phase where SERCA is active. Tau, which is the time constant of the rate of cytosolic Ca^{2+} removal, was also significantly improved with SAHA vs. vehicle (0.64 s ± 0.07 vs. 0.47 s ± 0.04; p = 0.0276) (Figure 1H). Taken together, SAHA increased contraction magnitude and relaxation velocity and accelerated cytosolic Ca^{2+} removal without altering the peak calcium transients.

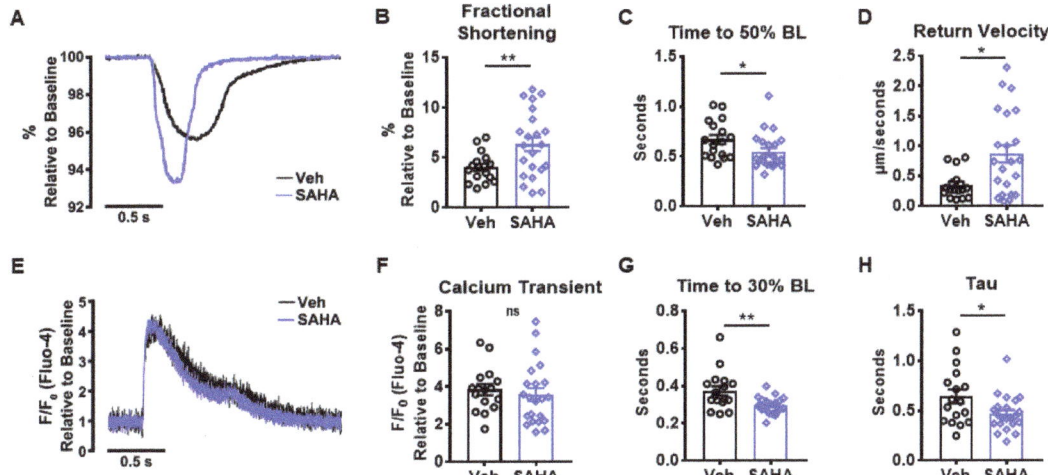

Figure 1. Effect of SAHA treatment on AFVM function. AFVM were isolated and incubated with SAHA or vehicle (2.5 µM) for 90 min, then incubated with Fluo-4am and Pluronic™ F-127 before functional measurements were acquired. (**A**) Representative contraction of SAHA treated vs. vehicle AFVM, which had an improvement in (**B**) fractional shortening, (**C**) Time to 50% baseline of contraction and (**D**) return velocity. (**E**) Representative calcium transient showing no difference between SAHA and vehicle-treated AFVM (**F**) peak calcium transient, but there was a decrease in (**G**) time to 30% baseline and (**H**) tau; n = 17–22 myocytes/parameter from 4 felines. Fractional shortening and tau were analyzed using two-sided Student's *t*-test. Time to 50% BL, return velocity, calcium transient, and time to 30% BL were analyzed using Mann–Whitney test. NS stands for not significant. * $p < 0.05$, ** $p < 0.01$. Data shown are means ± SEM.

3.2. SAHA Treatment Increases Myofilament Calcium Sensitivity

To assess the acute direct effect of SAHA on the sarcomere and differentiate myofilament from calcium cycling [25] effects, AFVM treated with 2.5 µM SAHA or vehicle for 90 min underwent a skinned myocyte isolation procedure. The membrane is exposed to triton detergent to chemically permeabilize all membranous structures including the nucleus, sarcolemma, sarcoplasmic reticulum, mitochondria, and other subcellular organelles, leaving only intact myofilaments [26]. This allows for direct assessment of myofilament function. Figure 2A shows average force–calcium relationship for SAHA and vehicle-treated skinned myocytes. There was a significant leftward shift with SAHA treatment. EC_{50} is the calcium concentration at which force is 50% of the maximum and representative of myofilament calcium sensitivity [23]. SAHA significantly reduced EC_{50} compared to veh (1.18 ± 0.07 µM vs. 0.95 ± 0.05 µM; $p = 0.0092$), indicating an increase in calcium sensitivity (Figure 2B). Maximal calcium-activated force (F_{max}) was also significantly increased with SAHA treatment (15.24 ± 1.11 mN/mm^2 vs. 20.68 ± 2.19 mN/mm^2; $p = 0.0397$) (Figure 2C). Furthermore, there was a significant decrease in passive stiffness at increasing sarcomere lengths (Figure 2D). These data indicate that SAHA treatment significantly altered several indices of myofilament function, including calcium sensitivity, F_{max}, and passive stiffness.

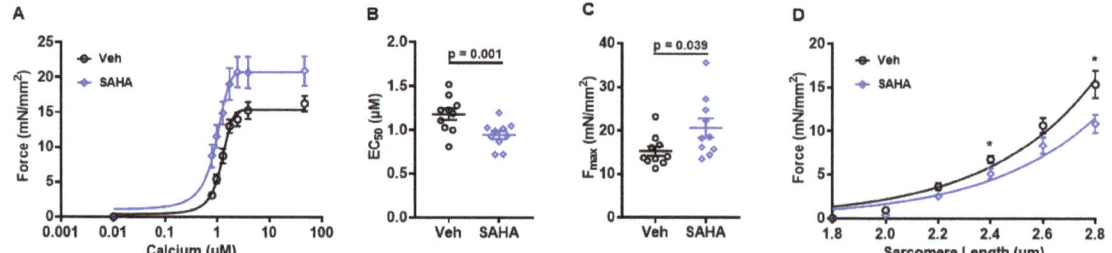

Figure 2. Effect of SAHA treatment on AFVM myofilament function. Skinned myocytes were isolated from AFVM to assess myofilament function. The (**A**) average force-calcium curves for SAHA and vehicle-treated skinned myocytes demonstrate a clear left shift with SAHA treatment. There was a decrease in the (**B**) EC_{50} with SAHA treatment, indicating an increase in myofilament calcium sensitivity and an increase in (**C**) maximal calcium-activated force (F_{max}); n = 10 myocytes from 3 felines for each group. There was a decrease in (**D**) passive stiffness at increasing sarcomere lengths. n = 8 vehicle treated myocytes from 3 felines, n = 10 SAHA-treated myocytes from 3 felines. All analysis was performed using a two-sided Student's *t*-test. * $p < 0.05$ Data shown are means ± SEM.

3.3. SAHA Treatment Alters Myosin Regulatory Light Chain Acetylation

Next, we aimed to assess the underlying mechanisms of SAHA-related effects and identify substrates for acetylation/deacetylation that influence cardiac function. As an HDAC inhibitor, SAHA blocks the removal of lysine acetyl groups. Based on the improvement in AFVM myofilament function with SAHA treatment, we hypothesized that myofilament acetylation would be increased as well. There was no significant difference in global AFVM myofilament acetylation between groups treated with vehicle or SAHA (Figure 3A,B). However, there was one distinct band at approximately 20 kDa that displayed significantly increased acetylation (1.00 ± 0.08 vs. 1.99 ± 0.20; $p = 0.0011$) (Figure 3C). To confirm the identity of this 20 kDa band, it was run on an SDS-PAGE/Coomassie gel, excised, and analyzed by mass spectrometry (MS) (Figure 3D). The band contained primarily myosin regulatory light chain (RLC, MYL2, MLC-2), which was significantly acetylated with SAHA treatment (0.04 ± 0.002 vs. 0.06 ± 0.004; $p = 0.0098$) (Figure 3E). One specific RLC site, lysine 115 (K115), had a significant increase in acetylation (0.002 ± 0.001 vs. 0.01 ± 0.002; $p = 0.0444$) (Figure 3F).

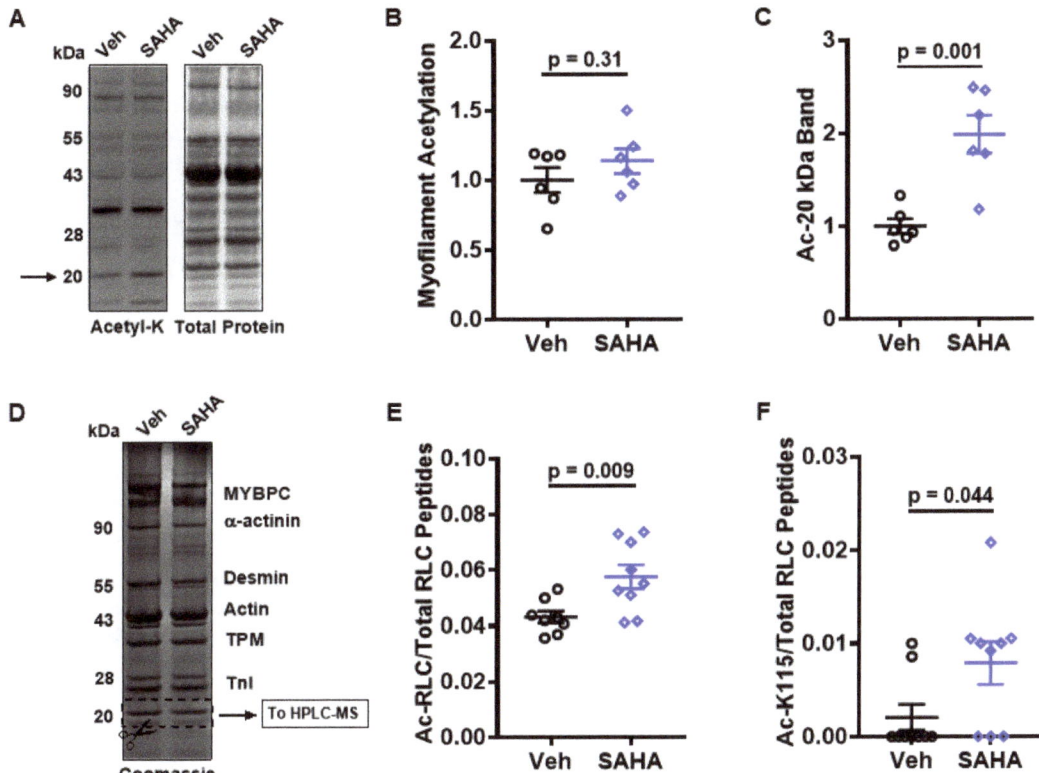

Figure 3. Effect of SAHA on myofilament acetylation. The myofilament acetylation was assessed in acutely treated AFVM (**A–F**). Western Blot analysis revealed that (**A,B**) total myofilament acetylation was not increased with SAHA treatment but there was significantly more (**C**) acetylation at a 20 kDa band (indicated with arrow in (**A**)); n = 6 felines per group. (**D**) Coomassie staining was performed, and the band was cut out for mass spectrometry analysis, which revealed that this 20 kDa band with (**E**) increased acetylation is the myosin regulatory light chain with one (**F**) specific residue (lysine 115) driving the increase in acetylation; n = 3 felines per group, 3 technical replicates per sample. All analysis was performed using a two-sided Student's *t*-test. Data shown are means ± SEM

3.4. SAHA Treatment Improves Developed Force and Diastolic Tension in Non-Failing Human Ventricular Myocardium

To validate the findings from AFVMs using a more translational approach, we repeated several experiments using left ventricle trabeculae isolated from non-failing human hearts. Trabeculae allow for the assessment of multicellular function in human intact myocardium [20,27–31]. For this study, trabeculae were used to assess the direct acute effects of SAHA. Ventricular trabeculae were isolated from non-failing human donor hearts, which were not suitable for transplantation (Table S1). SAHA-treated trabeculae had a less pronounced decrease in developed force over time (natural run down) (Figure 4A) with a similar systolic peak force (Figure S2A), although diastolic tension (Figure 4B) was significantly decreased. These findings are in line with the decreased passive stiffness we observed in vivo [5] and ex vivo. Furthermore, the maximum rate of force rise (dF/dt_{max}) normalized to diastolic tension was increased by SAHA treatment (Figure 4C). The maximum rate of force decay (dF/dt_{min}) was not different between groups (Figure S2B). These findings suggest increased contractility and decreased diastolic tension with SAHA treatment.

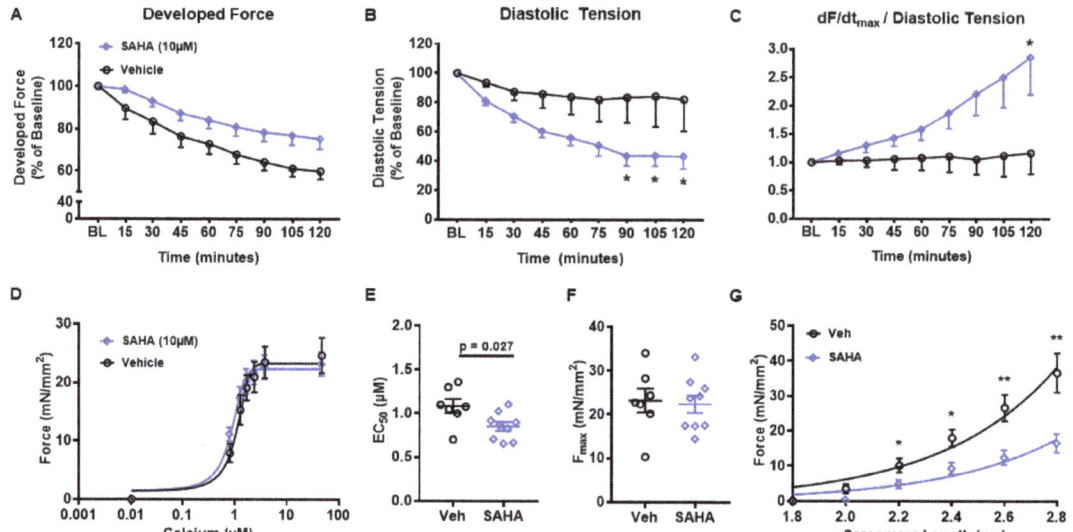

Figure 4. Effect of acute SAHA treatment on human trabeculae. Trabeculae were isolated from biopsies of non-failing human LV. There was an increase in (**A**) developed force and decreased (**B**) diastolic tension with SAHA treatment, with an increase in (**C**) dF/dt$_{max}$/diastolic tension; n = 5–13 trabeculae per parameter from 7 patients. Myofilaments were isolated from human LV trabeculae. There was a slight left shift in the (**D**) average force-calcium curve with SAHA treatment. SAHA-treated samples had a reduction in (**E**) EC$_{50}$, indicating an increase in myofilament calcium sensitivity but no difference in (**F**) F$_{max}$; n = 7 control myocytes from 3 patients, 9 SAHA from 3 patients. SAHA-treated samples had a decrease in (**G**) passive stiffness at increasing sarcomere lengths; n = 7 myocytes from 3 patients in each group. For trabeculae functional experiments (**A**–**C**), repeated measure two-way ANOVA was performed. For the myofilament functional experiments (**D**–**G**), analysis was performed using a two-sided Student's *t*-test. * $p < 0.05$, ** $p < 0.01$. Data shown are means ± SEM.

3.5. SAHA Treatment Enhances Myofilament Calcium Sensitivity in Non-Failing Human Ventricular Myocardium

Myofilaments were then isolated from the human trabeculae samples. Figure 4D shows the average force-calcium curves for SAHA and vehicle-treated samples. Just as in the SAHA-treated AFVM skinned myocytes, there was a significant decrease in EC$_{50}$ (1.08 ± 0.08 vs. 0.85 ± 0.05; p = 0.0266) (Figure 4E) with no change between groups for F$_{max}$ (Figure 4F). Consistent with our findings in AFVM, there was a significant decrease in passive stiffness at increasing sarcomere lengths with SAHA treatment (Figure 4G). Thus, SAHA treatment increases calcium sensitivity in human myocardium and at the same time reduces passive stiffness.

We assessed the protein abundance of key cardiac calcium-handling proteins in human myocardium to assess if they are involved in SAHA-mediated effects. There was no significant difference in protein abundance of phosphorylated calcium/calmodulin-dependent protein kinase (pCaMKII T286), CaMKII, sarcoendoplasmic reticulum calcium transport ATPase (SERCA), sodium-calcium exchanger 1 (NCX1), ryanodine receptor (Ryr), Ryr serine 2808, Cav1.2, Cav1.2 150 kDa, and Cav1.2 75 kDa. These findings suggest that improvemenst in cardiac function with SAHA treatment are not due to changes in the abundance or activity levels of these proteins (Figure 5A–J).

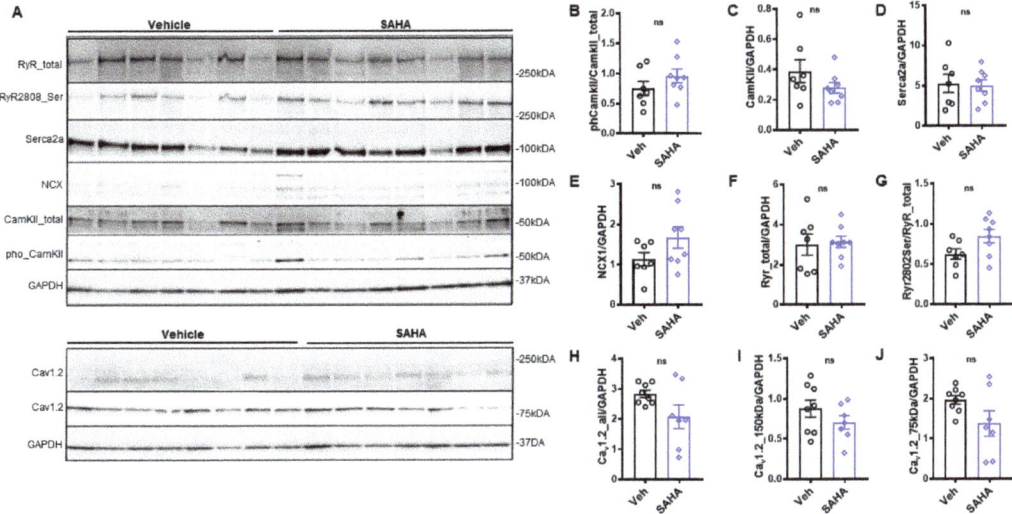

Figure 5. Effect of acute SAHA treatment on abundance of calcium handling proteins. Western Blots (**A**) of right atrium trabeculae after being treated with vehicle or SAHA. There was no change in protein abundance with SAHA treatment for (**B**) phosphorylated calcium/calmodulin-dependent protein kinase (pCaMKII T286), (**C**) CaMKII, (**D**) sarcoendoplasmic reticulum calcium transport ATPase (SERCA), (**E**) sodium–calcium exchanger 1 (NCX1), (**F**) ryanodine receptor (Ryr), (**G**) Ryr serine 2808, (**H**) Cav1.2, (**I**) Cav1.2 150 kDa, and (**J**) Cav1.2 75 kDa; n = 7–8 samples per protein from 8 patients. All analysis was performed using a two-sided Student's t-test. ns stands for not significant. Data shown are means ± SEM.

3.6. Isoform Selective HDAC Inhibition Increases Developed Force in Dose Dependent Manner

To harness the potential of HDACi to treat cardiovascular diseases, safer compounds may be required to enable long-term treatment. Therefore, more selective inhibitors of HDACs were explored to assess whether improved selectivity could maintain efficacy and minimize the dose-limiting toxicities, but with limited success so far [21]. Italfarmaco has designed new HDACi core scaffolds that maintain the inhibitory activity toward HDAC1 and HDAC2 and optimize the structure–activity relationship (SAR) for hematological safety in patients. In order to determine if this improvement in myocardial function is conserved with a more targeted approach, we evaluated the effect of these isoform selective HDAC inhibitors on non-failing human atrial trabeculae. Two class I-selective HDAC inhibitors, Rodin-A (inhibits HDAC 1 + 2) and IRBM-D (inhibits HDAC 1 + 2 + 3) were tested at high and low concentrations vs. vehicle (DMSO). The higher concentrations of Rodin-A and IRBM-D both caused a significant acute increase in developed force vs. the vehicle-treated group (Rodin-A: 94.5% ± 11.3%, n = 8; IRBM-D: 100.2% ± 7.7%, n = 7; veh: 70.7% ± 5.4%, n = 8; $p < 0.05$) (Figure 6A). There was also an increase in dF/dt$_{max}$ and dF/dt$_{min}$ with the higher concentration treatment (Figure 6B,C). This effect appears to be dose dependent as lower concentrations of Rodin-A and IRBM-D have blunted effects on developed force and kinetics (Figure 6D–F). This data provides proof of concept for the potential effectiveness of isoform selective HDAC inhibitors in human myocardium.

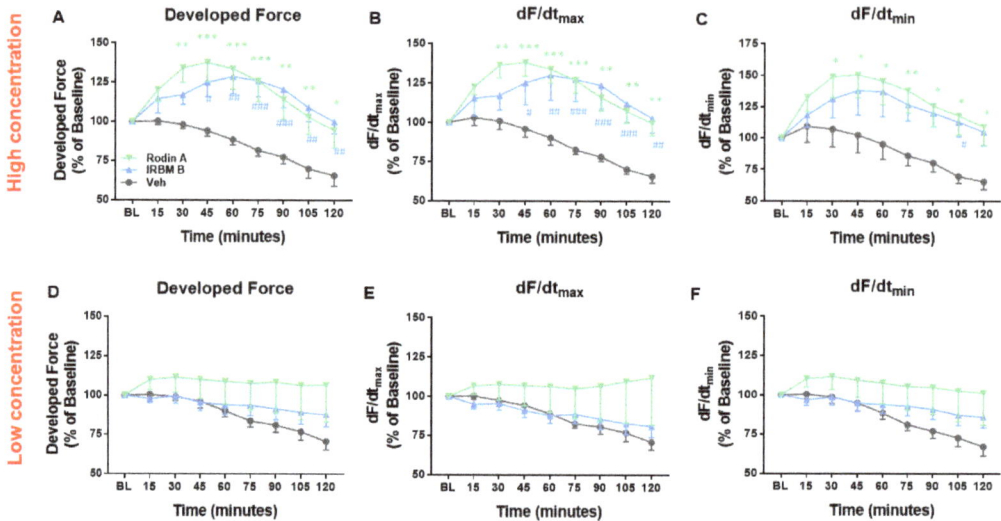

Figure 6. Effect of isoform selective HDAC inhibition on non-failing human trabeculae. Trabeculae were isolated from right atrial appendages (RAA) and treated with Rodin-A, IRBM-D, or vehicle at high or low concentrations. (**A**) Developed force, (**B**) dF/dt_{max}, and (**C**) dF/dt_{min} were all increased with high concentrations of Rodin-A and IRBM-D compared to vehicle treatment. There was no significant difference (**D**) developed force, (**E**) dF/dt_{max}, and (**F**) dF/dt_{min} in the lower concentration-treated groups compared to vehicle; high concentration: Rodin-A, n = 8 trabeculae; IRBM-D, n = 9 trabeculae; low concentration: Rodin-A, n = 7 trabeculae; IRBM-D, n = 13 trabeculae; vehicle, n = 8 trabeculae. RAA trabeculae were isolated from 30 patients. All analysis was performed using repeated measure two-way ANOVA. * $p < 0.05$, ** $p < 0.01$, *** $p < 0.001$ Rodin-A vs. vehicle, # $p < 0.05$, ## $p < 0.01$, ### $p < 0.001$ IRBM-D vs. vehicle. Data shown are means ± SEM.

4. Discussion

We previously [5] described the effects of SAHA in a large animal model of slow progressive pressure overload, recapitulating features of human HFpEF. We provided evidence supporting several potential mechanisms but there were many unanswered questions regarding how SAHA regulates cardiac function. This study was designed to develop a deeper understanding of how SAHA modulates function at the level of the cardiomyocyte and its contractile components. Furthermore, this study is the first to describe the effects of SAHA on human ventricular myocardium and extend these findings by performing parallel experiments using tissue derived from a large mammal with comparable physiological features. Using a systematic approach, we assessed the effect of SAHA on global cardiomyocyte function, myofilament function, and protein acetylation. Our study identified significant changes upon SAHA treatment in three cardiac properties—(1) increased contractility; (2) accelerated relaxation, and (3) decreased passive tension, suggestive of multiple sites of action on a cellular/molecular level.

4.1. SAHA Improves Contractility in Feline and Human Myocardium via Increasing Myofilament Calcium Sensitivity

In vivo SAHA treatment increased speckle-tracking-based global radial strain in our feline model [5]. In vitro data from the current study confirm these findings. SAHA increased fractional shortening in AFVMs and developed force in human non-failing myocardium. SAHA also induced a significant increase in the maximal rate of force rise (dF/dt_{max}) when normalized to diastolic tension. These findings suggest that SAHA treatment exerts positive inotropic effects, as the trabeculae generated similar peak systolic forces at lower diastolic tension (preload) compared to the vehicle-treated group [32].

In HFpEF patients, limited systolic reserve also affects diastolic function because recoil and suction forces during early diastole are attenuated [33], thus, improved contractility by SAHA may indirectly improve diastolic function. It is important to note that the increase in contractility is not mediated via an increase in calcium transients, which is an unfavorable mode of action in patients with heart failure. Several clinical trials have reported increased mortality and progression of heart failure among patients treated with inotropes, which alter intracellular calcium concentrations due to increased myocardial oxygen demand and arrhythmias. Emerging therapies to improve cardiac function via optimizing metabolism (mitotropes; e.g., SGLT2-inhibitors) or increasing sarcomere function (myotropes; e.g., omecamtiv mecarbil) may provide useful alternatives in the future [34]. In this regard, SAHA might be another promising candidate, since inotropy is mediated via calcium-independent mechanisms. In skinned myocyte experiments, we showed that ex-vivo acute treatment of AFVM and human myofilaments resulted in increased calcium sensitivity with SAHA treatment, reflected by a leftward shift of the force-calcium curve. Myofilament calcium sensitivity reflects the contractile response of the myofilaments to a given calcium concentration [35]. Troponin I (TnI) phosphorylation on multiple residues via protein kinase A contributes significantly to calcium-sensitive force production and myofilament relaxation. A single phosphorylation of TnI at serine 23 and 24 accelerates relaxation, but decreases contractility, thus enhancement in myocardial calcium sensitivity may slow down relaxation [36,37]. In our study we found a hastened relaxation and ruled out the contribution of classic key cardiac calcium handling proteins, suggesting alternative and several mechanisms underlying the effects of SAHA.

4.2. SAHA Increases Relaxation by Accelerating Cytosolic Calcium Removal

We previously described that in vivo SAHA treatment shortened the phase of linear relaxation duration on a myofibrillar level, which correlated with invasively measured indices of diastolic function (tau, LVEDP) [5]. While there is a growing body of evidence describing the impact of HDAC inhibition on the cardiovascular system, there is little evidence describing the effects of SAHA on cardiomyocyte function. The studies currently available in the literature describe the effect on cardiomyocytes isolated from rodents [13,14]. Meraviglia et al. reported increased SERCA2 acetylation and activity after SAHA treatment in cardiomyocytes isolated from healthy adult rats [13]. This study found no change in the amplitude or time to peak calcium transient between control and SAHA treated groups, in line with our findings. Tau, used as a surrogate for cytosolic calcium clearing, which was improved in the SAHA-treated cells, as was the time to 10%, 50%, and 90% decay in the fluorescence signal. We also found a shortening in tau and time to 30% BL, representing accelerated calcium reuptake. Meraviglia et al. also reported increased SERCA ATPase activity with SAHA treatment in microsomes isolated from both rat cardiomyocytes and HL-1 cells (AT-1 mouse atrial cardiomyocyte tumor lineage), which would be an explanation for increased rate of calcium removal [13]. However, they did not report differences in the contractility of the cell, with no change in fractional shortening or maximal rate of shortening but did note an increase in the maximal rate of re-lengthening. In our study, we saw a significant increase in fractional shortening with no difference in peak calcium in SAHA vs. veh-treated AFVMs, which is suggestive of increased myofilament calcium sensitivity. Bocchi et al. [14] assessed the effects of SAHA on cell contractility and calcium dynamics in unloaded ventricular myocytes isolated from the heart of control and diabetic rats. Although fractional shortening was unaltered, the maximal rate of shortening ($-dL/dt_{max}$) and time to peak calcium transient (TTP) were improved by SAHA. A potential explanation for the differences in results between this study and previous reports are differences in physiological properties between a rodent and a larger mammal, including prolonged action potential duration and myosin heavy chain composition (αMHC vs. βMHC) [15,16]. The physiological properties of felines more closely mimic those of humans, making the model highly valuable for translational research. We provide robust evidence of increased relaxation kinetics and cytosolic calcium removal with SAHA treatment. These effects together with improved myofibrillar relaxation (previously shown by our group) could explain the net improvements in in vivo diastolic function (reduction in LVEDP) seen in our model [5] despite an increase in myofilament calcium sensitivity.

The most consistent finding throughout the different aspects of this study is that SAHA decreases passive stiffness. Initially, diastolic tension was significantly decreased in intact trabeculae. Myofilaments isolated from treated AFVM and human trabeculae had a significant decrease in passive stiffness with SAHA treatment. The mechanism driving this beneficial functional change is unclear. We speculate that post-translational modification of the microtubule and/or titin may play a role.

4.3. Myosin Regulatory Light Chain Acetylation Is Increased with SAHA Treatment

Based on the evidence that HDACs can mediate post-translational modifications and the observed changes in myofilament function with SAHA treatment, assessing the myofilament for changes in acetylation was the clear next step. There was a significant increase in acetylation of a band at around 20 kDa, which mass spectrometry analysis revealed to be myosin regulatory light chain (RLC). More specifically, lysine 115 (K115) was heavily acetylated with SAHA treatment. The RLC and essential light chain (ELC) are part of the neck region of the myosin motor that is an essential part of muscle contraction [38]. Both the RLC and ELC can alter muscle contraction by mediating changes in myosin motor activity, again highlighting their importance in the function of muscle [38]. While few studies have looked at acetylation of myosin or the associated light chains, two proteomic-based reports have described cardiac acetylation of different species. The guinea pig cardiac lysine acetylome had similar acetylation to the AFVM in this study but did not note K115 [39]. In another study, top-down mass spectrometry was performed in both human and swine atrial and ventricular tissue. Both human and swine atrial RLC were found to be N^{α}-acetylated, but the significance of this finding was unclear and once again K115 was not noted [40]. Both studies described the proteome but did not report any functional findings to supplement the characterization. In this study, we narrowed our focus to the cardiomyocyte and myofilament to better understand how SAHA exerts its beneficial effects and provide evidence for a potential novel mechanism for pan-HDAC inhibition to directly impact cardiac function. Previous studies have reported co-localization of HDAC2 and myofibrils but did not report the substrate [41]. We provided evidence of a substrate via the acetylation of RLC K115. The current literature on cardiac acetylation is more descriptive and lacks functional analysis [39,40], but our study provides a functional assessment in addition to the proteomic data.

Since previous clinical trials using pan-HDAC inhibitors reported adverse effects such as leukocytopenia, thrombocytopenia, gastrointestinal symptoms, and QT interval prolongation [42], a more targeted approach may be needed to improve the safety profile of this class of drugs. Therefore, we assessed the functional effects of isoform-selective HDAC inhibitors, which are not commercially available. In this proof-of-concept study, we found a dose-dependent increase in developed force and twitch kinetics in human atrial tissue when inhibiting class 1 HDACs 1 + 2 using Rodin-A and HDACs 1 + 2 + 3 using IRBM-D. Future studies are warranted to delineate molecular and myofilament changes.

We report for the first time the effects of SAHA on human cardiac tissue and provide functional insights using live twitching human trabeculae. In the current study, we have provided evidence of a potential new mechanism for pan-HDAC inhibition improving cardiac function by improving myofilament calcium sensitivity. Importantly, we identified a potential substrate for hyperacetylation via SAHA that may be in direct control of cardiac contractility. The impact on relaxation is likely explained by (1) faster diastolic Ca^{2+} removal from the cytosol seen in isolated AFVMs; (2) improved myofibril relaxation [5] (recently reported by our group); and (3) improved contractility, which affects recoil and suction force during diastole (in vivo) [33]. We could not determine what underlying mechanisms are driving the improved passive tension, but it might be due to acetylation changes on myofilament proteins, titin, and/or microtubules as well.

Since the experiments described above were performed using a relatively acute period of HDAC inhibition treatment, the beneficial effects are likely due to post-translational modification by a direct effect of increased myofilament protein acetylation and not due to epigenetic effects (altering gene expression). It is important to point out, however, that we previously studied the effect of chronic SAHA treatment [5], which may lead to changes in gene expression and likely have broader cellular effects. Thus, we cannot rule out whether elevated RLC acetylation and myofilament calcium sensitivity is limited to the acute phase or if these are lasting changes. Future studies are needed to parse out the effects of acute and chronic SAHA administration.

These findings suggest that SAHA exerts multiple effects to culminate in improved cardiac function. The experiments performed were essential for laying the foundation for future studies that can have a more targeted focus on delineating mechanistic insights.

5. Limitations

Human HFpEF is a complex clinical syndrome and cannot be fully recapitulated in any animal model. However, the feline model used does capture several key clinical characteristics (i.e., elevated filing pressures, diastolic dysfunction, pulmonary hypertension, LV hypertrophy, LA dilation, and impaired function), making it a suitable platform for testing therapies. These animals are young (2 months of age at start of study) and have no metabolic comorbidities. Non-failing human cardiac tissue is rare and samples are available in limited quantities. This constrained the analyses that could be performed and did not allow for the development of an in-depth molecular component of the study using human cardiac tissue. Western blot analysis for abundance of key calcium handling proteins was performed using atrial tissue. While ventricular tissue would have been ideal, freshly harvested atrial tissue was available, and this allowed for us to assess the effect of SAHA compared to vehicle on live human myocardium. While we focused primarily on the myofilament, changes to titin or microtubules could also play a role in mediating the functional improvements observed. We did not perform any titin or microtubule-related experiments as they were beyond the scope of the study.

Supplementary Materials: The following supporting information can be downloaded at: https://www.mdpi.com/article/10.3390/pharmaceutics14071509/s1, Figure S1: Study Design; Figure S2: Effect of SAHA on trabeculae function; Table S1: Patient Characteristics.

Author Contributions: M.W., P.P.R., S.R.H. and J.A.K. conceived and designed the project. D.M.E., T.G.M., M.K., N.D., A.K., K.S., S.L.-H., M.P., T.K. and H.M. acquired the samples and data. D.M.E. and M.W. drafted the manuscript. T.G.M., D.V.L., A.Z., T.A.M., P.P.R., S.R.H. and J.A.K. critically revised the manuscript for key intellectual content. All authors have read and agreed to the published version of the manuscript.

Funding: This work was supported by the National Institute of Health [grant numbers HL147558 to S.R.H. and T.A.M., R01HL136737 to J.A.K.], the American Heart Association [grant number Predoctoral Fellowship 20PRE35170045 to T.G.M.], ERA-CVD (P.P.R.), Austrian Science Fund [grant number I 4168-B to P.P.R.], Medical University of Graz—Start Funding Program (M.W.), Austrian National Cardiac Society—Project Related Grant (M.W.).

Institutional Review Board Statement: All animal procedures were approved by the Lewis Katz School of Medicine Temple University Institutional Animal Care and Use Committee. The Ethical Committee of the Medical University of Graz approved the usage of human samples in this study. All experiments were conducted in accordance with the Declaration of Helsinki.

Informed Consent Statement: Informed consent was obtained for all atrial myocardium used. IRB approval was granted for use of ventricular myocardium collected from donor patients.

Data Availability Statement: Data is contained within the article or supplementary material.

Acknowledgments: We thank Christian Steinkuhler and Andrea Stevenazzi at Italfarmaco for providing the isoform selective HDAC inhibitors and for their assistance in designing the experiments using these compounds.

Conflicts of Interest: T.A.M. is on the SABs of Artemes Bio and Eikonizo Therapeutics, received funding from Italfarmaco for an unrelated project, and has a subcontract from Eikonizo Therapeutics for an SBIR grant from the National Institutes of Health (HL154959) J.A.K. received funding from Edgewise Therapeutics and Myokardia for unrelated projects.

References

1. Savarese, G.; Lund, L.H. Global Public Health Burden of Heart Failure. *Card. Fail. Rev.* **2017**, *3*, 7–11. [CrossRef]
2. Cao, D.J.; Wang, Z.V.; Battiprolu, P.K.; Jiang, N.; Morales, C.R.; Kong, Y.; Rothermel, B.A.; Gillette, T.G.; Hill, J.A. Histone deacetylase (HDAC) inhibitors attenuate cardiac hypertrophy by suppressing autophagy. *Proc. Natl. Acad. Sci. USA* **2011**, *108*, 4123–4128. [CrossRef] [PubMed]
3. Anker, S.D.; Butler, J.; Filippatos, G.; Ferreira, J.P.; Bocchi, E.; Böhm, M.; Brunner–La Rocca, H.-P.; Choi, D.-J.; Chopra, V.; Chuquiure-Valenzuela, E.; et al. Empagliflozin in Heart Failure with a Preserved Ejection Fraction. *N. Engl. J. Med.* **2021**, *385*, 1451–1461. [CrossRef]
4. Roh, J.; Houstis, N.; Rosenzweig, A. Why Don't We Have Proven Treatments for HFpEF? *Circ. Res.* **2017**, *120*, 1243–1245. [CrossRef]
5. Wallner, M.; Eaton, D.M.; Berretta, R.M.; Liesinger, L.; Schittmayer, M.; Gindlhuber, J.; Wu, J.; Jeong, M.Y.; Lin, Y.H.; Borghetti, G.; et al. HDAC inhibition improves cardiopulmonary function in a feline model of diastolic dysfunction. *Sci. Transl. Med.* **2020**, *12*, eaay7205. [CrossRef] [PubMed]
6. Wallner, M.; Eaton, D.M.; Berretta, R.M.; Borghetti, G.; Wu, J.; Baker, S.T.; Feldsott, E.A.; Sharp, T.E., 3rd; Mohsin, S.; Oyama, M.A.; et al. A Feline HFpEF Model with Pulmonary Hypertension and Compromised Pulmonary Function. *Sci. Rep.* **2017**, *7*, 16587. [CrossRef]
7. Ferrari, R.; Luscher, T.F. Reincarnated medicines: Using out-dated drugs for novel indications. *Eur. Heart J.* **2016**, *37*, 2571–2576. [CrossRef]
8. Grant, S.; Easley, C.; Kirkpatrick, P. Vorinostat. *Nat. Rev. Drug Discov.* **2007**, *6*, 21–22. [CrossRef]
9. McKinsey, T.A. Isoform-selective HDAC inhibitors: Closing in on translational medicine for the heart. *J. Mol. Cell. Cardiol.* **2011**, *51*, 491–496. [CrossRef]
10. McKinsey, T.A. Therapeutic potential for HDAC inhibitors in the heart. *Annu. Rev. Pharmacol. Toxicol.* **2012**, *52*, 303–319. [CrossRef]
11. Zhang, C.L.; McKinsey, T.A.; Chang, S.; Antos, C.L.; Hill, J.A.; Olson, E.N. Class II histone deacetylases act as signal-responsive repressors of cardiac hypertrophy. *Cell* **2002**, *110*, 479–488. [CrossRef]
12. Woulfe, K.C.; Ferrara, C.; Pioner, J.M.; Mahaffey, J.H.; Coppini, R.; Scellini, B.; Ferrantini, C.; Piroddi, N.; Tesi, C.; Poggesi, C.; et al. A Novel Method of Isolating Myofibrils From Primary Cardiomyocyte Culture Suitable for Myofibril Mechanical Study. *Front. Cardiovasc. Med.* **2019**, *6*, 12. [CrossRef] [PubMed]
13. Meraviglia, V.; Bocchi, L.; Sacchetto, R.; Florio, M.C.; Motta, B.M.; Corti, C.; Weichenberger, C.X.; Savi, M.; D'Elia, Y.; Rosato-Siri, M.D.; et al. HDAC Inhibition Improves the Sarcoendoplasmic Reticulum Ca(2+)-ATPase Activity in Cardiac Myocytes. *Int. J. Mol. Sci.* **2018**, *19*, 419. [CrossRef] [PubMed]
14. Bocchi, L.; Motta, B.M.; Savi, M.; Vilella, R.; Meraviglia, V.; Rizzi, F.; Galati, S.; Buschini, A.; Lazzaretti, M.; Pramstaller, P.P.; et al. The Histone Deacetylase Inhibitor Suberoylanilide Hydroxamic Acid (SAHA) Restores Cardiomyocyte Contractility in a Rat Model of Early Diabetes. *Int. J. Mol. Sci.* **2019**, *20*, 1873. [CrossRef]
15. Bers, D.M. Cardiac excitation-contraction coupling. *Nature* **2002**, *415*, 198–205. [CrossRef]
16. Marian, A.J.; Yu, Q.T.; Mann, D.L.; Graham, F.L.; Roberts, R. Expression of a mutation causing hypertrophic cardiomyopathy disrupts sarcomere assembly in adult feline cardiac myocytes. *Circ. Res.* **1995**, *77*, 98–106. [CrossRef]
17. Bailey, B.A.; Houser, S.R. Sarcoplasmic reticulum-related changes in cytosolic calcium in pressure-overload-induced feline LV hypertrophy. *Am. J. Physiol.* **1993**, *265*, H2009–H2016. [CrossRef]
18. Nuss, H.B.; Houser, S.R. Voltage dependence of contraction and calcium current in severely hypertrophied feline ventricular myocytes. *J. Mol. Cell. Cardiol.* **1991**, *23*, 717–726. [CrossRef]
19. Silver, L.H.; Hemwall, E.L.; Marino, T.A.; Houser, S.R. Isolation and morphology of calcium-tolerant feline ventricular myocytes. *Am. J. Physiol.* **1983**, *245*, H891–H896. [CrossRef]
20. Wallner, M.; Kolesnik, E.; Ablasser, K.; Khafaga, M.; Wakula, P.; Ljubojevic, S.; Thon-Gutschi, E.M.; Sourij, H.; Kapl, M.; Edmunds, N.J.; et al. Exenatide exerts a PKA-dependent positive inotropic effect in human atrial myocardium: GLP-1R mediated effects in human myocardium. *J. Mol. Cell. Cardiol.* **2015**, *89*, 365–375. [CrossRef]
21. Fuller, N.O.; Pirone, A.; Lynch, B.A.; Hewitt, M.C.; Quinton, M.S.; McKee, T.D.; Ivarsson, M. CoREST Complex-Selective Histone Deacetylase Inhibitors Show Prosynaptic Effects and an Improved Safety Profile To Enable Treatment of Synaptopathies. *ACS Chem. Neurosci.* **2019**, *10*, 1729–1743. [CrossRef] [PubMed]
22. Gallo, P.; Latronico, M.V.; Gallo, P.; Grimaldi, S.; Borgia, F.; Todaro, M.; Jones, P.; Gallinari, P.; De Francesco, R.; Ciliberto, G.; et al. Inhibition of class I histone deacetylase with an apicidin derivative prevents cardiac hypertrophy and failure. *Cardiovasc. Res.* **2008**, *80*, 416–424. [CrossRef]
23. Martin, T.G.; Myers, V.D.; Dubey, P.; Dubey, S.; Perez, E.; Moravec, C.S.; Willis, M.S.; Feldman, A.M.; Kirk, J.A. Cardiomyocyte contractile impairment in heart failure results from reduced BAG3-mediated sarcomeric protein turnover. *Nat. Commun.* **2021**, *12*, 2942. [CrossRef]
24. Eisner, D.A.; Caldwell, J.L.; Kistamas, K.; Trafford, A.W. Calcium and Excitation-Contraction Coupling in the Heart. *Circ. Res.* **2017**, *121*, 181–195. [CrossRef] [PubMed]

25. Lim, C.C.; Helmes, M.H.; Sawyer, D.B.; Jain, M.; Liao, R. High-throughput assessment of calcium sensitivity in skinned cardiac myocytes. *Am. J. Physiol.-Heart Circ. Physiol.* **2001**, *281*, H969–H974. [CrossRef] [PubMed]
26. Papadaki, M.; Holewinski, R.J.; Previs, S.B.; Martin, T.G.; Stachowski, M.J.; Li, A.; Blair, C.A.; Moravec, C.S.; Van Eyk, J.E.; Campbell, K.S.; et al. Diabetes with heart failure increases methylglyoxal modifications in the sarcomere, which inhibit function. *JCI Insight* **2018**, *3*, e121264. [CrossRef]
27. Goo, S.; Joshi, P.; Sands, G.; Gerneke, D.; Taberner, A.; Dollie, Q.; LeGrice, I.; Loiselle, D. Trabeculae carneae as models of the ventricular walls: Implications for the delivery of oxygen. *J. Gen. Physiol.* **2009**, *134*, 339–350. [CrossRef]
28. Rainer, P.P.; Primessnig, U.; Harenkamp, S.; Doleschal, B.; Wallner, M.; Fauler, G.; Stojakovic, T.; Wachter, R.; Yates, A.; Groschner, K.; et al. Bile acids induce arrhythmias in human atrial myocardium–implications for altered serum bile acid composition in patients with atrial fibrillation. *Heart* **2013**, *99*, 1685–1692. [CrossRef]
29. Sacherer, M.; Sedej, S.; Wakula, P.; Wallner, M.; Vos, M.A.; Kockskamper, J.; Stiegler, P.; Sereinigg, M.; von Lewinski, D.; Antoons, G.; et al. JTV519 (K201) reduces sarcoplasmic reticulum Ca(2)(+) leak and improves diastolic function in vitro in murine and human non-failing myocardium. *Br. J. Pharmacol.* **2012**, *167*, 493–504. [CrossRef]
30. Wallner, M.; Khafaga, M.; Kolesnik, E.; Vafiadis, A.; Schwantzer, G.; Eaton, D.M.; Curcic, P.; Kostenberger, M.; Knez, I.; Rainer, P.P.; et al. Istaroxime, a potential anticancer drug in prostate cancer, exerts beneficial functional effects in healthy and diseased human myocardium. *Oncotarget* **2017**, *8*, 49264–49274. [CrossRef]
31. Schwarzl, M.; Seiler, S.; Wallner, M.; von Lewinski, D.; Huber, S.; Maechler, H.; Steendijk, P.; Zelzer, S.; Truschnig-Wilders, M.; Obermayer-Pietsch, B.; et al. Mild hypothermia attenuates circulatory and pulmonary dysfunction during experimental endotoxemia. *Crit. Care Med.* **2013**, *41*, e401–e410. [CrossRef] [PubMed]
32. Delicce, A.V.; Makaryus, A.N. Physiology, Frank Starling Law. In *StatPearls*; StatPearls Publishing: Treasure Island, FL, USA, 2021.
33. Opdahl, A.; Remme, E.W.; Helle-Valle, T.; Lyseggen, E.; Vartdal, T.; Pettersen, E.; Edvardsen, T.; Smiseth, O.A. Determinants of Left Ventricular Early-Diastolic Lengthening Velocity. *Circulation* **2009**, *119*, 2578–2586. [CrossRef] [PubMed]
34. DesJardin, J.T.; Teerlink, J.R. Inotropic therapies in heart failure and cardiogenic shock: An educational review. *Eur. Heart J. Acute Cardiovasc. Care* **2021**, *10*, 676–686. [CrossRef] [PubMed]
35. Varian, K.D.; Raman, S.; Janssen, P.M. Measurement of myofilament calcium sensitivity at physiological temperature in intact cardiac trabeculae. *Am. J. Physiol. Heart Circ. Physiol.* **2006**, *290*, H2092–H2097. [CrossRef] [PubMed]
36. Salhi, H.E.; Hassel, N.C.; Siddiqui, J.K.; Brundage, E.A.; Ziolo, M.T.; Janssen, P.M.L.; Davis, J.P.; Biesiadecki, B.J. Myofilament Calcium Sensitivity: Mechanistic Insight into TnI Ser-23/24 and Ser-150 Phosphorylation Integration. *Front. Physiol.* **2016**, *7*, 567. [CrossRef] [PubMed]
37. Kobayashi, T.; Yang, X.; Walker, L.A.; Van Breemen, R.B.; Solaro, R.J. A non-equilibrium isoelectric focusing method to determine states of phosphorylation of cardiac troponin I: Identification of Ser-23 and Ser-24 as significant sites of phosphorylation by protein kinase C. *J. Mol. Cell. Cardiol.* **2005**, *38*, 213–218. [CrossRef]
38. Sitbon, Y.H.; Yadav, S.; Kazmierczak, K.; Szczesna-Cordary, D. Insights into myosin regulatory and essential light chains: A focus on their roles in cardiac and skeletal muscle function, development and disease. *J. Muscle Res. Cell Motil.* **2020**, *41*, 313–327. [CrossRef]
39. Foster, D.B.; Liu, T.; Rucker, J.; O'Meally, R.N.; Devine, L.R.; Cole, R.N.; O'Rourke, B. The cardiac acetyl-lysine proteome. *PLoS ONE* **2013**, *8*, e67513. [CrossRef]
40. Gregorich, Z.R.; Cai, W.; Lin, Z.; Chen, A.J.; Peng, Y.; Kohmoto, T.; Ge, Y. Distinct sequences and post-translational modifications in cardiac atrial and ventricular myosin light chains revealed by top-down mass spectrometry. *J. Mol. Cell. Cardiol.* **2017**, *107*, 13–21. [CrossRef]
41. Jeong, M.Y.; Lin, Y.H.; Wennersten, S.A.; Demos-Davies, K.M.; Cavasin, M.A.; Mahaffey, J.H.; Monzani, V.; Saripalli, C.; Mascagni, P.; Reece, T.B.; et al. Histone deacetylase activity governs diastolic dysfunction through a nongenomic mechanism. *Sci. Transl. Med.* **2018**, *10*, eaao0144. [CrossRef]
42. Badros, A.; Burger, A.M.; Philip, S.; Niesvizky, R.; Kolla, S.S.; Goloubeva, O.; Harris, C.; Zwiebel, J.; Wright, J.J.; Espinoza-Delgado, I.; et al. Phase I study of vorinostat in combination with bortezomib for relapsed and refractory multiple myeloma. *Clin. Cancer Res.* **2009**, *15*, 5250–5257. [CrossRef] [PubMed]

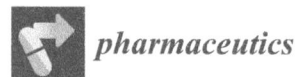

Review

The Role of Colchicine in Atherosclerosis: From Bench to Bedside

Leticia González [1,2], Juan Francisco Bulnes [3], María Paz Orellana [3], Paula Muñoz Venturelli [4,5] and Gonzalo Martínez Rodriguez [3,*]

1. Centro de Imágenes Biomédicas, Departamento de Radiología, Escuela de Medicina, Pontificia Universidad Católica de Chile, Santiago 8331150, Chile; leticia.gonzalez@uc.cl
2. Instituto Milenio de Ingeniería e Inteligencia Artificial para la Salud, iHEALTH, Pontificia Universidad Católica de Chile, Santiago 7820436, Chile
3. División de Enfermedades Cardiovasculares, Pontificia Universidad Católica de Chile, Santiago 8331150, Chile; jfbulnes@gmail.com (J.F.B.); mporella@uc.cl (M.P.O.)
4. Centro de Estudios Clínicos, Instituto de Ciencias e Innovación en Medicina (ICIM), Facultad de Medicina Clínica Alemana, Universidad del Desarrollo, Santiago 7610658, Chile; paumunoz@udd.cl
5. The George Institute for Global Health, Faculty of Medicine, University of New South Wales, Sydney, NSW 2042, Australia
* Correspondence: gmartinezr@med.puc.cl

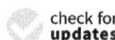

Citation: González, L.; Bulnes, J.F.; Orellana, M.P.; Muñoz Venturelli, P.; Martínez Rodriguez, G. The Role of Colchicine in Atherosclerosis: From Bench to Bedside. *Pharmaceutics* 2022, 14, 1395. https://doi.org/10.3390/pharmaceutics14071395

Academic Editors: Ionut Tudorancea and Radu Iliescu

Received: 9 June 2022
Accepted: 29 June 2022
Published: 1 July 2022

Publisher's Note: MDPI stays neutral with regard to jurisdictional claims in published maps and institutional affiliations.

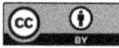

Copyright: © 2022 by the authors. Licensee MDPI, Basel, Switzerland. This article is an open access article distributed under the terms and conditions of the Creative Commons Attribution (CC BY) license (https://creativecommons.org/licenses/by/4.0/).

Abstract: Inflammation is a key feature of atherosclerosis. The inflammatory process is involved in all stages of disease progression, from the early formation of plaque to its instability and disruption, leading to clinical events. This strongly suggests that the use of anti-inflammatory agents might improve both atherosclerosis progression and cardiovascular outcomes. Colchicine, an alkaloid derived from the flower *Colchicum autumnale*, has been used for years in the treatment of inflammatory pathologies, including Gout, Mediterranean Fever, and Pericarditis. Colchicine is known to act over microtubules, inducing depolymerization, and over the NLRP3 inflammasome, which might explain its known anti-inflammatory properties. Recent evidence has shown the therapeutic potential of colchicine in the management of atherosclerosis and its complications, with limited adverse effects. In this review, we summarize the current knowledge regarding colchicine mechanisms of action and pharmacokinetics, as well as the available evidence on the use of colchicine for the treatment of coronary artery disease, covering basic, translational, and clinical studies.

Keywords: atherosclerosis; inflammation; colchicine; NLRP3 inflammasome; coronary artery disease; acute coronary syndrome

1. Introduction

Cardiovascular (CV) diseases remain the leading cause of mortality worldwide, accounting for up to one third of all registered deaths [1]. The main underlying cause behind cardiovascular disease is atherosclerosis, a chronic inflammatory disease targeting large and medium-sized arteries. In the USA alone, 400,000 people die of coronary artery atherosclerosis and over one million suffer from acute coronary syndrome each year [2]. Management of cardiovascular disease focuses on three main areas: (i) lipid lowering strategies, (ii) control of non-lipid risk factors (such as diabetes, hypertension, obesity, etc.) and (iii) stabilization of the atheromatous plaque, preventing rupture and thrombosis [3]. Current therapies, however, fail to prevent the reoccurrence of ischemic events, a phenomenon known as residual risk [4]. In a ten-year follow-up study of patients post ST elevation myocardial infarction (STEMI), 42% of patients presented with recurrent ischemic events, a risk that was highest during the first year (23.5% per patient/year) even when receiving currently recommended pharmacological treatment [5]. Therefore, the need for new therapies has shifted the focus towards anti-inflammatory drugs than can potentially target the chronic inflammation milieu of atherosclerotic plaques [6].

2. Methods

We conducted a full search of animal and human research, from basic studies to randomized clinical trials and meta-analyses, examining the use of colchicine for the treatment of atherosclerosis and/or coronary artery disease. Medline, Pubmed and Embase databases were searched until May 2022. Two researchers independently screened titles and abstracts of articles for full-text review. After data extraction, two researchers chose the most relevant articles and were in charge of elaborating the initial text, which was then sent to every author for further evaluation. If there were any discrepancies on a specific subject, the topic was re-analyzed, and a consensus was achieved. The final version of the manuscript was approved by every author.

3. Inflammation in Atherosclerosis

Inflammation plays a central role in the pathogenesis of atherosclerosis [7]. Both the innate and adaptive immune responses are involved in the process of atheroma formation, with monocyte/macrophages as key players throughout disease progression [8]. The development of the atherosclerotic plaque starts with the infiltration and accumulation of modified, apolipoprotein B-containing lipoproteins within the vessel wall [9]. Once in the intima layer, oxidized cholesterol in lipoproteins triggers the activation and production of inflammatory mediators in charge of recruiting circulating monocytes to the site of injury [9]. Within the vessel wall, monocytes differentiate to macrophages and engulf modified lipoproteins, becoming foam cells [9]. Foam cells continue to release inflammatory cytokines, in particular TNF-α and interleukin-1β (IL-1β) [10], exacerbating endothelial dysfunction and perpetuating the inflammatory response [11]. Advanced atherosclerotic plaques are characterized by a large lipid-rich core—composed of foam cells, cell debris and extracellular cholesterol—and a fibrous cap, formed by extracellular matrix and smooth muscle cells [12]. In later stages of the disease, macrophages within the plaque release matrix metalloproteinases that target the fibrous cap, destabilizing the plaque and setting the stage for plaque rupture and the consequent ischemic event [13,14] (Figure 1).

Neutrophils also participate in all stages of atherosclerosis development [15]. Indeed, circulating levels of neutrophils in humans predict future cardiovascular events [16], while in mice they correlate with the size of the developing plaque [17]. Myeloperoxidase (MPO), the main component of neutrophil granules, has been found in atherosclerotic plaques [18]. It has been shown that MPO-induced lipid peroxidation favors foam cell formation [19]. MPO can also activate metalloproteinases, inducing plaque disruption, by the release of reactive oxygen species (ROS) [20]. Similarly, neutrophils are known to release extracellular matrix proteinases that contribute to plaque destabilization [21], like elastase [22] and proteinase-3 [23], locating particularly in rupture-prone areas of the plaque [24,25]. Neutrophil depletion in apolipoprotein E knockout (ApoE KO) mice has been shown to reduce monocyte infiltration and plaque formation in the aorta [26]. In fact, neutrophils can affect monocyte recruitment through several mechanisms [27], including increased expression of adhesion molecules in the endothelium through the release of granule-proteins proteinase 3 and azurocidin [28]. Furthermore, neutrophil extracellular traps (NETs) are web-like structures made of genetic material, histones, MPO and others, which are released upon neutrophil activation [29]. The process of NETs formation is called NETosis and is introduced to discriminate this pathway from other types of cell death [30]. Of note, NETs have been found in atherosclerotic plaques of both mice and humans [31–33]. Increased levels of NETosis markers are associated with the severity of coronary atherosclerosis in patients [34]. Similarly, Mangold et al. have shown that the number of NETs and activated neutrophils in patients with acute coronary syndrome (ACS) is related to final infarct size [35]. Finally, autopsied disrupted plaques (i.e., with hemorrhage or erosion) from patients with ACS, presented significantly more neutrophils and NETs compared with plaques without those features [36].

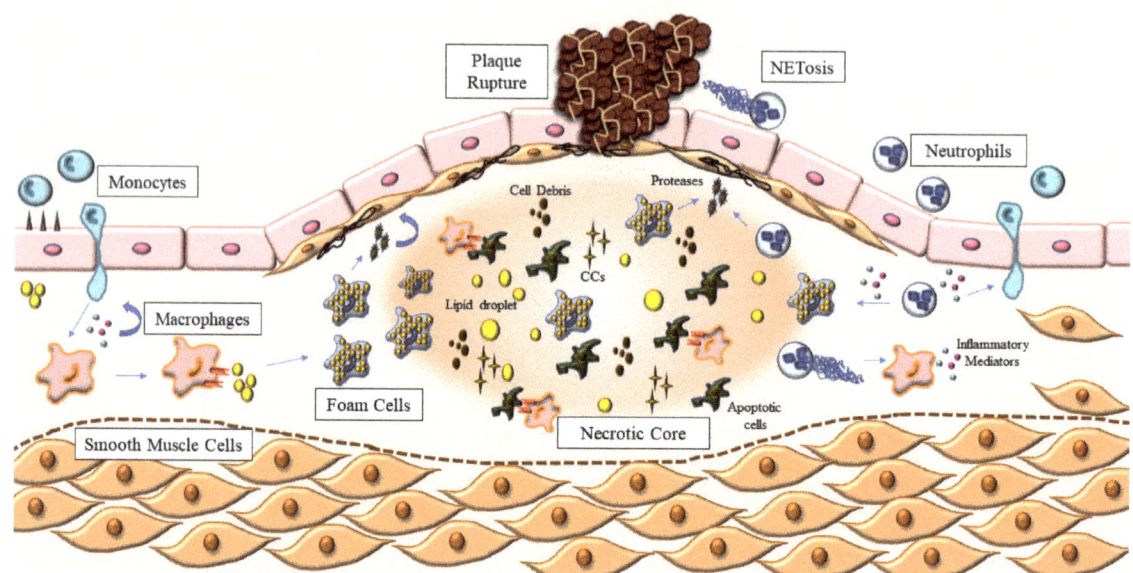

Figure 1. Atherosclerotic plaque development. Atherosclerosis starts with the accumulation of modified lipoproteins inside the vessel wall, which triggers the recruitment of leukocytes, monocytes and neutrophils from circulation. Once in the intima layer, monocytes differentiate into macrophages, which can now engulf the modified lipoproteins, becoming foam cells. Macrophages also continue to release inflammatory mediators—such as cytokines and chemokines—in response to the increased levels of cholesterol, further amplifying the response. Neutrophils also release pro-inflammatory mediators through granules and NETosis, contributing to an exacerbation of the inflammatory state within the vessel wall. Foam cells, apoptotic cells and cell debris, lipid droplets and extracellular cholesterol crystals (CCs) coalesce in the center of the growing plaque, forming the necrotic core, which is kept stable thanks to the fibrous cap: a structure made of smooth muscle cells and extracellular matrix proteins. The release of proteinases by macrophages and neutrophils weakens the fibrous cap, favoring plaque rupture and the exposure of the contents of the plaque to circulation, triggering blood coagulation and the clinical manifestations of atherosclerosis.

Cholesterol accumulates in atherosclerotic plaques not only in the form of intracellular cholesterol esters but also intra and extracellular cholesterol crystals (CCs) [37]. CCs have been found in all stages of atherosclerotic plaque development [38,39] and have been shown to be associated with plaque rupture [40]. CCs can induce NETosis, which can in turn prime macrophages to synthetize cytokine precursors, such as pro-IL-1β [31]. CCs can also directly activate the nucleotide-binding oligomerization domain-like receptor, pyrin domain-containing 3 (NLRP3) inflammasome in macrophages, resulting in the release of mature IL-1β, a key cytokine involved in the development and disruption of atherosclerotic plaques [37].

4. The NLRP3 Inflammasome

The innate immune system relies on a set of germline-encoded pattern recognition receptors (PRRs) to recognize pathogenic insults as well as defective cells [41]. PRRs detect the presence of pathogen-associated molecular patterns (PAMPs) or damage-associated molecular patterns (DAMPs), triggering downstream inflammatory pathways leading to removal of the insult and tissue repair [41]. The inflammasomes are cytosolic, multimeric protein complexes that respond to PAMPs and DAMPs [42]. Five members of the PRRs have been confirmed to form inflammasomes, key among them the NLRP3 inflammasome [43]. The NLRP3 inflammasome responds to a wide variety of activators including monosodium urate, extracellular adenosine triphosphate (ATP) and CCs [44]. The basal levels of the components of the NLRP3 inflammasome and their targets are very low [45]. As such, a two-step process of priming and activation is required [46,47]. The priming step is induced by the activation of Toll-like receptors (TLRs) and cytokine receptors, leading to upregulation of the transcription of NLRP3 and pro-IL-1β [48]. Afterwards, further stimuli will promote the inflammasome assembly, resulting in cytokine production [45]. Upon activation, the NLRP3 receptor oligomerizes and interacts with the adaptor protein apoptosis-associated speck-like protein containing a caspase-recruitment domain (ASC), to recruit and activate pro-caspase-1 [49,50]. Active caspase-1 can now cleave pro-IL-1β and pro-IL-18 into their biologically active, highly inflammatory forms [42].

In the context of atherosclerosis, CCs are considered a major driver of NLRP3 inflammasome activation [37]. It has been postulated that CCs activate the inflammasome in a process involving lysosomal damage after phagocytosis [51]. The inefficient clearance of CCs results in the leakage of cathepsin B into the cytoplasm, which in turn can activate the inflammasome complex [52]. Accordingly, the inflammatory response elicited by intraperitoneal CCs injection in WT mice is absent in mice deficient in NLRP3 inflammasome components [38]. Oxidized LDL has also been shown to induce NLRP3 activation through lysosomal disruption via interaction with CD36 [53]. As such, macrophages lacking CD36 fail to release IL-1β, indicating lack of NLRP3 activation [53].

The contribution of IL-1β to atherogenesis has been established by several animal studies, hinting at a role of the NLRP3 inflammasome in disease development [54–56]. Bone-marrow deficiency of ASC is associated with reduced vascular inflammation and neointimal formation in a mouse model of vascular injury [57]. LDLR KO mice receiving NLRP3, ASC or IL-1β deficient bone marrow developed significantly reduced atherosclerosis when challenged with an atherogenic diet [38]. Similarly, systemic or bone-marrow deficiency of caspase-1/11 is associated with a reduction in atherosclerotic lesions in both ApoE [58,59] and LDLR KO mice [60]. Conversely, bone marrow transplantation studies in ApoE KO mice have shown that lack of NLRP3, ASC or caspase-1 had no effect on atherosclerotic plaque size, plaque stability or macrophage infiltration [61]. Differences in experimental conditions might explain these contrasting results. In humans, high expression of NLRP3 inflammasome components has been detected in carotid atherosclerotic plaques [62] and high levels of expression of NLRP3 correlate with the severity of coronary artery atherosclerosis [63]. The inflammasome has been shown to be primed in peripheral monocytes from ACS patients compared with controls [64] and levels of NLRP3, IL-1β, IL-18 and other inflammasome components have been found to be elevated in ACS patients compared with controls [65]. Taken together, these studies highlight the important role of IL-1β and the NLRP3 inflammasome in atherosclerosis and mark them as possible targets for the development of new therapeutic strategies.

5. Colchicine

Colchicine is a botanical alkaloid derived from the flower *Colchicum autumnale*, first described as a medicinal plant in the Ebers papyrus of ancient Egypt in 1550 BC, where it was used for the management of pain and swelling [66]. The colchicine molecule, chemical name N-[(7S)-5,6,7,9-tetrahydro-1,2,3,10-tetramethoxy-9-oxobenzo(a)heptalen-7-yl)acetamide], is composed of three rings [67]. The A (trimethoxyphenyl moiety) and C ring (methoxytropone moiety) are highly involved in binding to tubulin and are maintained in a rigid configuration by B-rings [67]. Modifications to both the A and C rings significantly affect tubulin binding [67,68], while modifications on the B rings are associated with changes in activation energy of the binding and association/dissociation kinetics [69].

Nowadays, colchicine is widely used for the treatment of acute gout flares and Familial Mediterranean Fever (FMF) [70,71]. It has also been used in other inflammatory conditions such as calcium pyrophosphate disease, Adamantiades–Behcet's syndrome and—in the cardiovascular field—pericarditis [72]. Given the ease of access, low cost and favorable safety profile, colchicine has emerged as a potential oral treatment targeting the inflammatory component of atherosclerosis.

Mechanistically, colchicine acts by inhibiting tubulin polymerization, disrupting the cellular cytoskeleton, and impairing several processes including mitosis, intracellular transport, and phagocytosis [73]. Furthermore, colchicine inhibits neutrophil chemotaxis and adhesion to the inflamed endothelium [74]. At nanoconcentrations, colchicine alters E-selectin distribution on endothelial cells, affecting neutrophil adhesion [75]. On the µM level, colchicine induces L-selectin shedding, preventing recruitment [75]. Paschke and colleagues have also shown that colchicine affects human neutrophil deformability and motility, affecting a key step in inflammatory processes, cell extravasation [76]. Monosodium urate (MSU)-induced superoxide production in neutrophils in vitro is also affected by colchicine treatment [77]. Superoxide production inhibition has also been reported in vivo in MSU-treated peritoneal macrophages, at a dosage significantly lower than the required to affect neutrophil infiltration [78]. Colchicine also modulates TNF-α synthesis by rat liver macrophages [79] and downregulates TNF receptors in both macrophages and endothelial cells [80].

Platelets play a key role in atherosclerosis complications [12]. Early reports have suggested that colchicine might also affect platelet aggregation [81] through mechanisms involving inhibition of cofilin and LIM domain kinase 1 [82]. In FMF patients, colchicine reduced β-thromboglobulin levels, a protein released during platelet activation, with no effect on mean platelet volume, a marker of platelet activity [83]. A more recent experiment by Shah and colleagues showed that colchicine administration to healthy subjects at a clinically relevant dose (1.8 mg single dose) reduced leukocyte-platelet aggregation (both monocyte and neutrophil) as well as levels of surface markers of platelet activity, such as p-selectin and PAC-1 (activated GP IIb/IIIa), with no effect on homotypic platelet aggregation [84]. Likewise, Raju and colleagues have also showed that oral colchicine at a dose of 1 mg did not affect platelet aggregation in response to several stimuli, in patients with acute coronary syndrome [85]. It is possible then that the anti-inflammatory action of colchicine on neutrophils could impact platelet function. NETs can facilitate thrombosis by promoting platelet adhesion, activation, and aggregation, and also the accumulation of prothrombotic factors such as von Willebrand factor and fibrinogen [86]. Interestingly, colchicine has been shown to reduce NETosis induced by CC [87], in neutrophils isolated from individuals with Behcet's disease [88] and in patients with ACS [89].

6. Colchicine and the NLRP3 Inflammasome

Several studies have confirmed that colchicine limits NLRP3 inflammasome activity. Martinon and colleagues first described inactivation of the NLRP3 inflammasome by colchicine in THP1 cells treated with monosodium urate crystals [90]. In patients with FMF colchicine suppressed IL-1β release from both bone marrow-derived macrophages where the inflammasome was constitutively activated and peripheral blood monocytes [91]. Misawa and colleagues also reported a dose-dependent effect of colchicine on IL-1β production in J774 macrophages treated with various inducers of the NLRP3 inflammasome, including MSU and ATP [92]. Furthermore, colchicine has been described as inhibiting the intracellular transport of ASC, preventing co-localization of NLRP3 components and thus the consequent release of active IL-1β [92]. The pathway through which colchicine inhibits the NLRP3 inflammasome is not clear, however some mechanisms have been proposed. In a model of small intestinal injury, Otani and colleagues showed that colchicine inhibited protein expression of cleaved caspase-1 and IL-1β, without affecting mRNA levels of NLRP3 or IL-1β. Monocyte caspase-1 inhibition has been detected in ACS patients as well [64]. Very recently, using molecular dynamic simulation in a mouse model, it has been proposed that colchicine could interact with the ATP binding region of the NLRP3-NACHT domain, thus potentially precluding inflammasome activation [93]. Similarly, in

ATP-mediated NLRP3 inflammasome activation, formation of P2X7 pores is a key step [94]. In this context, Marques-da-Silva et al. demonstrated that colchicine is a strong inhibitor of pore formation in mouse peritoneal macrophages after ATP-induced ethidium bromide permeability, resulting in the release of lower levels of ROS and IL-1β [95]. The same results were also seen in vivo, in mice inoculated with lipopolysaccharide and ATP [95].

The ability of colchicine to interfere with the activation of the NLRP3 inflammasome, in addition to its effect on microtubule formation and neutrophil-mediated inflammation, points towards the use of colchicine as a potential strategy to target the inflammatory component of atherosclerosis.

7. Pharmacokinetics and Safety

Colchicine is rapidly absorbed by the jejunum and ileum with a bioavailability that fluctuates between 24 to 88% [96]. Peak plasma concentrations occur within 0.5–2 h after oral administration, although it can be detected in leukocytes up to 10 days after ingestion [97]. In circulation, approximately 40% is conjugated to plasmatic proteins and the establishment of colchicine–protein complexes in tissues contributes to its large volume distribution [67]. Colchicine is rapidly distributed to peripheral leukocytes and concentration in these cells may exceed those detected in plasma [98]. Most of the drug undergoes enterohepatic recirculation, leading to a second peak in plasma within 6 h of ingestion, and is eliminated through feces and bile [97]. Around 20% of colchicine is eliminated in the urine at 2 h and 30% after 24 h [97]. Colchicine average elimination half-life is 20 h, which can be prolonged by certain pathologies including renal failure and hepatic cirrhosis [99].

Gastrointestinal (GI) intolerance (diarrhea, abdominal pain, vomiting) is the most common side effect of colchicine, affecting around 20% of patients, followed by myalgias [100]. Most of these side effects can be managed with lower daily doses (around 0.5 mg/day) or long-term treatments [100]. Regarding safety, the first meta-analysis that looked at the safety of colchicine use only reported an 83% increased risk of GI side effects, with no evidence of significant serious adverse effects over 824 patient-years [101]. Similar results have been recently reported by Stewart and colleagues in a meta-analysis of 35 randomized controlled trials [102]. Colchicine significantly increased diarrhea (RR 2.4, 95% confidence interval (CI) 1.6–3.7) and other GI events (RR 1.7, 95% CI 1.3–2.3). No increased rate of other adverse events was detected, including infection, hepatic, hematological, muscular, and sensorial events [102]. On the other hand, a pooled analysis of randomized clinical trials comparing low dose colchicine versus placebo showed that colchicine was associated with a significantly higher risk of non-CV death (OR 1.55; 95% CI 1.10 to 2.17; $p = 0.01$) compared with the placebo group [103]. However, few studies were included and, as stated by the authors, the events reported were low, indicating that the data should be considered with caution [103]. In line with this, a recent retrospective cohort of 24,410 patients with gout showed that colchicine use resulted in an increased risk of pneumonia (adjusted HR, 1.42; 95% CI 1.32–1.53; $p < 0.05$), related to use duration and accumulated dose [104].

Colchicine interacts with two main proteins that impact its pharmacokinetics and pharmacodynamics: cytochrome P450 3A4 (CYP3A4) and P-glycoprotein. Intestinal and hepatic CYP3A4 metabolize colchicine by demethylation, producing 2- and 3-demethylcolchicine [97]. P-glycoprotein, on the other hand, limits GI availability by extruding colchicine from the GI tract [67]. Adverse reactions have been reported by patients consuming either CYP3A4 inhibitors or P-glycoprotein inhibitors, resulting in altered colchicine metabolism and toxicity [67]. Dose adjustment is recommended in these situations. Some cases of myopathy and/or rhabdomyolysis have been reported for instances when colchicine was used in conjunction with statins, however, they are in general well tolerated when used simultaneously [105]. Death due to colchicine administration has been reported when used in conjunction with clarithromycin, particularly in patients with renal insufficiency [106].

8. Colchicine in Atherosclerosis

8.1. Pre-Clinical Studies

The first animal studies looking at the potential use of colchicine for atherosclerosis showed rather conflicting results. Colchicine administration of high-lipid diet-fed rabbits resulted in a reduction of circulating lipids, restoration of normal triglyceride levels and a protective effect on plaque development in the aorta [107]. On the other hand, colchicine administration on a swine model of balloon-induced atherosclerosis showed the opposite effect, with a mild worsening of plaque development [108]. Though the models used were different, the inconclusive results might have tampered the interest in the usage of this drug for atherosclerosis management. Early in vitro experiments in smooth muscle cells isolated from human atherosclerotic plaques showed that colchicine affected proliferation and migration, which could potentially impact atherosclerosis development [109]. More recently, Huang and colleagues have shown that colchicine administration to hyperlipidemic rats resulted in a reduction in circulating levels of C-reactive protein and lipoprotein associated phospholipase A2, while elevating nitric oxide production, pointing to an improvement in endothelial function. Interestingly, this effect was further enhanced by the concomitant administration of atorvastatin [110]. While Kaminiotis and colleagues have shown that oral administration of colchicine in high-cholesterol diet-fed rabbits showed no effects on atherosclerosis progression [111], Mylonas and colleagues have shown in the same model that colchicine-based anti-inflammatory therapies significantly diminished de novo atherogenesis, decreased triglyceride levels [112,113] and also tampered Krüppel-like factor 4—a transcription factor involved in atheromatosis—overexpression in thoracic aortas [113].

The effect of colchicine in acute myocardial infarction has also been explored. Intraperitoneal administration of colchicine in a mouse model of ischemia/reperfusion resulted in a significant reduction in infarct size 24 h after injury, when administered before reperfusion had been established [114]. Significant improvement in hemodynamic parameters and cardiac fibrosis were also reported [114]. Colchicine has also been shown to be protective when administered after ischemia/reperfusion injury, reducing macrophage infiltration, cardiac remodeling, and dysfunction in a rat model of left coronary artery (LCA) ligation [115]. Similarly, in a mouse model of MI induced by permanent LCA ligation, short-term colchicine administration post MI significantly improved survival, cardiac function and heart failure [116]. This improvement in cardiac performance was associated with a reduction in monocyte and neutrophil infiltration, mRNA expression of inflammatory cytokines and components of the NLRP3 inflammasome 24 h after injury [116]. In SRBI KO/ApoeR61$^{h/h}$ mice, orally administered colchicine resulted in improved survival after feeding with atherogenic diet, however, neither inflammatory markers nor aortic plaque volume were different between the treated and untreated groups (González L, Martínez G, unpublished data).

Finally, the role of colchicine in plaque stabilization has been recently explored by Cecconi and colleagues [117], where atherosclerosis was induced by a high cholesterol diet and balloon endothelial denudation in rabbits. Colchicine treatment reduced the relative increase in aortic wall volume, measured as normalized wall index, and inflammation, measured as 18F-FDG uptake in PET/CT imaging, which could potentially help stabilize the plaque. This effect, however, was only seen in animals with high levels of circulating cholesterol [117]. Table 1 summarizes the available pre-clinical data on colchicine and atherosclerosis.

Table 1. Pre-clinical studies.

Study	Animal Model	Disease Induction	Colchicine Dosage *	Length of Intervention	Main Findings
Wojcicki et al., 1986 [107]	Rabbit	High-lipid diet	0.2 mg/kg i.p. twice a week	3 months	Reduction of circulating lipids, restoration of normal triglyceride levels and a protective effect on plaque development in the aorta
Lee et al., 1976 [108]	Yorkshire Swine	Balloon-induced denudation of aortic endothelium plus hypercholesterolemic diet	0.2 mg/kg/day	6 months	Slight worsening of atherosclerosis development in the aorta. No effect on serum cholesterol levels
Huang et al., 2014 [110]	Sprague–Dawley rats	High fat, high cholesterol diet for 6 weeks	0.5 mg/kg body weight/day i.p.	2 weeks	Reduction in circulating levels of C-reactive protein and lipoprotein associated phospholipase A2. Elevation of nitric oxide production. Effect was enhanced when administered along atorvastatin
Kaminiotis et al., 2017 [111]	New Zealand White rabbits	High cholesterol diet (1% w/w)	2 mg/kg body weight	7 weeks	No effect of colchicine on atherosclerosis or IL-18 levels. Slight effect on triglyceride levels
Spartalis et al., 2021 [112]	New Zealand White rabbits	High cholesterol diet (1% w/w)	2 mg/kg body weight plus 250 mg/kg body weight/day fenofibrate or 15 mg/kg body weight/day N-acetylcysteine (NAC)	7 weeks	Colchicine reduced aortic atherosclerosis especially when combined with NAC. Reduction in IL-6 and lower triglyceride levels were also reported
Mylonas et al., 2022 [113]	New Zealand White rabbits	High cholesterol diet (1% w/w)	2 mg/kg body weight plus 250 mg/kg body weight/day fenofibrate or 15 mg/kg body weight/day NAC	7 weeks	Reduction in de novo atherogenesis in the aorta and reduction of KLF4 expression in thoracic aortas
Akodad et al., 2017 [114]	C57BL/6 mice	Ligation of left coronary artery followed by reperfusion	400 µg/kg i.p.	25 min before reperfusion	Significant reduction of infarct size. Improvement of hemodynamic parameters. Decreased cardiac fibrosis

Table 1. Cont.

Study	Animal Model	Disease Induction	Colchicine Dosage *	Length of Intervention	Main Findings
Mori et al., 2021 [115]	Wistar Rats	Ligation of left coronary artery followed by reperfusion	0.4 mg/kg/day i.p.	7 days	Reduction in post acute MI inflammation, ventricular remodeling, and dysfunction
Fujisue et al., 2017 [116]	C57BL/6J mice	Permanent ligation of left descending coronary artery	0.1 mg/kg/day	7 days port MI	Attenuation of pro-inflammatory cytokines and NLRP3 inflammasome components. Improved cardiac function, heart function and survival.
Cecconi et al., 2021 [117]	New Zealand White Rabbit	balloon endothelial denudation plus high cholesterol diet	0.2 mg/kg/day, 5 days/week, SQ	18 weeks	Reduction of the increase in aortic wall volume and inflammation

* Oral administration unless stated otherwise; i.p: intraperitoneal; NAC: N-acetylcysteine; NLRP3: nucleotide-binding oligomerization domain-like receptor, pyrin domain-containing 3; SQ: subcutaneous.

8.2. Translational Studies

In a pilot study including 64 patients with stable coronary artery disease (CAD), Nidorf and colleagues showed that colchicine in low doses decreased high-sensitivity C-reactive protein (hsCRP) levels, a biomarker of inflammation, with no significant side effects [118]. However, the same protective effect was not seen in a pilot randomized controlled trial including patients with acute coronary syndrome (ACS) or stroke, where colchicine failed to reduce hsCRP levels [85]. The different results could be explained by the cause behind hsCRP elevation, which might not be sensitive to colchicine treatment, the dosage used and the context in which the drug was used—acute vs chronic inflammation. A local approach was then used by our group, in which the effect of colchicine on inflammatory cytokine production was assessed in blood samples collected from the coronary sinus [119]. ACS patients were recruited and randomized to receive either colchicine or placebo on top of standard therapy and levels of IL-1β, IL-18 and IL-6 were quantified. Acute colchicine administration resulted in a significant reduction in transcoronary cytokine gradients, suggesting a local intracardiac effect on the NLRP3 inflammasome [119]. In a follow-up study in a different cohort of ACS patients, a significant reduction in the release of IL-1β was observed with colchicine treatment in stimulated peripheral blood monocytes [64]. This reduction was associated with a suppression of monocyte caspase-1 activity. Colchicine was also able to reduce transcoronary and monocyte production of chemokines in treated ACS patients compared with control, which could also positively impact CV outcomes [120]. Furthermore, colchicine treatment suppressed NET production post percutaneous coronary intervention in ACS patients, a process that has been associated with periprocedural MI [89]. Tumor necrosis factor (TNF)-related apoptosis-inducing ligand (TRAIL) is a cytokine belonging to the TNF family of ligands. Evidence shows that a deficiency in circulating TRAIL is associated with atherosclerotic plaque development, probably by inducing a more dysfunctional type of macrophage, with less migratory capacity, and impaired reverse cholesterol efflux and efferocytosis [121]. Research from our group shows that acute colchicine treatment significantly increases plasma TRAIL levels, purportedly regulating the inhibitory effect of IL-18 upon TRAIL [122].

The anti-inflammatory potential of colchicine in chronic CAD has been recently reevaluated. Colchicine—either alone or in combination with methotrexate—did not improve coronary endothelial function in patients with stable CAD, measured through non-invasive MRI [123]. In a proteomics study, serum samples from CAD patients were compared before and 30 days after colchicine treatment. The expression of a total of 37 proteins was reduced, including members of the NLRP3 inflammasome pathway (IL-18, IL-1 receptor antagonist and IL-6), adaptative immune system proteins (C-C motif chemokine 17, CD40 ligand, pro-IL-6) and proteins involved in neutrophil degranulation (myeloperoxidase, myeloblastin and azurocidin among others) [124]. A reduction in median hsCRP has also been reported [124]. In the same cohort of patients, colchicine reportedly affected some biomarkers of inflammation. Colchicine treatment for a year resulted in a reduction of extracellular vesicle (EV) NLRP3 protein but no changes in serum NLRP3 protein levels [125]. Lower levels of hsCRP were also detected but this reduction was not related to EV NLRP3 protein levels [125]. MicroRNAs are known to be involved in multiple pathways driving atherosclerosis development. Barraclough and colleagues recently studied the microRNA signature in ACS patients and how colchicine might affect its expression [126]. Plasma samples collected from the aorta, coronary sinus and right atrium were collected from control, ACS standard therapy and ACS standard therapy plus colchicine patients. A total of 30 miRNAs were significantly elevated in the ACS group compared with controls. In patients with ACS, 12 miRNAs were lower when patients received colchicine and seven of these returned to control levels after colchicine treatment. More importantly, three miRNAs suppressed by colchicine are known to be regulators of inflammatory pathways, indicating that levels of miRNAs could potentially be used to track treatment effectiveness [126].

8.3. Phase 2 Clinical Studies

Colchicine has been shown to be protective in the context of ischemia/reperfusion, in accordance with pre-clinical results. The perioperative administration of colchicine to patients undergoing coronary bypass grafting resulted in a reduction in postoperative levels of myocardial injury biomarkers such as high-sensitivity troponin T (hsTrop) and creatine kinase-myocardial brain fraction (CKmb) [127]. Deftereos and colleagues have also reported beneficial effects of colchicine administration to STEMI patients treated with percutaneous coronary intervention [128]. Colchicine significantly reduced CKmb concentrations as well as infarct size when compared with placebo group [128]. However, the anti-inflammatory effect of colchicine could not be demonstrated in another study including STEMI patients, where hsCRP levels remained unaffected by the treatment [129]. Oral administration of high dose colchicine also demonstrated no effect on infarct size (assessed by cardiac magnetic resonance) in STEMI patients, when administered at reperfusion and for five consecutive days [130].

The anti-inflammatory effect of colchicine treatment in ACS patients seems to be associated with positive changes at atherosclerotic plaque level. In a prospective nonrandomized observational study including 80 patients with recent ACS, colchicine administration was associated with a reduction in low attenuation plaque volume (LAPV)—a measure of plaque instability and predictor of future coronary events [131]. A positive correlation between LAPV and reduced hsCRP levels has also been reported [131]. Furthermore, the addition of colchicine on top of standard therapy in ACS patients (0.5 mg daily for six months) positively impacted the occurrence of major adverse cardiovascular events, improving overall survival in a randomized, placebo-control trial [132]. Reduction in inflammatory markers (hsCRP, IL-6) after colchicine treatment has been reported in chronic coronary artery disease as well [133].

The Colchicine–PCI randomized trial evaluated the effect of colchicine administration before (1–2 h, 1.8 mg) percutaneous coronary intervention on post-PCI myocardial injury, in patients with stable angina (SA) and ACS [134]. Shah and colleagues have reported that preprocedural colchicine did not protect against PCI-related myocardial injury (including PCI-related MI and MACE at 30 days), despite a reduction in IL-6 and hsCRP levels (22–24 h post-PCI) [134]. Dissimilar results have been reported by Cole and colleagues in a similar pilot study, evaluating SA and ACS patients [135]. Colchicine administration prior to PCI intervention (1.5 mg, 6–24 h) significantly reduced major and minor periprocedural MI and injury, especially in NSTEMI patients [135]. Colchicine also significantly reduced pre-PCI inflammatory cytokine levels (IL-6, IL-1β, TNF-α, IFN-γ) and white blood cell counts, with no differences in post-PCI values [136]. Absolute Troponin change was also reportedly lower in the colchicine group [136]. The difference in results might be influenced by both the population studied and, very importantly, the time of colchicine administration.

8.4. Phase 3 Clinical Studies and Meta-Analyses

In the setting of ACS, the COLCOT trial randomized 4745 patients to receive colchicine (0.5 mg BID) or placebo within 30 days post-MI [137]. Colchicine led to a significant reduction of the primary outcome (a composite of death from cardiovascular causes, resuscitated cardiac arrest, myocardial infarction, stroke, or urgent hospitalization for angina leading to coronary revascularization) by 23% (HR 0.77; 95% CI 0.61–0.96; $p = 0.02$). This was mainly driven by a significant reduction in the incidence of stroke (HR 0.26; 95% CI 0.10–0.70) and urgent hospitalization for angina leading to coronary revascularization (HR 0.50; 95% CI 0.31–0.81) [137]. Interestingly, in a post-hoc analysis of COLCOT, time-to-treatment initiation (i.e., length of time between the index MI and the initiation of colchicine) was inversely correlated with colchicine clinical benefit. Indeed, when administered in-hospital within the first three days after the event, colchicine was associated with a 48% reduction in the risk of ischemic events; which contrasted with a lack of benefit when started later (four to seven days, and seven to thirty days) [138]. The other RCT in the ACS setting, the COPS trial, was an Australian-based study that randomly assigned 795 patients diagnosed with MI or unstable angina to receive colchicine (0.5 mg BID for one month, then 0.5 mg QD for eleven months) vs. placebo [139]. Although the original trial failed to demonstrate a benefit on the one-year primary outcome, an extended 24-month follow-up did show a significant 40% reduction in the composite of all-cause mortality, ACS, ischemia-driven-unplanned-urgent revascularization, and non-cardioembolic ischemic stroke. Of note, just as in COLCOT, the main outcome was driven by a significant reduction in urgent revascularization (HR, 0.19; 95% CI 0.05–0.66; $p = 0.009$) [140].

In the setting of chronic CAD, the LoDoCo trial randomized 532 patients to receive colchicine 0.5 mg or no colchicine, using an open label design [141]. Colchicine led to a reduction of the primary outcome (composite of ACS, out-of-hospital cardiac arrest, or non-cardioembolic ischemic stroke) of 67% (HR 0.33; 95% CI 0.18–0.59; $p < 0.001$), due to a significant reduction in the risk of ACS (HR 0.33; 95% CI 0.18–0.63; $p < 0.001$). This same group published, seven years later, the LoDoCo 2 trial, using a more robust—double blinded, placebo controlled—study design and a 10-fold higher number of patients [142]. In this landmark trial, colchicine led to a reduction in the primary outcome (a composite of cardiovascular death, spontaneous (nonprocedural) myocardial infarction, ischemic stroke, or ischemia-driven coronary revascularization) of 31% (HR 0.69; 95% CI 0.57–0.83; $p < 0.001$), which was due, again, to a significant reduction of MI (HR 0.7; 95% CI 0.53–0.93; $p = 0.01$) and also of ischemia-driven coronary revascularization (HR 0.75; 95% CI 0.60–0.94; $p = 0.01$) [142].

The analysis of the components of ACS in LoDoCo suggested that colchicine reduced the probability of acute coronary events unrelated to stent disease (i.e., in native segments), with lack of effect in the prevention of stent-related disease (i.e., acute stent thrombosis or stent restenosis) [141]. However, in a previous study that included diabetic patients undergoing PCI with bare metal stents, six-month angiographic restenosis rates were reduced by 62% in the group of patients randomized to colchicine as compared with patients in the control group (16% vs. 33%; OR 0.38, 95% CI 0.18–0.79; $p = 0.007$) [143]. These results may suggest that, along with atheroma plaque stabilization in native coronary arteries, the anti-inflammatory and anti-mitotic effects of colchicine may be equally effective in the prevention of neointimal hyperplasia, the central process in the pathophysiology of in-stent restenosis. However, the effects of colchicine preventing stent related disease in the era of new generation drug eluting stents may be unclear, as the rates of restenosis have decreased significantly [144].

As individual trials suffer from significant heterogeneity regarding the clinical setting (acute versus chronic CAD), treatment (colchicine dose and length of follow-up) and end point definitions, several systematic reviews and meta-analysis have been conducted to the summarize clinical effects of colchicine [145–148]. In one of these, by Fiolet and colleagues, inclusion criteria were restricted to RCT's with a minimum follow-up of three months, thus including the five trials mentioned above. In their analysis, colchicine reduced the risk for the primary endpoint—a composite of MI, stroke, or cardiovascular death—by 25% (RR 0.75; 95% CI 0.61–0.92; $p = 0.005$) with a low between-trial heterogeneity ($I^2 = 23.9\%$). Colchicine led to a significant reduction of the individual endpoints MI by 22% (RR 0.78; 95% CI 0.64–0.94; $p = 0.010$), stroke by 46% (RR 0.54; 95% CI 0.34–0.86; $p = 0.009$), and coronary revascularization by 23% (RR 0.77; 95% CI 0.66–0.90; $p < 0.001$) [145]. In subgroup analysis the benefit observed with colchicine was consistent in both acute and chronic coronary syndrome and irrespective of gender [145]. It is noteworthy that the magnitude of the benefit obtained with colchicine in patients with CAD is comparable to that achieved by each of the mainstay therapies for the secondary prevention of CAD—such as antiplatelet agents and statins [149,150]—and has been achieved against a background of optimal treatment with these therapies.

The applicability of these findings may depend upon specific patient subsets. For example, the observed benefit of colchicine may be even higher in patients with diabetes mellitus. In a meta-analysis conducted by Kuzemczak and colleagues, in patients with CAD, the absolute risk reduction of the composite endpoint of MACE achieved by colchicine in patients with diabetes was greater than in patients without diabetes (absolute risk reduction of 3.94% vs. 2.32%, $p < 0.001$) [151]. On the other hand, as most trials have excluded patients with heart failure and chronic kidney disease, the effects of colchicine for the treatment of CAD in these important populations remain unknown.

Despite these favorable effects seen with colchicine, some trials have documented concerning results regarding non-CV mortality. In the COPS trial the rate of all-cause death was higher in the colchicine group compared with placebo (HR 8.20; 95% CI 1.03–65.61; $p = 0.047$) due to an increase in non-cardiovascular deaths, which were mostly due to sepsis [139]. Likewise, in the LoDoCo 2 trial there was an increase in non-cardiovascular deaths (HR 1.51; 95% CI 0.99–2.31), but without a parallel increase in severe infections, new cancer diagnosis or severe gastrointestinal adverse effects [142]. Meta-analyses have shown a non-significant lower incidence of cardiovascular mortality (RR 0.82; 95% CI 0.55–1.23; $p = 0.339$) counterbalanced by a non-significant higher incidence of non-cardiovascular deaths (RR 1.38; 95% CI 0.99–1.92; $p = 0.060$), with no difference in all-cause mortality (RR 1.08; 95% CI 0.71–1.62; $p = 0.726$) [145].

Taken together, RCTs show a consistent beneficial effect of colchicine by limiting new cardiovascular events and stroke. However, some barriers remain before a widespread use of colchicine in clinical practice can be adopted. Firstly, and as discussed above, its net effect on mortality is still under scrutiny, with a possible increase in non-cardiovascular deaths, which needs to be clarified in future trials. Secondly, in the era of precision medicine, a more individualized approach may be adopted to target specific populations where colchicine can produce a maximum benefit, such as in those patients with (i) persistent inflammation after the index event (i.e., persistently high hsCRP); (ii) particular markers of excess NLRP3 inflammasome activity (i.e., carriers of the rs10754555 gene variant); or (iii) high-risk of recurrence (such as diabetics). And finally, in the setting of secondary prevention of coronary artery disease, incorporating an additional drug to patients who are already under treatment with multiple medications with proven benefit brings forth the problem of poor adherence, as well as the risk of aggravating polypharmacy in an increasingly elderly and frail population. Table 2 summarizes the available phase 2 and phase 3 data on colchicine and atherosclerosis.

Table 2. Phase 2 and 3 clinical studies.

Trials	Setting	Key Inclusion Criteria	No. of Participants	Treatment	Main Results	Follow Up (Mean)
Giannopoulos et al. (2015) [127]	CABG	Patients undergoing CABG	59	Colchicine 0.5 mg BID vs. placebo	↓ 62% hsTnT and ↓ 52% CK-MB concentration	48 h after surgery
Deftereos et al. (2015) [128]	STEMI	STEMI ≤ 12 h from pain onset (treated with PCI)	151	Colchicine loading dose of 2 mg plus 0.5 mg BID vs. placebo	↓ 49% of CK-MB and ↓ 57% of hsTnT AUC concentration ↓ 25% MI volume (MRI)	9 days
COLIN (2017) [129]	STEMI	STEMI with one main coronary artery occluded	44	Colchicine 1 mg QD vs. placebo	No significant effect on: - hsCRP peak value	During hospitalization
Mewton et al. (2021) [130]	STEMI	STEMI referred for PCI	192	Colchicine 2 mg loading dose plus 0.5 mg BID vs. placebo	No significant effect on: - Infarct size at 5 days (MRI) - LV end-diastolic volume change at 3 months (MRI)	3 months
Vaidya et al. (2018) [131]	ACS	ACS (<1 month)	80	Colchicine 0.5 mg QD plus OMT vs. OMT alone	↓ Low attenuation plaque volume in CCTA (↓ 40.9% vs. ↓ 17%) hsCRP (↓ 37.3% vs. ↓ 14.6%)	12 months
Akrami et al. (2021) [132]	ACS	ACS (with medical therapy or PCI)	249	Colchicine 0.5 mg QD vs. placebo	↓ 71% MACE ↓ 84% ACS No significant effect on: - Decompensated HF - Death from any cause - Cardiovascular death	6 months
Fiolet et al. (2020) [133]	CCS	CCS and hsCRP ≥ 2 mg/L	138	Colchicine 0.5 mg QD	↓ 41% hsCRP levels ↓ 16% IL-6 levels	30 days
Colchicine-PCI (2020) [134]	PCI	Subjects referred for PCI (ACS or CCS)	400	Colchicine 1.8 mg pre-procedural	No significant effect on: - PCI-related myocardial injury - 30-day MACE (Death from any cause, MI, revascularization)	30 days
COPE-PCI (2021) [135]	PCI	Patients undergoing PCI (CCS or NSTEMI)	196	Colchicine 1.5 mg pre-procedural	↓ 41% Periprocedural myocardial injury	24 hrs
COLCOT (2019) [138]	ACS	MI (treated with PCI) within 30 days	4745	Colchicine 0.5 mg BID vs. placebo	↓ 23% MACE ↓ 84% Stroke ↓ 50% urgent hospitalization for angina leading to coronary revascularization No significant effect on: - Cardiovascular death - Resuscitated cardiac arrest - MI	19.5 months

Table 2. Cont.

Trials	Setting	Key Inclusion Criteria	No. of Participants	Treatment	Main Results	Follow Up (Mean)
COPS (2020) [139]	ACS	ACS treated with PCI or optimal medical therapy	795	Colchicine 0.5 mg BID for one month, then 0.5 mg QD for 11 months vs. placebo	↓ 84% Ischemia-driven urgent revascularization ↓ Death from any cause (8 vs. 1 patients) No significant effect on: - MACE - ACS - Stroke (ischemic, non-cardioembolic)	12 months
COPS (2021) [139]	ACS	ACS treated with PCI or optimal medical therapy	795	Same as above, no colchicine or placebo from months 13 to 24.	↓ 41% MACE ↓ 81% Ischemia-driven urgent revascularization No significant effect on: - Death from any cause - ACS - Stroke (ischemic, non-cardioembolic)	24 months
LoDoCo (2013) [141]	CCS	CCS, clinically stable for >6 months	532	Colchicine 0.5 mg QD vs. no colchicine	↓ 67% MACE ↓ 67% ACS No significant effect on: - Cardiac arrest - Stroke (ischemic, non-cardioembolic)	36 months
LoDoCo2 (2020) [142]	CCS	CCS, clinically stable for >6 months	5522	Colchicine 0.5 mg QD vs. placebo	↓ 31% MACE ↓ 30% MI (spontaneous, nonprocedural) ↓ 25% ischemia-driven coronary revascularization No significant effect on: - Cardiovascular death - Stroke (ischemic)	28.6 months
Deftereos S, et al. (2013) [143]	ACS/CCS	Diabetic patients undergoing PCI with BMS	196	Colchicine 0.5 mg BID vs. placebo	↓ 62% Angiographic in stent restenosis↓ 58% IVUS in stent restenosis	6 months

↓: indicates reduction of measured outcome. ACS: Acute coronary syndrome; AUC: area under the curve; BID: twice daily; BMS: bare-metal stent; CABG: coronary artery bypass grafting; CCS: chronic coronary syndrome; CCTA: coronary computed tomography angiography; CKMB: creatine kinase-MB; HF: heart failure; hsCRP: high-sensitive C reactive protein; hsTnT: high-sensitive Troponin T; IVUS: intravascular ultrasound; LV: left ventricle; MACE: Major adverse cardiovascular events, refers to the composite primary endpoint of each study, including all the individual outcomes listed in the box.; MI: myocardial infarction; MRI: magnetic resonance imaging; NSTEMI: non-ST-elevation MI; OMT: optimal medical therapy; PCI: percutaneous coronary intervention; QD: once daily; STEMI: ST-elevation MI; UA: unstable angina.

9. Conclusions

The inflammatory component of atherosclerosis pathogenesis offers new avenues through which novel therapies can be used and/or developed. Though around for decades, only recently has colchicine been in the eye of scientists and clinicians looking for new therapies for the management of coronary artery disease complications. The intracellular effects of colchicine directly impact key cellular players of inflammation, resulting in protective effects against atherosclerosis development (Figure 2). Translational research and phase 2 and 3 clinical trials have predominantly shown a beneficial effect of colchicine by modulating many underlying processes related to athero-inflammation and resulting in less clinical events. However, the net clinical effect upon mortality is still unclear and new trials must address this issue to be able to finally introduce this long-waited drug into the therapeutic toolkit to treat coronary artery disease.

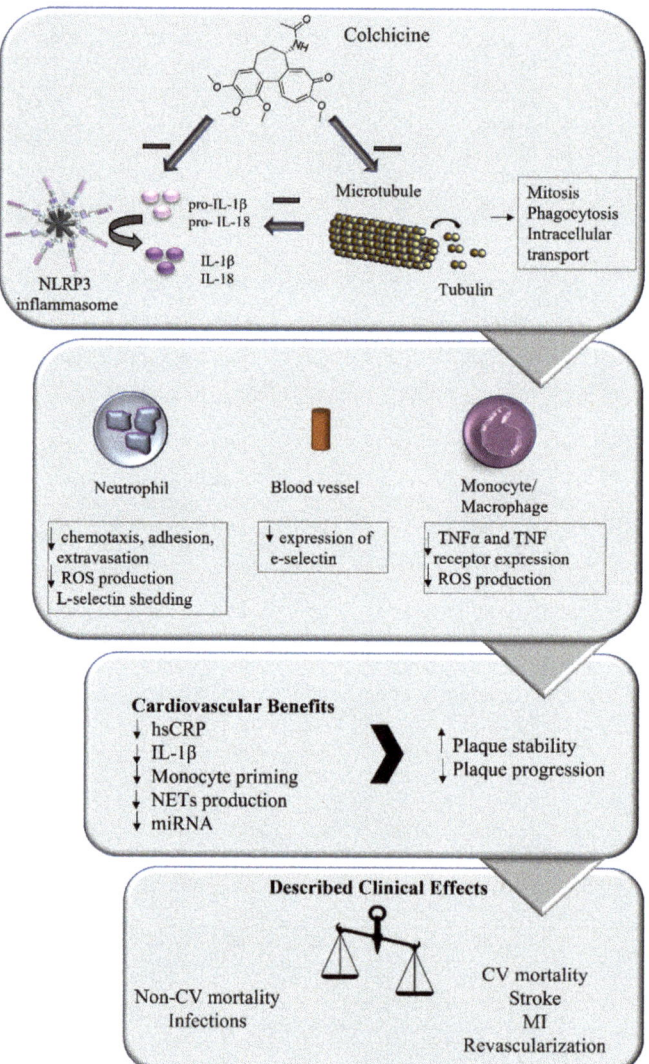

Figure 2. Role of colchicine in coronary artery disease treatment. Colchicine has been described to affect microtubule stability, impacting several intracellular processes including mitosis, phagocytosis, and intracellular transport. It has also been reported that colchicine affects NLRP3 inflammasome activation, impacting inflammatory cytokines production, both directly and through its action on microtubules. These intracellular effects directly impact the inflammatory response of neutrophils, monocyte/macrophages, and blood vessels, which translates into several cardiovascular benefits. The overall effect on plaque stability and progression impacts the clinical manifestations of atherosclerosis, reducing the incidence of major adverse cardiovascular effects, suggesting that the addition of colchicine to the management of coronary artery disease might be beneficial.

Author Contributions: G.M.R. and P.M.V. designed the study. G.M.R. and L.G. screened the available literature. L.G. and J.F.B. wrote the original draft. G.M.R., M.P.O. and P.M.V. reviewed and edited the manuscript. All authors have read and agreed to the published version of the manuscript.

Funding: GM: MPO: Fondo Nacional de Desarrollo Científico y Tecnológico (FONDECYT) de la Agencia Nacional de Investigación y Desarrollo (ANID)-Proyecto FONDECYT Regular 1210655, LG: ANID, Programa Iniciativa Científica Milenio–ICN2021_004.

Institutional Review Board Statement: Not applicable.

Informed Consent Statement: Not applicable.

Data Availability Statement: Not applicable.

Conflicts of Interest: The authors declare no conflict of interest.

References

1. World Health Organization. The World Health Report 1999: Making a difference. *Health Millions* **1999**, *25*, 3–5.
2. Roger, V.L.; Go, A.S.; Lloyd-Jones, D.M.; Benjamin, E.J.; Berry, J.D.; Borden, W.B.; Bravata, D.M.; Dai, S.; Ford, E.S.; Fox, C.S.; et al. Heart disease and stroke statistics—2012 update: A report from the American Heart Association. *Circulation* **2012**, *125*, e2–e220. [CrossRef] [PubMed]
3. Vaidya, K.; Martinez, G.; Patel, S. The Role of Colchicine in Acute Coronary Syndromes. *Clin. Ther.* **2019**, *41*, 11–20. [CrossRef] [PubMed]
4. Reith, C.; Armitage, J. Management of residual risk after statin therapy. *Atherosclerosis* **2016**, *245*, 161–170. [CrossRef]
5. Huynh, T.; Montigny, M.; Iftikhar, U.; Gagnon, R.; Eisenberg, M.; Lauzon, C.; Mansour, S.; Rinfret, S.; Afilalo, M.; Nguyen, M.; et al. Recurrent Cardiovascular Events in Survivors of Myocardial Infarction with ST-Segment Elevation (from the AMI-QUEBEC Study). *Am. J. Cardiol.* **2018**, *121*, 897–902. [CrossRef]
6. Khan, R.; Spagnoli, V.; Tardif, J.C.; L'Allier, P.L. Novel anti-inflammatory therapies for the treatment of atherosclerosis. *Atherosclerosis* **2015**, *240*, 497–509. [CrossRef]
7. Geovanini, G.R.; Libby, P. Atherosclerosis and inflammation: Overview and updates. *Clin. Sci.* **2018**, *132*, 1243–1252. [CrossRef]
8. Hansson, G.K.; Libby, P.; Schonbeck, U.; Yan, Z.Q. Innate and adaptive immunity in the pathogenesis of atherosclerosis. *Circ. Res.* **2002**, *91*, 281–291. [CrossRef]
9. Libby, P. Inflammation in atherosclerosis. *Nature* **2002**, *420*, 868–874. [CrossRef]
10. Stewart, C.R.; Stuart, L.M.; Wilkinson, K.; van Gils, J.M.; Deng, J.; Halle, A.; Rayner, K.J.; Boyer, L.; Zhong, R.; Frazier, W.A.; et al. CD36 ligands promote sterile inflammation through assembly of a Toll-like receptor 4 and 6 heterodimer. *Nat. Immunol.* **2010**, *11*, 155–161. [CrossRef]
11. De Winther, M.P.; Kanters, E.; Kraal, G.; Hofker, M.H. Nuclear factor kappaB signaling in atherogenesis. *Arterioscler. Thromb. Vasc. Biol.* **2005**, *25*, 904–914. [CrossRef] [PubMed]
12. Libby, P.; Ridker, P.M.; Hansson, G.K. Progress and challenges in translating the biology of atherosclerosis. *Nature* **2011**, *473*, 317–325. [CrossRef] [PubMed]
13. Sukhova, G.K.; Schonbeck, U.; Rabkin, E.; Schoen, F.J.; Poole, A.R.; Billinghurst, R.C.; Libby, P. Evidence for increased collagenolysis by interstitial collagenases-1 and -3 in vulnerable human atheromatous plaques. *Circulation* **1999**, *99*, 2503–2509. [CrossRef] [PubMed]
14. Deguchi, J.O.; Aikawa, E.; Libby, P.; Vachon, J.R.; Inada, M.; Krane, S.M.; Whittaker, P.; Aikawa, M. Matrix metalloproteinase-13/collagenase-3 deletion promotes collagen accumulation and organization in mouse atherosclerotic plaques. *Circulation* **2005**, *112*, 2708–2715. [CrossRef]
15. Silvestre-Roig, C.; Braster, Q.; Ortega-Gomez, A.; Soehnlein, O. Neutrophils as regulators of cardiovascular inflammation. *Nat. Rev. Cardiol.* **2020**, *17*, 327–340. [CrossRef]
16. Guasti, L.; Dentali, F.; Castiglioni, L.; Maroni, L.; Marino, F.; Squizzato, A.; Ageno, W.; Gianni, M.; Gaudio, G.; Grandi, A.M.; et al. Neutrophils and clinical outcomes in patients with acute coronary syndromes and/or cardiac revascularisation. A systematic review on more than 34,000 subjects. *Thromb. Haemost.* **2011**, *106*, 591–599. [CrossRef]
17. Drechsler, M.; Megens, R.T.; van Zandvoort, M.; Weber, C.; Soehnlein, O. Hyperlipidemia-triggered neutrophilia promotes early atherosclerosis. *Circulation* **2010**, *122*, 1837–1845. [CrossRef]
18. Malle, E.; Waeg, G.; Schreiber, R.; Grone, E.F.; Sattler, W.; Grone, H.J. Immunohistochemical evidence for the myeloperoxidase/ H_2O_2/halide system in human atherosclerotic lesions: Colocalization of myeloperoxidase and hypochlorite-modified proteins. *Eur. J. Biochem.* **2000**, *267*, 4495–4503. [CrossRef]
19. Podrez, E.A.; Febbraio, M.; Sheibani, N.; Schmitt, D.; Silverstein, R.L.; Hajjar, D.P.; Cohen, P.A.; Frazier, W.A.; Hoff, H.F.; Hazen, S.L. Macrophage scavenger receptor CD36 is the major receptor for LDL modified by monocyte-generated reactive nitrogen species. *J. Clin. Investig.* **2000**, *105*, 1095–1108. [CrossRef]

20. Fu, X.; Kassim, S.Y.; Parks, W.C.; Heinecke, J.W. Hypochlorous acid oxygenates the cysteine switch domain of pro-matrilysin (MMP-7). A mechanism for matrix metalloproteinase activation and atherosclerotic plaque rupture by myeloperoxidase. *J. Biol. Chem.* **2001**, *276*, 41279–41287. [CrossRef]
21. Dorweiler, B.; Torzewski, M.; Dahm, M.; Kirkpatrick, C.J.; Lackner, K.J.; Vahl, C.F. Subendothelial infiltration of neutrophil granulocytes and liberation of matrix-destabilizing enzymes in an experimental model of human neo-intima. *Thromb. Haemost.* **2008**, *99*, 373–381. [CrossRef] [PubMed]
22. Henriksen, P.A.; Sallenave, J.M. Human neutrophil elastase: Mediator and therapeutic target in atherosclerosis. *Int. J. Biochem. Cell Biol.* **2008**, *40*, 1095–1100. [CrossRef] [PubMed]
23. Pezzato, E.; Dona, M.; Sartor, L.; Dell'Aica, I.; Benelli, R.; Albini, A.; Garbisa, S. Proteinase-3 directly activates MMP-2 and degrades gelatin and Matrigel; differential inhibition by (-)epigallocatechin-3-gallate. *J. Leukoc. Biol.* **2003**, *74*, 88–94. [CrossRef] [PubMed]
24. Rotzius, P.; Soehnlein, O.; Kenne, E.; Lindbom, L.; Nystrom, K.; Thams, S.; Eriksson, E.E. ApoE(-/-)/lysozyme M(EGFP/EGFP) mice as a versatile model to study monocyte and neutrophil trafficking in atherosclerosis. *Atherosclerosis* **2009**, *202*, 111–118. [CrossRef] [PubMed]
25. Ionita, M.G.; van den Borne, P.; Catanzariti, L.M.; Moll, F.L.; de Vries, J.P.; Pasterkamp, G.; Vink, A.; de Kleijn, D.P. High neutrophil numbers in human carotid atherosclerotic plaques are associated with characteristics of rupture-prone lesions. *Arterioscler. Thromb. Vasc. Biol.* **2010**, *30*, 1842–1848. [CrossRef]
26. Zernecke, A.; Bot, I.; Djalali-Talab, Y.; Shagdarsuren, E.; Bidzhekov, K.; Meiler, S.; Krohn, R.; Schober, A.; Sperandio, M.; Soehnlein, O.; et al. Protective role of CXC receptor 4/CXC ligand 12 unveils the importance of neutrophils in atherosclerosis. *Circ. Res.* **2008**, *102*, 209–217. [CrossRef]
27. Soehnlein, O.; Lindbom, L.; Weber, C. Mechanisms underlying neutrophil-mediated monocyte recruitment. *Blood* **2009**, *114*, 4613–4623. [CrossRef]
28. Rasmuson, J.; Kenne, E.; Wahlgren, M.; Soehnlein, O.; Lindbom, L. Heparinoid sevuparin inhibits Streptococcus-induced vascular leak through neutralizing neutrophil-derived proteins. *FASEB J.* **2019**, *33*, 10443–10452. [CrossRef]
29. Doring, Y.; Soehnlein, O.; Weber, C. Neutrophil Extracellular Traps in Atherosclerosis and Atherothrombosis. *Circ. Res.* **2017**, *120*, 736–743. [CrossRef]
30. Brinkmann, V.; Reichard, U.; Goosmann, C.; Fauler, B.; Uhlemann, Y.; Weiss, D.S.; Weinrauch, Y.; Zychlinsky, A. Neutrophil extracellular traps kill bacteria. *Science* **2004**, *303*, 1532–1535. [CrossRef]
31. Warnatsch, A.; Ioannou, M.; Wang, Q.; Papayannopoulos, V. Inflammation. Neutrophil extracellular traps license macrophages for cytokine production in atherosclerosis. *Science* **2015**, *349*, 316–320. [CrossRef] [PubMed]
32. Megens, R.T.; Vijayan, S.; Lievens, D.; Doring, Y.; van Zandvoort, M.A.; Grommes, J.; Weber, C.; Soehnlein, O. Presence of luminal neutrophil extracellular traps in atherosclerosis. *Thromb. Haemost.* **2012**, *107*, 597–598. [CrossRef] [PubMed]
33. Quillard, T.; Araujo, H.A.; Franck, G.; Shvartz, E.; Sukhova, G.; Libby, P. TLR2 and neutrophils potentiate endothelial stress, apoptosis and detachment: Implications for superficial erosion. *Eur. Heart J.* **2015**, *36*, 1394–1404. [CrossRef] [PubMed]
34. Borissoff, J.I.; Joosen, I.A.; Versteylen, M.O.; Brill, A.; Fuchs, T.A.; Savchenko, A.S.; Gallant, M.; Martinod, K.; Ten Cate, H.; Hofstra, L.; et al. Elevated levels of circulating DNA and chromatin are independently associated with severe coronary atherosclerosis and a prothrombotic state. *Arterioscler. Thromb. Vasc. Biol.* **2013**, *33*, 2032–2040. [CrossRef] [PubMed]
35. Mangold, A.; Alias, S.; Scherz, T.; Hofbauer, M.; Jakowitsch, J.; Panzenbock, A.; Simon, D.; Laimer, D.; Bangert, C.; Kammerlander, A.; et al. Coronary neutrophil extracellular trap burden and deoxyribonuclease activity in ST-elevation acute coronary syndrome are predictors of ST-segment resolution and infarct size. *Circ. Res.* **2015**, *116*, 1182–1192. [CrossRef]
36. Pertiwi, K.R.; van der Wal, A.C.; Pabittei, D.R.; Mackaaij, C.; van Leeuwen, M.B.; Li, X.; de Boer, O.J. Neutrophil Extracellular Traps Participate in All Different Types of Thrombotic and Haemorrhagic Complications of Coronary Atherosclerosis. *Thromb. Haemost.* **2018**, *118*, 1078–1087. [CrossRef]
37. Grebe, A.; Latz, E. Cholesterol crystals and inflammation. *Curr. Rheumatol. Rep.* **2013**, *15*, 313. [CrossRef]
38. Duewell, P.; Kono, H.; Rayner, K.J.; Sirois, C.M.; Vladimer, G.; Bauernfeind, F.G.; Abela, G.S.; Franchi, L.; Nunez, G.; Schnurr, M.; et al. NLRP3 inflammasomes are required for atherogenesis and activated by cholesterol crystals. *Nature* **2010**, *464*, 1357–1361. [CrossRef]
39. Small, D.M. George Lyman Duff memorial lecture. Progression and regression of atherosclerotic lesions. Insights from lipid physical biochemistry. *Arteriosclerosis* **1988**, *8*, 103–129. [CrossRef]
40. Abela, G.S. Cholesterol crystals piercing the arterial plaque and intima trigger local and systemic inflammation. *J. Clin. Lipidol.* **2010**, *4*, 156–164. [CrossRef]
41. Takeuchi, O.; Akira, S. Pattern recognition receptors and inflammation. *Cell* **2010**, *140*, 805–820. [CrossRef] [PubMed]
42. Sharma, B.R.; Kanneganti, T.D. NLRP3 inflammasome in cancer and metabolic diseases. *Nat. Immunol.* **2021**, *22*, 550–559. [CrossRef] [PubMed]
43. Sharma, D.; Kanneganti, T.D. The cell biology of inflammasomes: Mechanisms of inflammasome activation and regulation. *J. Cell Biol.* **2016**, *213*, 617–629. [CrossRef] [PubMed]
44. Pope, R.M.; Tschopp, J. The role of interleukin-1 and the inflammasome in gout: Implications for therapy. *Arthritis Rheum.* **2007**, *56*, 3183–3188. [CrossRef]
45. Stutz, A.; Golenbock, D.T.; Latz, E. Inflammasomes: Too big to miss. *J. Clin. Investig.* **2009**, *119*, 3502–3511. [CrossRef]

46. Christgen, S.; Kanneganti, T.D. Inflammasomes and the fine line between defense and disease. *Curr. Opin. Immunol.* **2020**, *62*, 39–44. [CrossRef]
47. Franchi, L.; Munoz-Planillo, R.; Nunez, G. Sensing and reacting to microbes through the inflammasomes. *Nat. Immunol.* **2012**, *13*, 325–332. [CrossRef]
48. Mathur, A.; Hayward, J.A.; Man, S.M. Molecular mechanisms of inflammasome signaling. *J. Leukoc. Biol.* **2018**, *103*, 233–257. [CrossRef]
49. Vajjhala, P.R.; Mirams, R.E.; Hill, J.M. Multiple binding sites on the pyrin domain of ASC protein allow self-association and interaction with NLRP3 protein. *J. Biol. Chem.* **2012**, *287*, 41732–41743. [CrossRef]
50. Fernandes-Alnemri, T.; Wu, J.; Yu, J.W.; Datta, P.; Miller, B.; Jankowski, W.; Rosenberg, S.; Zhang, J.; Alnemri, E.S. The pyroptosome: A supramolecular assembly of ASC dimers mediating inflammatory cell death via caspase-1 activation. *Cell Death Differ* **2007**, *14*, 1590–1604. [CrossRef]
51. Hornung, V.; Bauernfeind, F.; Halle, A.; Samstad, E.O.; Kono, H.; Rock, K.L.; Fitzgerald, K.A.; Latz, E. Silica crystals and aluminum salts activate the NALP3 inflammasome through phagosomal destabilization. *Nat. Immunol.* **2008**, *9*, 847–856. [CrossRef] [PubMed]
52. Weber, K.; Schilling, J.D. Lysosomes integrate metabolic-inflammatory cross-talk in primary macrophage inflammasome activation. *J. Biol. Chem.* **2014**, *289*, 9158–9171. [CrossRef]
53. Sheedy, F.J.; Grebe, A.; Rayner, K.J.; Kalantari, P.; Ramkhelawon, B.; Carpenter, S.B.; Becker, C.E.; Ediriweera, H.N.; Mullick, A.E.; Golenbock, D.T.; et al. CD36 coordinates NLRP3 inflammasome activation by facilitating intracellular nucleation of soluble ligands into particulate ligands in sterile inflammation. *Nat. Immunol.* **2013**, *14*, 812–820. [CrossRef] [PubMed]
54. Kirii, H.; Niwa, T.; Yamada, Y.; Wada, H.; Saito, K.; Iwakura, Y.; Asano, M.; Moriwaki, H.; Seishima, M. Lack of interleukin-1beta decreases the severity of atherosclerosis in ApoE-deficient mice. *Arterioscler. Thromb. Vasc. Biol.* **2003**, *23*, 656–660. [CrossRef] [PubMed]
55. Alexander, M.R.; Moehle, C.W.; Johnson, J.L.; Yang, Z.; Lee, J.K.; Jackson, C.L.; Owens, G.K. Genetic inactivation of IL-1 signaling enhances atherosclerotic plaque instability and reduces outward vessel remodeling in advanced atherosclerosis in mice. *J. Clin. Investig.* **2012**, *122*, 70–79. [CrossRef] [PubMed]
56. Libby, P. Interleukin-1 Beta as a Target for Atherosclerosis Therapy: Biological Basis of CANTOS and Beyond. *J. Am. Coll. Cardiol.* **2017**, *70*, 2278–2289. [CrossRef]
57. Yajima, N.; Takahashi, M.; Morimoto, H.; Shiba, Y.; Takahashi, Y.; Masumoto, J.; Ise, H.; Sagara, J.; Nakayama, J.; Taniguchi, S.; et al. Critical role of bone marrow apoptosis-associated speck-like protein, an inflammasome adaptor molecule, in neointimal formation after vascular injury in mice. *Circulation* **2008**, *117*, 3079–3087. [CrossRef]
58. Gage, J.; Hasu, M.; Thabet, M.; Whitman, S.C. Caspase-1 deficiency decreases atherosclerosis in apolipoprotein E-null mice. *Can. J. Cardiol.* **2012**, *28*, 222–229. [CrossRef]
59. Usui, F.; Shirasuna, K.; Kimura, H.; Tatsumi, K.; Kawashima, A.; Karasawa, T.; Hida, S.; Sagara, J.; Taniguchi, S.; Takahashi, M. Critical role of caspase-1 in vascular inflammation and development of atherosclerosis in Western diet-fed apolipoprotein E-deficient mice. *Biochem. Biophys. Res. Commun.* **2012**, *425*, 162–168. [CrossRef]
60. Hendrikx, T.; Jeurissen, M.L.; van Gorp, P.J.; Gijbels, M.J.; Walenbergh, S.M.; Houben, T.; van Gorp, R.; Pottgens, C.C.; Stienstra, R.; Netea, M.G.; et al. Bone marrow-specific caspase-1/11 deficiency inhibits atherosclerosis development in Ldlr(-/-) mice. *FEBS J.* **2015**, *282*, 2327–2338. [CrossRef]
61. Menu, P.; Pellegrin, M.; Aubert, J.F.; Bouzourene, K.; Tardivel, A.; Mazzolai, L.; Tschopp, J. Atherosclerosis in ApoE-deficient mice progresses independently of the NLRP3 inflammasome. *Cell Death Dis* **2011**, *2*, e137. [CrossRef] [PubMed]
62. Shi, X.; Xie, W.L.; Kong, W.W.; Chen, D.; Qu, P. Expression of the NLRP3 Inflammasome in Carotid Atherosclerosis. *J. Stroke Cerebrovasc. Dis.* **2015**, *24*, 2455–2466. [CrossRef] [PubMed]
63. Paramel Varghese, G.; Folkersen, L.; Strawbridge, R.J.; Halvorsen, B.; Yndestad, A.; Ranheim, T.; Krohg-Sorensen, K.; Skjelland, M.; Espevik, T.; Aukrust, P.; et al. NLRP3 Inflammasome Expression and Activation in Human Atherosclerosis. *J. Am. Heart Assoc.* **2016**, *5*, e003031. [CrossRef] [PubMed]
64. Robertson, S.; Martinez, G.J.; Payet, C.A.; Barraclough, J.Y.; Celermajer, D.S.; Bursill, C.; Patel, S. Colchicine therapy in acute coronary syndrome patients acts on caspase-1 to suppress NLRP3 inflammasome monocyte activation. *Clin. Sci.* **2016**, *130*, 1237–1246. [CrossRef] [PubMed]
65. Altaf, A.; Qu, P.; Zhao, Y.; Wang, H.; Lou, D.; Niu, N. NLRP3 inflammasome in peripheral blood monocytes of acute coronary syndrome patients and its relationship with statins. *Coron. Artery Dis.* **2015**, *26*, 409–421. [CrossRef] [PubMed]
66. Dasgeb, B.; Kornreich, D.; McGuinn, K.; Okon, L.; Brownell, I.; Sackett, D.L. Colchicine: An ancient drug with novel applications. *Br. J. Dermatol.* **2018**, *178*, 350–356. [CrossRef]
67. D'Amario, D.; Cappetta, D.; Cappannoli, L.; Princi, G.; Migliaro, S.; Diana, G.; Chouchane, K.; Borovac, J.A.; Restivo, A.; Arcudi, A.; et al. Colchicine in ischemic heart disease: The good, the bad and the ugly. *Clin. Res. Cardiol.* **2021**, *110*, 1531–1542. [CrossRef]
68. Cortese, F.; Bhattacharyya, B.; Wolff, J. Podophyllotoxin as a probe for the colchicine binding site of tubulin. *J. Biol. Chem.* **1977**, *252*, 1134–1140. [CrossRef]
69. Pyles, E.A.; Hastie, S.B. Effect of the B ring and the C-7 substituent on the kinetics of colchicinoid-tubulin associations. *Biochemistry* **1993**, *32*, 2329–2336. [CrossRef]

70. Pascart, T.; Richette, P. Colchicine in Gout: An Update. *Curr. Pharm. Des.* **2018**, *24*, 684–689. [CrossRef]
71. Portincasa, P. Colchicine, Biologic Agents and More for the Treatment of Familial Mediterranean Fever. The Old, the New, and the Rare. *Curr. Med. Chem.* **2016**, *23*, 60–86. [CrossRef] [PubMed]
72. Deftereos, S.G.; Beerkens, F.J.; Shah, B.; Giannopoulos, G.; Vrachatis, D.A.; Giotaki, S.G.; Siasos, G.; Nicolas, J.; Arnott, C.; Patel, S.; et al. Colchicine in Cardiovascular Disease: In-Depth Review. *Circulation* **2022**, *145*, 61–78. [CrossRef] [PubMed]
73. Taylor, E.W. The Mechanism of Colchicine Inhibition of Mitosis. I. Kinetics of Inhibition and the Binding of H3-Colchicine. *J. Cell Biol.* **1965**, *25*, 145–160. [CrossRef]
74. Asako, H.; Kubes, P.; Baethge, B.A.; Wolf, R.E.; Granger, D.N. Colchicine and methotrexate reduce leukocyte adherence and emigration in rat mesenteric venules. *Inflammation* **1992**, *16*, 45–56. [CrossRef] [PubMed]
75. Cronstein, B.N.; Molad, Y.; Reibman, J.; Balakhane, E.; Levin, R.I.; Weissmann, G. Colchicine alters the quantitative and qualitative display of selectins on endothelial cells and neutrophils. *J. Clin. Investig.* **1995**, *96*, 994–1002. [CrossRef] [PubMed]
76. Paschke, S.; Weidner, A.F.; Paust, T.; Marti, O.; Beil, M.; Ben-Chetrit, E. Technical advance: Inhibition of neutrophil chemotaxis by colchicine is modulated through viscoelastic properties of subcellular compartments. *J. Leukoc. Biol.* **2013**, *94*, 1091–1096. [CrossRef] [PubMed]
77. Roberge, C.J.; Gaudry, M.; de Medicis, R.; Lussier, A.; Poubelle, P.E.; Naccache, P.H. Crystal-induced neutrophil activation. IV. Specific inhibition of tyrosine phosphorylation by colchicine. *J. Clin. Investig.* **1993**, *92*, 1722–1729. [CrossRef]
78. Chia, E.W.; Grainger, R.; Harper, J.L. Colchicine suppresses neutrophil superoxide production in a murine model of gouty arthritis: A rationale for use of low-dose colchicine. *Br. J. Pharmacol.* **2008**, *153*, 1288–1295. [CrossRef]
79. Viktorov, A.V.; Yurkiv, V.A. Albendazole and colchicine modulate LPS-induced secretion of inflammatory mediators by liver macrophages. *Bull. Exp. Biol. Med.* **2011**, *151*, 683–685. [CrossRef]
80. Ding, A.H.; Porteu, F.; Sanchez, E.; Nathan, C.F. Downregulation of tumor necrosis factor receptors on macrophages and endothelial cells by microtubule depolymerizing agents. *J. Exp. Med.* **1990**, *171*, 715–727. [CrossRef]
81. Menche, D.; Israel, A.; Karpatkin, S. Platelets and microtubules. Effect of colchicine and D2O on platelet aggregation and release induced by calcium ionophore A23187. *J. Clin. Investig.* **1980**, *66*, 284–291. [CrossRef] [PubMed]
82. Cimmino, G.; Tarallo, R.; Conte, S.; Morello, A.; Pellegrino, G.; Loffredo, F.S.; Cali, G.; De Luca, N.; Golino, P.; Trimarco, B.; et al. Colchicine reduces platelet aggregation by modulating cytoskeleton rearrangement via inhibition of cofilin and LIM domain kinase 1. *Vascul. Pharmacol.* **2018**, *111*, 62–70. [CrossRef] [PubMed]
83. Abanonu, G.B.; Daskin, A.; Akdogan, M.F.; Uyar, S.; Demirtunc, R. Mean platelet volume and beta-thromboglobulin levels in familial Mediterranean fever: Effect of colchicine use? *Eur. J. Intern. Med.* **2012**, *23*, 661–664. [CrossRef] [PubMed]
84. Shah, B.; Allen, N.; Harchandani, B.; Pillinger, M.; Katz, S.; Sedlis, S.P.; Echagarruga, C.; Samuels, S.K.; Morina, P.; Singh, P.; et al. Effect of Colchicine on Platelet-Platelet and Platelet-Leukocyte Interactions: A Pilot Study in Healthy Subjects. *Inflammation* **2016**, *39*, 182–189. [CrossRef] [PubMed]
85. Raju, N.C.; Yi, Q.; Nidorf, M.; Fagel, N.D.; Hiralal, R.; Eikelboom, J.W. Effect of colchicine compared with placebo on high sensitivity C-reactive protein in patients with acute coronary syndrome or acute stroke: A pilot randomized controlled trial. *J. Thromb. Thrombolysis* **2012**, *33*, 88–94. [CrossRef]
86. Moschonas, I.C.; Tselepis, A.D. The pathway of neutrophil extracellular traps towards atherosclerosis and thrombosis. *Atherosclerosis* **2019**, *288*, 9–16. [CrossRef]
87. Munoz, L.E.; Boeltz, S.; Bilyy, R.; Schauer, C.; Mahajan, A.; Widulin, N.; Gruneboom, A.; Herrmann, I.; Boada, E.; Rauh, M.; et al. Neutrophil Extracellular Traps Initiate Gallstone Formation. *Immunity* **2019**, *51*, 443–450.e4. [CrossRef]
88. Safi, R.; Kallas, R.; Bardawil, T.; Mehanna, C.J.; Abbas, O.; Hamam, R.; Uthman, I.; Kibbi, A.G.; Nassar, D. Neutrophils contribute to vasculitis by increased release of neutrophil extracellular traps in Behcet's disease. *J. Dermatol. Sci.* **2018**, *92*, 143–150. [CrossRef]
89. Vaidya, K.; Tucker, B.; Kurup, R.; Khandkar, C.; Pandzic, E.; Barraclough, J.; Machet, J.; Misra, A.; Kavurma, M.; Martinez, G.; et al. Colchicine Inhibits Neutrophil Extracellular Trap Formation in Patients with Acute Coronary Syndrome After Percutaneous Coronary Intervention. *J. Am. Heart Assoc.* **2021**, *10*, e018993. [CrossRef]
90. Martinon, F.; Petrilli, V.; Mayor, A.; Tardivel, A.; Tschopp, J. Gout-associated uric acid crystals activate the NALP3 inflammasome. *Nature* **2006**, *440*, 237–241. [CrossRef]
91. Park, Y.H.; Wood, G.; Kastner, D.L.; Chae, J.J. Pyrin inflammasome activation and RhoA signaling in the autoinflammatory diseases FMF and HIDS. *Nat. Immunol.* **2016**, *17*, 914–921. [CrossRef] [PubMed]
92. Misawa, T.; Takahama, M.; Kozaki, T.; Lee, H.; Zou, J.; Saitoh, T.; Akira, S. Microtubule-driven spatial arrangement of mitochondria promotes activation of the NLRP3 inflammasome. *Nat. Immunol.* **2013**, *14*, 454–460. [CrossRef] [PubMed]
93. Lai, H.T.T.; Do, H.M.; Nguyen, T.T. Evaluation of Colchicine's interaction with the ATP-binding region of mice NLRP3-NACHT domain using molecular docking and dynamics simulation. *J. Phys. Conf. Ser.* **2022**, *2269*, 12012. [CrossRef]
94. Schroder, K.; Tschopp, J. The inflammasomes. *Cell* **2010**, *140*, 821–832. [CrossRef]
95. Marques-da-Silva, C.; Chaves, M.M.; Castro, N.G.; Coutinho-Silva, R.; Guimaraes, M.Z. Colchicine inhibits cationic dye uptake induced by ATP in P2X2 and P2X7 receptor-expressing cells: Implications for its therapeutic action. *Br. J. Pharmacol.* **2011**, *163*, 912–926. [CrossRef]
96. Sabouraud, A.; Chappey, O.; Dupin, T.; Scherrmann, J.M. Binding of colchicine and thiocolchicoside to human serum proteins and blood cells. *Int. J. Clin. Pharmacol. Ther.* **1994**, *32*, 429–432.
97. Niel, E.; Scherrmann, J.M. Colchicine today. *Jt. Bone Spine* **2006**, *73*, 672–678. [CrossRef]

98. Terkeltaub, R.A. Colchicine update: 2008. *Semin. Arthritis Rheum.* **2009**, *38*, 411–419. [CrossRef]
99. Putterman, C.; Ben-Chetrit, E.; Caraco, Y.; Levy, M. Colchicine intoxication: Clinical pharmacology, risk factors, features, and management. *Semin. Arthritis Rheum.* **1991**, *21*, 143–155. [CrossRef]
100. Andreis, A.; Imazio, M.; Avondo, S.; Casula, M.; Paneva, E.; Piroli, F.; De Ferrari, G.M. Adverse events of colchicine for cardiovascular diseases: A comprehensive meta-analysis of 14 188 patients from 21 randomized controlled trials. *J. Cardiovasc. Med.* **2021**, *22*, 637–644. [CrossRef]
101. Hemkens, L.G.; Ewald, H.; Gloy, V.L.; Arpagaus, A.; Olu, K.K.; Nidorf, M.; Glinz, D.; Nordmann, A.J.; Briel, M. Colchicine for prevention of cardiovascular events. *Cochrane Database Syst. Rev.* **2016**, *1*, CD011047. [CrossRef] [PubMed]
102. Stewart, S.; Yang, K.C.K.; Atkins, K.; Dalbeth, N.; Robinson, P.C. Adverse events during oral colchicine use: A systematic review and meta-analysis of randomised controlled trials. *Arthritis Res. Ther.* **2020**, *22*, 28. [CrossRef] [PubMed]
103. Galli, M.; Princi, G.; Crea, F.; D'Amario, D. Response-letter to the editor: Colchicine and risk of non-cardiovascular death in patients with coronary artery disease: A pooled analysis underlying possible safety concerns. *Eur. Heart J. Cardiovasc Pharmacother* **2021**, *7*, e72–e73. [CrossRef]
104. Tsai, T.L.; Wei, J.C.; Wu, Y.T.; Ku, Y.H.; Lu, K.L.; Wang, Y.H.; Chiou, J.Y. The Association Between Usage of Colchicine and Pneumonia: A Nationwide, Population-Based Cohort Study. *Front. Pharmacol.* **2019**, *10*, 908. [CrossRef] [PubMed]
105. Schwier, N.C.; Cornelio, C.K.; Boylan, P.M. A systematic review of the drug-drug interaction between statins and colchicine: Patient characteristics, etiologies, and clinical management strategies. *Pharmacotherapy* **2022**, *42*, 320–333. [CrossRef] [PubMed]
106. Hung, I.F.; Wu, A.K.; Cheng, V.C.; Tang, B.S.; To, K.W.; Yeung, C.K.; Woo, P.C.; Lau, S.K.; Cheung, B.M.; Yuen, K.Y. Fatal interaction between clarithromycin and colchicine in patients with renal insufficiency: A retrospective study. *Clin. Infect. Dis.* **2005**, *41*, 291–300. [CrossRef] [PubMed]
107. Wojcicki, J.; Hinek, A.; Jaworska, M.; Samochowiec, L. The effect of colchicine on the development of experimental atherosclerosis in rabbits. *Pol. J. Pharmacol. Pharm.* **1986**, *38*, 343–348.
108. Lee, W.M.; Morrison, E.S.; Scott, R.F.; Lee, K.T.; Kroms, M. Effects of methyl prednisolone and colchicine on the development of aortic atherosclerosis in swine. *Atherosclerosis* **1976**, *25*, 213–224. [CrossRef]
109. Bauriedel, G.; Ganesh, S.; Uberfuhr, P.; Welsch, U.; Hofling, B. Growth-inhibiting effect of colchicine on cultured vascular wall myocytes from arteriosclerotic lesions. *Z. Kardiol.* **1992**, *81*, 92–98.
110. Huang, C.; Cen, C.; Wang, C.; Zhan, H.; Ding, X. Synergistic effects of colchicine combined with atorvastatin in rats with hyperlipidemia. *Lipids Health Dis.* **2014**, *13*, 67. [CrossRef]
111. Kaminiotis, V.V.; Agrogiannis, G.; Konstantopoulos, P.; Androutsopoulou, V.; Korou, L.M.; Vlachos, I.S.; Dontas, I.A.; Perrea, D.; Iliopoulos, D.C. Per os colchicine administration in cholesterol fed rabbits: Triglycerides lowering effects without affecting atherosclerosis progress. *Lipids Health Dis.* **2017**, *16*, 184. [CrossRef] [PubMed]
112. Spartalis, M.; Siasos, G.; Mastrogeorgiou, M.; Spartalis, E.; Kaminiotis, V.V.; Mylonas, K.S.; Kapelouzou, A.; Kontogiannis, C.; Doulamis, I.P.; Toutouzas, K.; et al. The effect of per os colchicine administration in combination with fenofibrate and N-acetylcysteine on triglyceride levels and the development of atherosclerotic lesions in cholesterol-fed rabbits. *Eur. Rev. Med. Pharmacol. Sci.* **2021**, *25*, 7765–7776. [CrossRef]
113. Mylonas, K.S.; Kapelouzou, A.; Spartalis, M.; Mastrogeorgiou, M.; Spartalis, E.; Bakoyiannis, C.; Liakakos, T.; Schizas, D.; Iliopoulos, D.; Nikiteas, N. KLF4 Upregulation in Atherosclerotic Thoracic Aortas: Exploring the Protective Effect of Colchicine-based Regimens in a Hyperlipidemic Rabbit Model. *Ann. Vasc. Surg.* **2022**, *78*, 328–335. [CrossRef] [PubMed]
114. Akodad, M.; Fauconnier, J.; Sicard, P.; Huet, F.; Blandel, F.; Bourret, A.; de Santa Barbara, P.; Aguilhon, S.; LeGall, M.; Hugon, G.; et al. Interest of colchicine in the treatment of acute myocardial infarct responsible for heart failure in a mouse model. *Int. J. Cardiol.* **2017**, *240*, 347–353. [CrossRef] [PubMed]
115. Mori, H.; Taki, J.; Wakabayashi, H.; Hiromasa, T.; Inaki, A.; Ogawa, K.; Shiba, K.; Kinuya, S. Colchicine treatment early after infarction attenuates myocardial inflammatory response demonstrated by (14)C-methionine imaging and subsequent ventricular remodeling by quantitative gated SPECT. *Ann. Nucl. Med.* **2021**, *35*, 253–259. [CrossRef] [PubMed]
116. Fujisue, K.; Sugamura, K.; Kurokawa, H.; Matsubara, J.; Ishii, M.; Izumiya, Y.; Kaikita, K.; Sugiyama, S. Colchicine Improves Survival, Left Ventricular Remodeling, and Chronic Cardiac Function After Acute Myocardial Infarction. *Circ. J.* **2017**, *81*, 1174–1182. [CrossRef]
117. Cecconi, A.; Vilchez-Tschischke, J.P.; Mateo, J.; Sanchez-Gonzalez, J.; Espana, S.; Fernandez-Jimenez, R.; Lopez-Melgar, B.; Fernandez Friera, L.; Lopez-Martin, G.J.; Fuster, V.; et al. Effects of Colchicine on Atherosclerotic Plaque Stabilization: A Multimodality Imaging Study in an Animal Model. *J. Cardiovasc. Transl. Res.* **2021**, *14*, 150–160. [CrossRef]
118. Nidorf, M.; Thompson, P.L. Effect of colchicine (0.5 mg twice daily) on high-sensitivity C-reactive protein independent of aspirin and atorvastatin in patients with stable coronary artery disease. *Am. J. Cardiol.* **2007**, *99*, 805–807. [CrossRef]
119. Martinez, G.J.; Robertson, S.; Barraclough, J.; Xia, Q.; Mallat, Z.; Bursill, C.; Celermajer, D.S.; Patel, S. Colchicine Acutely Suppresses Local Cardiac Production of Inflammatory Cytokines in Patients with an Acute Coronary Syndrome. *J. Am. Heart Assoc.* **2015**, *4*, e002128. [CrossRef]
120. Tucker, B.; Kurup, R.; Barraclough, J.; Henriquez, R.; Cartland, S.; Arnott, C.; Misra, A.; Martinez, G.; Kavurma, M.; Patel, S. Colchicine as a Novel Therapy for Suppressing Chemokine Production in Patients with an Acute Coronary Syndrome: A Pilot Study. *Clin. Ther.* **2019**, *41*, 2172–2181. [CrossRef]

121. Cartland, S.P.; Genner, S.W.; Martinez, G.J.; Robertson, S.; Kockx, M.; Lin, R.C.; O'Sullivan, J.F.; Koay, Y.C.; Manuneedhi Cholan, P.; Kebede, M.A.; et al. TRAIL-Expressing Monocyte/Macrophages Are Critical for Reducing Inflammation and Atherosclerosis. *iScience* **2019**, *12*, 41–52. [CrossRef] [PubMed]
122. Cartland, S.P.; Lin, R.C.Y.; Genner, S.; Patil, M.S.; Martinez, G.J.; Barraclough, J.Y.; Gloss, B.; Misra, A.; Patel, S.; Kavurma, M.M. Vascular transcriptome landscape of Trail(-/-) mice: Implications and therapeutic strategies for diabetic vascular disease. *FASEB J.* **2020**, *34*, 9547–9562. [CrossRef]
123. Hays, A.G.; Schar, M.; Barditch-Crovo, P.; Bagchi, S.; Bonanno, G.; Meyer, J.; Afework, Y.; Streeb, V.; Stradley, S.; Kelly, S.; et al. A randomized, placebo-controlled, double-blinded clinical trial of colchicine to improve vascular health in people living with HIV. *AIDS* **2021**, *35*, 1041–1050. [CrossRef] [PubMed]
124. Opstal, T.S.J.; Hoogeveen, R.M.; Fiolet, A.T.L.; Silvis, M.J.M.; The, S.H.K.; Bax, W.A.; de Kleijn, D.P.V.; Mosterd, A.; Stroes, E.S.G.; Cornel, J.H. Colchicine Attenuates Inflammation Beyond the Inflammasome in Chronic Coronary Artery Disease: A LoDoCo2 Proteomic Substudy. *Circulation* **2020**, *142*, 1996–1998. [CrossRef] [PubMed]
125. Silvis, M.J.M.; Fiolet, A.T.L.; Opstal, T.S.J.; Dekker, M.; Suquilanda, D.; Zivkovic, M.; Duyvendak, M.; The, S.H.K.; Timmers, L.; Bax, W.A.; et al. Colchicine reduces extracellular vesicle NLRP3 inflammasome protein levels in chronic coronary disease: A LoDoCo2 biomarker substudy. *Atherosclerosis* **2021**, *334*, 93–100. [CrossRef] [PubMed]
126. Barraclough, J.Y.; Joglekar, M.V.; Januszewski, A.S.; Martinez, G.; Celermajer, D.S.; Keech, A.C.; Hardikar, A.A.; Patel, S. A MicroRNA Signature in Acute Coronary Syndrome Patients and Modulation by Colchicine. *J. Cardiovasc. Pharmacol. Ther.* **2020**, *25*, 444–455. [CrossRef]
127. Giannopoulos, G.; Angelidis, C.; Kouritas, V.K.; Dedeilias, P.; Filippatos, G.; Cleman, M.W.; Panagopoulou, V.; Siasos, G.; Tousoulis, D.; Lekakis, J.; et al. Usefulness of colchicine to reduce perioperative myocardial damage in patients who underwent on-pump coronary artery bypass grafting. *Am. J. Cardiol.* **2015**, *115*, 1376–1381. [CrossRef]
128. Deftereos, S.; Giannopoulos, G.; Angelidis, C.; Alexopoulos, N.; Filippatos, G.; Papoutsidakis, N.; Sianos, G.; Goudevenos, J.; Alexopoulos, D.; Pyrgakis, V.; et al. Anti-Inflammatory Treatment with Colchicine in Acute Myocardial Infarction: A Pilot Study. *Circulation* **2015**, *132*, 1395–1403. [CrossRef]
129. Akodad, M.; Lattuca, B.; Nagot, N.; Georgescu, V.; Buisson, M.; Cristol, J.P.; Leclercq, F.; Macia, J.C.; Gervasoni, R.; Cung, T.T.; et al. COLIN trial: Value of colchicine in the treatment of patients with acute myocardial infarction and inflammatory response. *Arch. Cardiovasc. Dis.* **2017**, *110*, 395–402. [CrossRef]
130. Mewton, N.; Roubille, F.; Bresson, D.; Prieur, C.; Bouleti, C.; Bochaton, T.; Ivanes, F.; Dubreuil, O.; Biere, L.; Hayek, A.; et al. Effect of Colchicine on Myocardial Injury in Acute Myocardial Infarction. *Circulation* **2021**, *144*, 859–869. [CrossRef]
131. Vaidya, K.; Arnott, C.; Martinez, G.J.; Ng, B.; McCormack, S.; Sullivan, D.R.; Celermajer, D.S.; Patel, S. Colchicine Therapy and Plaque Stabilization in Patients with Acute Coronary Syndrome: A CT Coronary Angiography Study. *JACC Cardiovasc. Imaging* **2018**, *11*, 305–316. [CrossRef] [PubMed]
132. Akrami, M.; Izadpanah, P.; Bazrafshan, M.; Hatamipour, U.; Nouraein, N.; Drissi, H.B.; Manafi, A. Effects of colchicine on major adverse cardiac events in next 6-month period after acute coronary syndrome occurrence; a randomized placebo-control trial. *BMC Cardiovasc. Disord.* **2021**, *21*, 583. [CrossRef]
133. Fiolet, A.T.L.; Silvis, M.J.M.; Opstal, T.S.J.; Bax, W.A.; van der Horst, F.A.L.; Mosterd, A.; de Kleijn, D.; Cornel, J.H. Short-term effect of low-dose colchicine on inflammatory biomarkers, lipids, blood count and renal function in chronic coronary artery disease and elevated high-sensitivity C-reactive protein. *PLoS ONE* **2020**, *15*, e0237665. [CrossRef] [PubMed]
134. Shah, B.; Pillinger, M.; Zhong, H.; Cronstein, B.; Xia, Y.; Lorin, J.D.; Smilowitz, N.R.; Feit, F.; Ratnapala, N.; Keller, N.M.; et al. Effects of Acute Colchicine Administration Prior to Percutaneous Coronary Intervention: COLCHICINE-PCI Randomized Trial. *Circ. Cardiovasc. Interv.* **2020**, *13*, e008717. [CrossRef] [PubMed]
135. Cole, J.; Htun, N.; Lew, R.; Freilich, M.; Quinn, S.; Layland, J. Colchicine to Prevent Periprocedural Myocardial Injury in Percutaneous Coronary Intervention: The COPE-PCI Pilot Trial. *Circ. Cardiovasc. Interv.* **2021**, *14*, e009992. [CrossRef]
136. Cole, J.; Htun, N.; Lew, R.; Freilich, M.; Quinn, S.; Layland, J. COlchicine to Prevent PeriprocEdural Myocardial Injury in Percutaneous Coronary Intervention (COPE-PCI): A Descriptive Cytokine Pilot Sub-Study. *Cardiovasc. Revasc. Med.* **2022**, *39*, 84–89. [CrossRef]
137. Tardif, J.C.; Kouz, S.; Waters, D.D.; Bertrand, O.F.; Diaz, R.; Maggioni, A.P.; Pinto, F.J.; Ibrahim, R.; Gamra, H.; Kiwan, G.S.; et al. Efficacy and Safety of Low-Dose Colchicine after Myocardial Infarction. *N. Engl. J. Med.* **2019**, *381*, 2497–2505. [CrossRef]
138. Bouabdallaoui, N.; Tardif, J.C.; Waters, D.D.; Pinto, F.J.; Maggioni, A.P.; Diaz, R.; Berry, C.; Koenig, W.; Lopez-Sendon, J.; Gamra, H.; et al. Time-to-treatment initiation of colchicine and cardiovascular outcomes after myocardial infarction in the Colchicine Cardiovascular Outcomes Trial (COLCOT). *Eur. Heart J.* **2020**, *41*, 4092–4099. [CrossRef]
139. Tong, D.C.; Quinn, S.; Nasis, A.; Hiew, C.; Roberts-Thomson, P.; Adams, H.; Sriamareswaran, R.; Htun, N.M.; Wilson, W.; Stub, D.; et al. Colchicine in Patients with Acute Coronary Syndrome: The Australian COPS Randomized Clinical Trial. *Circulation* **2020**, *142*, 1890–1900. [CrossRef]
140. Tong, D.C.; Bloom, J.E.; Quinn, S.; Nasis, A.; Hiew, C.; Roberts-Thomson, P.; Adams, H.; Sriamareswaran, R.; Htun, N.M.; Wilson, W.; et al. Colchicine in Patients with Acute Coronary Syndrome: Two-Year Follow-Up of the Australian COPS Randomized Clinical Trial. *Circulation* **2021**, *144*, 1584–1586. [CrossRef]
141. Nidorf, S.M.; Eikelboom, J.W.; Budgeon, C.A.; Thompson, P.L. Low-dose colchicine for secondary prevention of cardiovascular disease. *J. Am. Coll. Cardiol.* **2013**, *61*, 404–410. [CrossRef] [PubMed]

142. Nidorf, S.M.; Fiolet, A.T.L.; Mosterd, A.; Eikelboom, J.W.; Schut, A.; Opstal, T.S.J.; The, S.H.K.; Xu, X.F.; Ireland, M.A.; Lenderink, T.; et al. Colchicine in Patients with Chronic Coronary Disease. *N. Engl. J. Med.* **2020**, *383*, 1838–1847. [CrossRef] [PubMed]
143. Deftereos, S.; Giannopoulos, G.; Raisakis, K.; Kossyvakis, C.; Kaoukis, A.; Panagopoulou, V.; Driva, M.; Hahalis, G.; Pyrgakis, V.; Alexopoulos, D.; et al. Colchicine treatment for the prevention of bare-metal stent restenosis in diabetic patients. *J. Am. Coll. Cardiol.* **2013**, *61*, 1679–1685. [CrossRef]
144. Kereiakes, D.J.; Smits, P.C.; Kedhi, E.; Parise, H.; Fahy, M.; Serruys, P.W.; Stone, G.W. Predictors of death or myocardial infarction, ischaemic-driven revascularisation, and major adverse cardiovascular events following everolimus-eluting or paclitaxel-eluting stent deployment: Pooled analysis from the SPIRIT II, III, IV and COMPARE trials. *EuroIntervention* **2011**, *7*, 74–83. [CrossRef]
145. Fiolet, A.T.L.; Opstal, T.S.J.; Mosterd, A.; Eikelboom, J.W.; Jolly, S.S.; Keech, A.C.; Kelly, P.; Tong, D.C.; Layland, J.; Nidorf, S.M.; et al. Efficacy and safety of low-dose colchicine in patients with coronary disease: A systematic review and meta-analysis of randomized trials. *Eur. Heart J.* **2021**, *42*, 2765–2775. [CrossRef] [PubMed]
146. Aimo, A.; Pascual Figal, D.A.; Bayes-Genis, A.; Emdin, M.; Georgiopoulos, G. Effect of low-dose colchicine in acute and chronic coronary syndromes: A systematic review and meta-analysis. *Eur. J. Clin. Investig.* **2021**, *51*, e13464. [CrossRef] [PubMed]
147. Kofler, T.; Kurmann, R.; Lehnick, D.; Cioffi, G.M.; Chandran, S.; Attinger-Toller, A.; Toggweiler, S.; Kobza, R.; Moccetti, F.; Cuculi, F.; et al. Colchicine in Patients With Coronary Artery Disease: A Systematic Review and Meta-Analysis of Randomized Trials. *J. Am. Heart Assoc.* **2021**, *10*, e021198. [CrossRef]
148. Samuel, M.; Tardif, J.C.; Bouabdallaoui, N.; Khairy, P.; Dubé, M.P.; Blondeau, L.; Guertin, M.C. Colchicine for Secondary Prevention of Cardiovascular Disease: A Systematic Review and Meta-analysis of Randomized Controlled Trials. *Can. J. Cardiol.* **2021**, *37*, 776–785. [CrossRef]
149. Antithrombotic Trialists, C.; Baigent, C.; Blackwell, L.; Collins, R.; Emberson, J.; Godwin, J.; Peto, R.; Buring, J.; Hennekens, C.; Kearney, P.; et al. Aspirin in the primary and secondary prevention of vascular disease: Collaborative meta-analysis of individual participant data from randomised trials. *Lancet* **2009**, *373*, 1849–1860. [CrossRef]
150. Cholesterol Treatment Trialists, C.; Baigent, C.; Blackwell, L.; Emberson, J.; Holland, L.E.; Reith, C.; Bhala, N.; Peto, R.; Barnes, E.H.; Keech, A.; et al. Efficacy and safety of more intensive lowering of LDL cholesterol: A meta-analysis of data from 170,000 participants in 26 randomised trials. *Lancet* **2010**, *376*, 1670–1681. [CrossRef]
151. Kuzemczak, M.; Ibrahem, A.; Alkhalil, M. Colchicine in Patients with Coronary Artery Disease with or Without Diabetes Mellitus: A Meta-analysis of Randomized Clinical Trials. *Clin. Drug Investig.* **2021**, *41*, 667–674. [CrossRef] [PubMed]

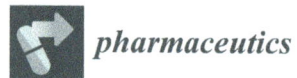

Review

Novel Pharmaceutical and Nutraceutical-Based Approaches for Cardiovascular Diseases Prevention Targeting Atherogenic Small Dense LDL

Jelena Vekic [1], Aleksandra Zeljkovic [1], Aleksandra Stefanovic [1], Natasa Bogavac-Stanojevic [1], Ioannis Ilias [2], José Silva-Nunes [3,4,5], Anca Pantea Stoian [6], Andrej Janez [7] and Manfredi Rizzo [6,8,*]

1. Department of Medical Biochemistry, University of Belgrade-Faculty of Pharmacy, 11000 Belgrade, Serbia; jelena.vekic@pharmacy.bg.ac.rs (J.V.); aleksandra.zeljkovic@pharmacy.bg.ac.rs (A.Z.); aleksandra.stefanovic@pharmacy.bg.ac.rs (A.S.); natasa.bogavac@pharmacy.bg.ac.rs (N.B.-S.)
2. Department of Endocrinology, Diabetes and Metabolism, Elena Venizelou Hospital, 11521 Athens, Greece; iiliasmd@yahoo.com
3. Department of Endocrinology, Diabetes and Metabolism, Centro Hospitalar Universitário Lisboa Central, 1069-166 Lisbon, Portugal; silva.nunes@nms.unl.pt
4. Nova Medical School, Faculdade de Ciencias Medicas, Universidade Nova de Lisboa, 1169-056 Lisbon, Portugal
5. Health and Technology Research Center (HTRC), Escola Superior de Tecnologia da Saude de Lisboa, 1990-096 Lisbon, Portugal
6. Faculty of Medicine, Diabetes, Nutrition and Metabolic Diseases, Carol Davila University, 050474 Bucharest, Romania; ancastoian@yahoo.com
7. Department of Endocrinology, Diabetes and Metabolic Diseases, University Medical Centre, University of Ljubljana, 1000 Ljubljana, Slovenia; andrej.janez@kclj.si
8. Department of Health Promotion, Mother and Child Care, Internal Medicine and Medical Specialties, University of Palermo, 90100 Palermo, Italy
* Correspondence: manfredi.rizzo@unipa.it

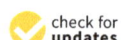

Citation: Vekic, J.; Zeljkovic, A.; Stefanovic, A.; Bogavac-Stanojevic, N.; Ilias, I.; Silva-Nunes, J.; Stoian, A.P.; Janez, A.; Rizzo, M. Novel Pharmaceutical and Nutraceutical-Based Approaches for Cardiovascular Diseases Prevention Targeting Atherogenic Small Dense LDL. *Pharmaceutics* **2022**, *14*, 825. https://doi.org/10.3390/pharmaceutics14040825

Academic Editors: Ionut Tudorancea, Radu Iliescu and Yasumasa Ikeda

Received: 27 February 2022
Accepted: 7 April 2022
Published: 9 April 2022

Publisher's Note: MDPI stays neutral with regard to jurisdictional claims in published maps and institutional affiliations.

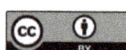

Copyright: © 2022 by the authors. Licensee MDPI, Basel, Switzerland. This article is an open access article distributed under the terms and conditions of the Creative Commons Attribution (CC BY) license (https://creativecommons.org/licenses/by/4.0/).

Abstract: Compelling evidence supports the causative link between increased levels of low-density lipoprotein cholesterol (LDL-C) and atherosclerotic cardiovascular disease (CVD) development. For that reason, the principal aim of primary and secondary cardiovascular prevention is to reach and sustain recommended LDL-C goals. Although there is a considerable body of evidence that shows that lowering LDL-C levels is directly associated with CVD risk reduction, recent data shows that the majority of patients across Europe cannot achieve their LDL-C targets. In attempting to address this matter, a new overarching concept of a lipid-lowering approach, comprising of even more intensive, much earlier and longer intervention to reduce LDL-C level, was recently proposed for high-risk patients. Another important concern is the residual risk for recurrent cardiovascular events despite optimal LDL-C reduction, suggesting that novel lipid biomarkers should also be considered as potential therapeutic targets. Among them, small dense LDL particles (sdLDL) seem to have the most significant potential for therapeutic modulation. This paper discusses the potential of traditional and emerging lipid-lowering approaches for cardiovascular prevention by targeting sdLDL particles.

Keywords: lipids; lipoproteins; small dense LDL; cholesterol; prevention; therapy

1. Introduction

The pathogenesis of atherosclerotic cardiovascular disease (CVD) involves the interplay of multiple pathophysiological processes, exposing a complex network of emerging risk factors and therapeutic targets. Nevertheless, elevated low-density lipoprotein-cholesterol (LDL-C) has been recognized as one of the few risk factors with a fundamental causative role in CVD [1]. However, today, it is widely accepted that routine quantification of LDL-C level does not provide an insight into the quality of circulating LDL pool, which is composed of a mixture of particles, differing in lipid content, density, size, electric charge, and potential proatherogenic properties [2]. Among them, the assessment of small dense LDL (sdLDL) particles is of particular importance since it is established that they have the greatest atherogenic potential [2]. Nevertheless, the complexity of techniques for measuring sdLDL seems to be the major obstacle for wider application of this biomarker in clinical practice [3]. Similarly, although statins remain a cornerstone of current lipid-lowering therapy [1], a clear benefit of introducing innovative therapeutic approaches [4] and nutraceuticals [5] in the lipid management of high-risk patients should not be neglected.

Small dense LDL particles, being profoundly involved in atherosclerosis development, are highly important as a target for modern pharmacological and non-pharmacological therapy. In recent years, novel therapeutics with great potential for sdLDL reduction, beyond of that achieved by traditional lipid-lowering medications, have been approved. Furthermore, the results of intervention studies using nutraceuticals have pointed to several prospective candidates with a favorable impact on these atherogenic particles. This paper will review the effects of current and emerging therapeutic options for the modulation of sdLDL particles.

2. Small Dense LDL and Cardiovascular Risk

One of the main clinically important consequences of plasma LDL heterogeneity is that a considerable proportion of patients might develop CVD despite optimal LDL-C concentrations. This phenomenon is attributed to the differences in cholesterol content within LDL particles among individuals exhibiting similar LDL-C levels [6]. Indeed, numerous studies have confirmed that smaller LDL particle size, increased sdLDL proportion, and/or elevated cholesterol concentration carried by sdLDL (sdLDL-C) are associated with the onset of CVD, independently of LDL-C level [7–9]. These data clearly indicate the superiority of LDL quality over LDL quantity in CVD risk prediction. Of note, it has been suggested that electric charge can also affect the atherogenic properties of LDL. Namely, it has been demonstrated that more electronegative LDL subfractions are present in a higher extent in the plasma of hypercholesterolemic subjects [10]. Moreover, previous studies have shown that these particles induce apoptosis and inhibit the differentiation of endothelial cells [10,11]. Recent evidence pointed toward the proatherogenic role of electronegative LDL, which is accomplished through the promotion of inflammation, macrophage differentiation, and triglyceride (TG) accumulation in lipid droplets [12]. However, as recently reviewed by Rivas-Urbina et al. [13], a full spectrum of biological roles of electronegative LDL in various pathological conditions remains to be elucidated. Interestingly, it has been shown that the amount of electronegative LDL subfractions determined by capillary isotachophoresis correlates negatively with LDL particle size, thus suggesting that electronegative LDL is accumulated in the sdLDL fraction [14]. In addition, Zhang et al. [15] demonstrated that rosuvastatin treatment significantly reduced the electronegative LDL contained in both large and sdLDL, thereby implying another pleiotropic effect of statins. Bearing in mind an obvious similarity in the biological effects of electronegative LDL and sdLDL particles, the question of their association and potential synergistic activity during atherosclerosis development deserves further investigation.

Insulin resistance is a well-studied metabolic alteration that serves as a driving force for increased sdLDL formation. In brief, an insulin-resistant state favors production and simultaneously delays catabolism of very-low density lipoprotein (VLDL), which results in hypertriglyceridemia [16]. Further activation of cholesterol-ester transfer protein (CETP) stimulates the exchange of triglycerides and cholesterol-esters (CE) between VLDL and LDL particles. The cascade of events culminates through the hydrolysis of TG-rich LDL particles by hepatic lipase, which converts them into sdLDL [17]. Of note, high-density lipoproteins (HDL) also undergo similar modification, which ultimately leads to a reduction in HDL-C level [3]. Therefore, insulin-resistant individuals are usually characterized by a specific form of atherogenic dyslipidemia, comprising elevated TG, low HDL-C level, and preponderance of sdLDL particles [18].

A crucial step in atherosclerotic plaque formation is cholesterol accumulation in macrophages and their transition to lipid-rich foam cells in the arterial wall. SdLDL particles are recognized as the main origin of deposited cholesterol in atherosclerotic plaque. Compared to larger LDL subfractions, sdLDL particles possess considerably higher atherogenic capacity due to delayed clearance from plasma and easier accumulation in the subendothelial space [2]. In addition, sdLDL particles are more prone to structural modifications, which further increase their proaterogenic properties. Adverse modifications of sdLDL particles include oxidation, desialylation, glycation, and alterations of protein components [19]. Clinically, the most important consequence of sdLDL accumulation in plasma and subendothelial space is their subsequent transformation into oxidized LDL particles (oxLDL). These particles have a central role in foam cell formation, but also possess potent biological effects in terms of promoting endothelial dysfunction, inflammation, oxidative stress, cell proliferation, and thrombosis, thereby further contributing to plaque progression and destabilization [20]. Hence, several categories of patients with this specific metabolic disorder, intimately associated with increased CVD risk, could benefit from sdLDL measurement and therapeutic modulation (Figure 1).

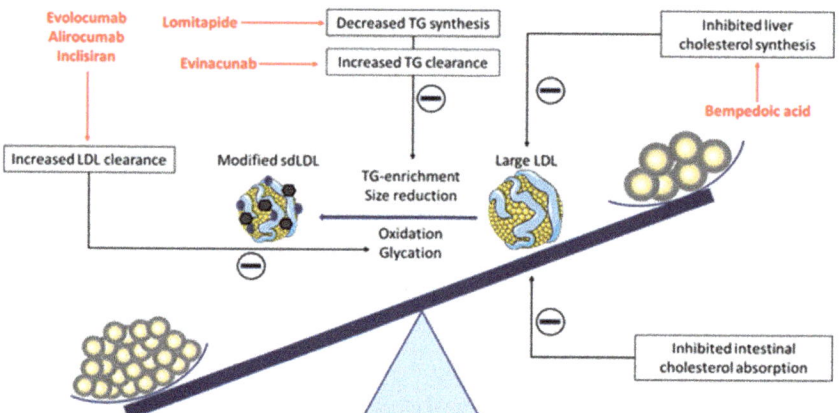

Figure 1. Therapeutic approaches for the reduction in sdLDL particles.

To summarize, screening for sdLDL should be advised to a wide range of high-risk subjects including those with multiple risk factors, particularly metabolic syndrome, patients with type 2 diabetes mellitus, but also patients who need secondary prevention, in attempting to reduce the residual risk. Although lipid guidelines, as the framework for CVD risk assessment, recommend standard lipid screening, advanced lipid testing might identify individuals with hidden cardiovascular risk by assessing the alterations of a wide range of lipid biomarkers. In this manner, assessment of LDL heterogeneity including sdLDL or LDL particle number (LDL-P) can be achieved by employing ultracentrifugation, gradient gel electrophoresis, HPLC, NMR, and ion mobility techniques [21]. Aside from these sophisticated methods, homogeneous assays for cholesterol content within sdLDL (sdLDL-C) have become available in routine laboratories, thus offering the possibility of a personalized approach in CVD prevention as well as of therapeutic individualization.

3. The Effect of Novel Lipid-Lowering Therapies on sdLDL Particles

Currently, the effects of novel lipid-lowering therapies on sdLDL reduction have been less explored, mainly because these medications were only recently approved. Therefore, this section will discuss their potential beneficial effects on sdLDL, based on the pharmacological mechanisms and available data gathered from observational studies and clinical trials.

3.1. PCSK9-Targeted Therapies

Proprotein convertase subtilisin/kexin type 9 (PCSK9) is a serine protease that enhances the degradation of hepatic LDL receptors, thus abolishing the clearance of LDL particles by the liver [22]. So far, two innovative approaches for targeting PCSK9 including inhibition of its activity or synthesis have emerged as effective and safe interventions for LDL-C lowering and cardiovascular prevention. In particular, two monoclonal anti-PCSK9 antibodies, evolocumab and alirocumab, are able to bind PCSK9 in plasma and antagonize its action while inclisiran, a small interfering ribonucleic acid (siRNA), prevents the translation of PCSK9 mRNA [4]. Both strategies aim to re-establish cholesterol homeostasis by increasing the expression of LDL receptors, which will consequently promote the clearance of LDL particles by the liver. Convincing data from the FOURIER [23] and ODYSSEY OUTCOMES [24] trials demonstrated substantial LDL-C level reduction by 50% with evolocumab and alirocumab, respectively. At present, PCSK9 inhibitors are recommended for patients with familial hypercholesterolemia and secondary prevention of high-risk patients who fail to reach the LDL-target despite optimal treatment or those intolerant to statins [4].

Regarding inclisiran, data from phase III trials (Orion 10 and 11) showed that LDL-C level reduction of 50% can be achieved by two doses per year [25,26]. In late 2020, inclisiran was authorized in the EU for the treatment of patients with primary hypercholesterolemia and the secondary prevention for patients who require additional LDL-C lowering [27]. Toward the end of 2021, inclisiran was also approved by FDA.

Several observational studies have shown a positive correlation of plasma PCSK9 and sdLDL levels in high-risk patients [28,29]. Thus, targeting PCSK9 might also be a promising strategy to control the level of circulating sdLDL particles. Analysis of the data from the DESCARTES trial showed that addition of evolocumab to statin therapy in patients with hyperlipidema significantly reduced concentrations of TG-rich lipoproteins and both large and small LDL particles [29]. Similarly, a post hoc analysis of phase II alirocumab trials showed a significant reduction in cholesterol content in all atherogenic lipoproteins including small dense LDL subclasses [30]. In addition, recent studies in patients with familial hypercholesterolemia suggest that beneficial effects of PCSK9 inhibitor therapy on sdLDL particles are associated with an improvement in endothelial function [31] and carotid stiffness [32]. While exploring the potential benefit of PCSK9 targeting for sdLDL reduction, one should not neglect that inclisiran is also efficient in reducing atherogenic lipoproteins (i.e., non-HDL-cholesterol and Lp(a) levels) [26,33,34]. However, the effects on sdLDL are yet to be determined.

3.2. Bempedoic Acid

An innovative approach of LDL-C lowering by bempedoic acid offers an additional option for targeting sdLDL particles. Namely, bempedoic acid attenuates the activity of ATP-citrate lyase (ACL), an enzyme responsible for the generation of acetyl-coenzyme A, the central building unit for lipogenesis and steroidogenesis [35]. Since bempedoic acid inhibits cholesterol synthesis at an earlier point than HMG-CoA reductase, it is useful as an add-on therapy to statins and/or ezetimibe. By inhibiting cholesterol synthesis, bempedoic acid causes the upregulation of hepatic LDL receptors and consequent clearance of LDL particles, thus lowering plasma LDL-C levels alone by 15–25%, while in combination with ezetimibe, more than 30% [36]. Bempedoic acid was authorized in the U.S. and the EU for primary prevention of patients with heterozygous familial hypercholesterolemia and for secondary prevention of CVD patients who require additional lowering of the LDL-C level [37].

Data from clinical trials showed that the beneficial effects of bempedoic acid are also reflected in the improvement in other lipid status parameters such as non-HDL-C and apolipoprotein B (apo B), but also on the level of high-sensitivity C-reactive protein (hsCRP), a marker of subclinical inflammation [38]. A meta-analysis of phase II and phase III trials showed that bempedoic acid significantly reduced the LDL particle number (LDL-P), but had no effects on VLDL particle number and TG level [39]. It also has a beneficial effect on serum glucose level by activating liver AMP-kinase [40]. Notably, in a recent analysis of pooled data from phase III trials, the use of bempedoic acid was not associated with the risk for diabetes onset or worsening metabolic control in patients with diabetes [41]. Hence, bempedoic acid seems to be safe for insulin-resistant subjects. This specific category of patients would also be expected to benefit the most from sdLDL reduction by bempedoic acid, but this effect remains to be tested in the future.

3.3. Lomitapide

Lomitapide is a small molecule that binds and inhibits microsomal triglyceride transfer protein (MTP) in the liver and intestine. Since MTP facilitates the transfer of TG, phospholipids, and CE to apoB during the assembling processes of chylomicrons and VLDL particles [42], inhibition of its activity reduces the levels of TG-rich lipoproteins in plasma. One of the first MTP inhibitors, tested in the animal model of human homozygous familial hypercholesterolemia, demonstrated a reduction in plasma apoB-containing lipoproteins without alterations of liver enzymes [43]. However, since inhibition of MTP induced accumulation of TG in hepatic and intestinal cells, further research was abandoned due to the possible adverse effects [44]. Lomitapide was evaluated in a phase III study in homozygous familial hypercholesterolemia patients with ongoing lipid-lowering therapy and apheresis. It was found that LDL-C level decrease was dose-dependent and that most patients achieved a LDL-C reduction of more than 50% [45]. The efficacy of lomitapide was confirmed by the results of a long-term extension study [46] as well as by another clinical study [47] and real-world data [48]. The treatment also reduced TG and non-HDL-C levels [46]. However, high doses were associated with adverse effects such as steatorrhea, gastrointestinal symptoms, or liver steatosis. At present, lomitapide has been approved only for the management of homozygous familial hypercholesterolemia [49].

Despite beneficial effects on serum TG level, there is no convincing data to conclude whether lomitapide could be considered for the management of atherogenic dyslipidemia. Based on the data from a phase III clinical study, lomitapide treatment was associated with a moderate decrease in HDL-C levels [45]. However, Yahya et al. [50] showed that such a reduction in HDL-C was followed by the shift of the HDL subclass distribution toward more extensive, more buoyant HDL 2 particles, without significant impact on cholesterol efflux capacity (i.e., HDL functionality). Currently, no available data have demonstrated the effects of lomitapide on the sdLDL particles. Observational data suggest that a common polymorphism $-492G/T$ within the promoter of the *MTP* gene is not associated with variations in LDL size and subclass distribution [51]. However, these findings do not exclude targeting of MTP as a potential strategy for the modulation of sdLDL, and the potential effects of lomitapide need to be evaluated in further studies.

3.4. Evinacumab

Angiopoietin-like protein 3 (ANGPTL3) is a member of the ANGPTL family of proteins with numerous functions in lipid metabolism, inflammation, glucose homeostasis, and cancer [52]. ANGPTL3 primarily regulates lipid metabolism by modulating the availability of TG for adipose, heart, and skeletal muscles throughout the inhibition of lipoprotein (LPL) and endothelial lipase (EL) [53]. The deficiency of ANGPTL3 enhances the clearance of TG-rich lipoproteins and carriers of *ANGPTL3* mutations have lower plasma TG, LDL-C and HDL-C levels, and reduced CVD risk [54]. Thus, ANGPTL3 is recognized as an emerging therapeutic target for dyslipidemia.

Evinacumab is a fully human monoclonal antibody directed against ANGPTL3. It binds the N-terminal domain of ANGPTL3 and abolishes the inhibition of LPL and EL [55]. Evinacumab demonstrated a dose-dependent reduction in LDL-C, TG, non-HDL-C, HDL-C, total cholesterol, apoB, and Lp(a) levels in a randomized, double-blind, placebo-controlled trial including subjects with moderately elevated LDL-C levels [56]. In the phase III ELIPSE HoFH study, evinacumab administration was associated with a reduction in LDL-C and

TG levels by 49% and 50%, respectively [57]. A proof-of-concept study showed that the addition of evinacumab to standard lipid-lowering therapy of familial hypercholesterolemia further reduced LDL-C levels [58]. The effect on LDL-C level reduction is likely to be mediated by an increased catabolic rate of apoB within the LDL particles and their precursors [59]. Evinacumab has been authorized for the treatment of homozygous familial hypercholesterolemia by FDA and EMA since 2021 [60].

Recent studies in apparently healthy subjects [61] and patients with diabetes [62] have reported a positive association between increased plasma ANGPTL3 and sdLDL particles. These findings suggest possible beneficial effects of ANGPTL3 inhibition on sdLDL, which should be verified in the future. Aside from evinacumab, two additional approaches for the silencing of ANGPTL3 synthesis by antisense oligonucleotides (ANGPTL3-RLX) and siRNA (ARO-ANG3) are currently being investigated in clinical trials. Furthermore, Fukami et al. [63] recently developed a peptide vaccine for the targeting of ANGPTL3 and demonstrated a reduction in sdLDL-C level in a preclinical study, offering a promising new approach to the treatment of atherogenic dyslipidemia.

4. The Effect of Nutraceuticals on sdLDL Particles

Dietary supplements and functional food are recommended for lowering LDL-C concentrations in individuals with high cholesterol concentrations and intermediate or low cardiovascular risk who are not candidates for pharmacotherapy as well as in patients with high and very high cardiovascular risk but with inadequate response to pharmacotherapy [1]. The LDL-C lowering effects of nutraceuticals rise from their capability to modulate basic processes of exogenous cholesterol absorption, endogenous cholesterol synthesis, its metabolism, and elimination (Figure 1). By affecting these and several other processes within lipoprotein metabolism, nutraceuticals can also modulate sdLDL particles. However, scientific research still needs to fully confirm clinical evidence of the nutraceuticals' efficacy and evaluate its safety and tolerability.

4.1. Phytosterols

Primary food sources of phytosterols are vegetable oil, vegetable margarine, cereal products, vegetables, nuts, and legumes. Dominant phytosterols from food are β-sitosterol, campesterol, stigmasterol, and campestanol [64]. Approximate daily intake is between 250 mg/day in Northern Europe to 500 mg/day in Mediterranean countries [1]. Phytosterols directly compete with exogenous intestinal cholesterol for the Neimann-Pick C1-Like 1 (NPC1L1) transporter on enterocytes and thus reduce cholesterol absorption. A compensatory increase in hepatic LDL receptor expression follows diminished intestinal cholesterol uptake, which altogether results in a decrease in plasma LDL-C concentration [65]. Daily intake of 2 g of phytosterols can decrease the total cholesterol (TC) and LDL-C levels up to 10%, with little or no effects on HDL-C and TG concentrations [1,66]. Regarding the qualitative and quantitative characteristics of LDL particles, the results of previous studies showed that intake of phytosterols has positive effects [67,68]. In patients with metabolic syndrome, two months of supplementation with four g/day of phytosterols resulted in reduced TC, LDL-C, and sdLDL-C levels [69]. Furthermore, the results of Garoufi et al. [70] showed that daily consumption of 2 g of plant sterols decreased sdLDL-C levels in children with hypercholesterolemia. On the other hand, 12 weeks of supplementation with 2.6 g/day of phytosterol esters showed no effects on the proportion of LDL subclasses and mean LDL diameter in hypercholesterolemic adults who were not taking lipid-lowering therapy [70]. Nevertheless, recent scientific findings support the view that adequate daily phytosterol supplementation can lower cardiovascular risk in hypercholesterolemic individuals by reducing sdLDL particles [1]. Current European recommendations endorse a supplementation with more than two g/day of phytosterols in hypercholesterolemic individuals with low or intermediate cardiovascular risk and adults and children with familial hypercholesterolemia [1]. Daily phytosterol intake is also recommended for high- and very high-risk patients who fail to achieve recommended LDL-C goals with statin therapy [1]. Possible adverse effects of phytosterol supplementation are related to potential lower intestinal absorption of fat-soluble vitamins [71]. Notably, these nutraceuticals are not recommended for individuals with sitosterolemia, a metabolic disorder resulting from a mutation in genes that encode ABCG5/G8 transporters and subsequent retention of phytosterols [72].

4.2. Dietary Fiber

Dietary fiber, soluble and non-soluble, mainly found in vegetables, fruits, grains, and legumes, are nutraceuticals resistant to digestion in the small intestine with beneficial effects on cholesterol metabolism. The mechanisms of action of dietary fiber (pectin, β-glucans, psyllium) with respect to cholesterol metabolism are not completely resolved, but their main effect is attributed to the ability to boost the excretion of bile acids and fecal cholesterol [73,74]. In this way, dietary fiber indirectly modifies LDL receptor expression and enhances the clearance of LDL particles [75]. A systematic review and meta-analysis of randomized controlled trials showed that daily intake of approximately 3.5 g of β-glucan significantly reduced LDL-C concentration [76]. Shrestha et al. [77] showed that daily intake of a combination of psyllium and phytosterols reduced LDL-C concentration, but also reduced the medium and small LDL particles and increased LDL size. Current ESC/EAS guidelines recommend a daily intake of 3 to 10 g of dietary fiber to achieve a relevant reduction of 3–5% in LDL-C concentration [1].

4.3. Monacolin K

Being the main source of LDL-C in plasma, liver cholesterol synthesis also affects the amount of every LDL subclass. However, in contrast to the well-studied beneficial effects of pharmacological agents HMG-CoA reductase inhibitors on the size and distribution of LDL subclasses, only scarce evidence is available regarding natural products with similar activity. Red yeast rice's major bioactive constituent monacolin K, also known as lovastatin, is renowned for its beneficial hypolipemic effects [78]. To the best of our knowledge, no studies have analyzed the effects of isolated monacolin K on sdLDL particles. However, a recent study of Galletti et al. [79] revealed a significant increase in LDL particle size in patients with metabolic syndrome after 24-week treatment with a combination of lipid-lowering nutraceuticals containing monacolin K, berberine, and policosanol. Administration of the same nutraceuticals reportedly caused a reduction in the relative proportion of sdLDL particles in a group of 30 patients with familial combined hyperlipidemia [80]. However, it should be appreciated that other components of the mentioned nutraceutical combination also exhibit hypocholesterolemic effects. Specifically, policosanol, a long-chained alcohol derived from various fruits, nuts, sugarcane etc., also acts as an inhibitor of cholesterol synthesis as well as a stimulator of LDL uptake and cholesterol excretion [81]. Similarly, berberine can enhance LDL uptake by upregulation of LDL receptors and inhibition of PCSK9 [82,83]. Therefore, it remains to be established how these nutraceuticals separately affect plasma sdLDL and whether they act synergistically when combined. Regarding the safety of the supplementation, monacolin K adverse effects mostly arise from its analogy with statins; possible rhabdomyolysis is the major concern. However, available evidence suggests that administration of 3–10 mg/day of monacolin K has minimal side effects, so it is generally considered safe [84].

4.4. Polyphenols

Flavonoids are among the best-studied polyphenols in terms of hypolipemic activity. However, their precise effects on the redistribution of lipoprotein particles are largely unexplored. However, there is evidence of the specific influence of several flavonoids on sdLDL particles. For example, it has been demonstrated that citrus flavonoids such as naringin and hesperidin exhibit lipid-lowering effects by inhibiting HMG-CoA reductase and acyl-CoA:cholesterol O-acyltransferase (ACAT) activities in rats [85]. Likewise, bergamot (*Citrus bergamia*) flavonoids reportedly possess statin-like effects [5]. It has also been shown that the administration of bergamot flavonoid extract (neoeriocitrin, neohesperidin and naringin) for six months resulted in a significant increase in large, alongside a concomitant decrease in small LDL subclass proportions, in subjects with hypercholesterolemia [86]. Similar results were reported for the soluble derivative of hesperidin, which is an abundant flavonoid in citrus fruit peel. Namely, it was demonstrated that the 24-week long administration of 500 mg/day of glucosyl-hesperidin to hypertriglyceridemic patients caused an increase in LDL particle size [87]. Furthermore, in general, citrus flavonoids have a good safety profile and minimal side effects [88], so they could be promising agents in ameliorating LDL subclass distribution, and can ultimately be used for the prevention and treatment of cardiovascular disease [88].

Soy isoflavones such as genistein are capable of the downregulation of HMG-CoA activity [89]. Accordingly, a meta-analysis showed that soy isoflavones significantly reduce TC and LDL-C concentrations [90]. In contrast, any beneficial influence of isolated soy isoflavone administration on sdLDL particles was not proven in postmenopausal women [91]. It should also be appreciated that several concerns were raised concerning the safety of soy isoflavones. Namely, due to their estrogen-like effects, it is necessary to clarify whether using these compounds could be associated with an increased risk for specific types of cancer [92].

Other polyphenols also affect cholesterol synthesis. It has been shown that curcuminoids, bioactive polyphenolic compounds of turmeric (*Curcuma longa*), cause a decrease in the enzymatic activity of HMG-CoA reductase, among other effects [93,94]. Although the impact of curcuminoids on serum lipid profile has been confirmed [95], Moohebati et al. [96] reported that short-term (four weeks) supplementation with 1 g/day of curcuminoids did not provide any changes in sdLDL-C. Similarly, Panahi et al. [97] found no differences in sdLDL-C after eight weeks of prolonged curcuminoid supplementation in patients with metabolic syndrome.

4.5. Omega-3 Long-Chain Polyunsaturated Fatty Acids

It has long been documented that omega-3 long-chain polyunsaturated fatty acids (n-3 LCPUFA) can significantly modulate the lipid profile, mainly by reducing TG levels [5]. The two most intensively studied n-3 LCPUFA, relevant to human health are eicosapentaenoic acid (EPA) and docosahexaenoic acid (DHA). Many previous studies have explored the influence of n-3 LCPUFA administration on sdLDL. Bearing in mind the contribution of hypertriglyceridemia in sdLDL genesis, it was reasonable to assume that n-3 LCPUFA, by their TG-lowering activity, can indirectly affect sdLDL particles. Indeed, it has been shown that DHA supplementation (3 g/day) for 90 days improved LDL subclass distribution in both fasting and postprandial plasma of patients with hypertriglyceridemia [98]. Similar results were obtained after six week long administration of 1.52 g/day of DHA in subjects with decreased HDL-C [99]. Regarding EPA, Satoh et al. [100] demonstrated that purified EPA (1.8 g/day for three months) provoked a decrease in the proportion of sdLDL-C and sdLDL particles as well as in CETP activity. Moreover, a recent in vitro study showed that EPA is highly potent in preventing the oxidation of sdLDL [101].

The combined effects of EPA and DHA have been examined in various clinical studies. Thus, it has been shown that the concentration of large LDL particles increased and the concentration of sdLDL decreased in type 2 diabetes patients after 12 weeks of supplementation with 4 g/day of n-3 LCPUFA, in parallel with their standard treatment [102]. Similarly, as reported by Agouridis et al. [103], combined therapy of low-dose rosuvastatin and n-3 LCPUFA (2 g/day) was equally effective in raising LDL particle size, along with high-dose rosuvastatin in patients with mixed dyslipidemia and metabolic syndrome. Considering the significant side effects of high-dose statins, these results might be of interest for the individualization of hypolipemic therapy in subjects with an inadequate response to statins. In addition, a recent randomized, open-label phase 4 study demonstrated that 8-week treatment with n-3 LCPUFA (2 g/twice-daily) in combination with statins yielded a significant increase in LDL particle size in dyslipidemic patients [104]. Interestingly,

3-month administration of 1.7 g/day of n-3 LCPUFA did not cause any changes in sdLDL percentage in patients with end-stage renal disease [105].

Other n-3 PUFAs might also be of interest regarding their putative effects on atherogenic dyslipidemia. Kawakami et al. [106] demonstrated that 12-week supplementation with flaxseed oil, as an abundant source of alpha-linolenic acid (ALA), is associated with a significant decrease in sdLDL-C concentration in healthy adult Japanese men. In contrast, Wilkinson et al. [107] demonstrated that 12-week dietary intake of flaxseed oil did not cause significant changes in LDL subclass distribution when compared to the supplementation with fish oil in healthy male adults. Interestingly, Tuccinardi et al. [108] demonstrated that walnut consumption decreased the concentration of sdLDL particles in obese individuals. Walnuts (*Juglans regia*) are rich in polyphenols and fiber, but especially in ALA. However, it should be noted that sample size in the majority of these studies was rather small, so larger studies are needed, either to confirm or to rule out any contribution of ALA to the amelioration of LDL subfraction profile.

A meta-analysis of 21 randomized controlled trials [109] has shown that n-3 LCPUFA containing products are well tolerated, although several side effects are present including fishy taste, dermatological and gastrointestinal problems as well as alterations of biochemical parameters. However, these adverse effects were mild in general. Recently, it has been suggested that the genetic background might be responsible for individual susceptibility to adverse reactions after supplementation with n-3 LCPUFA [110] and this could have important consequences in terms of an individualized approach during the administration of these nutraceuticals.

4.6. Other Nutriceuticals

Prickly pear (*Opuntia ficus indica*) is a plant from the Cactaceae family that is distributed worldwide including in the Americas, Africa, Australia, and the Mediterranean. The prickly pear pulp, peel, seeds, and cladodes are rich in PUFA, phytosterols, and phenolic compounds, and this plant is traditionally recognized by its beneficial health effects [111]. It has been shown that a 4-week regular intake of pasta containing Opuntia ficus extract decreased the percentage of sdLDL particles in subjects with at least one criterion for metabolic syndrome fulfilled [112]. These findings advocate for a wider use of prickly pear as part of a nutraceutical approach to dyslipidemia.

Oolong tea is a moderately fermented extract of the leaves of *Camellia sinensis*, which is a mixture of polyphenolic compounds, catechins, and their polymeric derivatives theaflavins and arubigins [113]. The main oolong tea antiatherogenic effect is most likely a reduction in TC and LDL-C concentrations. Proposed mechanisms of action involve the polyphenols' antioxidative properties, activation of the AMPK signaling pathway, inhibition of HMG-CoA reductase, interaction with cholesterol absorption, and inhibition of bile acid reabsorption [114,115]. In addition, Shimada et al. [116] showed that oolong tea consumption affected the atherosclerosis progression in patients with coronary artery disease by improving the lipid profile and slightly increasing the LDL particle size.

It has been found that biologically active soy proteins and peptides could be involved in the regulation of LDL receptor activity [117], reduction in intestinal cholesterol absorption [118], cholesterol biosynthesis rate, and increase in bile salt fecal excretion [119]. Clinical evidence for these effects of soy proteins has been recently published in a meta-analysis of 46 studies [120]. The authors concluded that soy proteins significantly reduced TC and LDL-C concentrations in adults and supported plant protein dietary intake [120]. Furthermore, Desroches et al. [121] showed that soy protein consumption shifted LDL particle distribution toward a less atherogenic pattern in hypercholesterolemic individuals older than 50 years.

Although not nutraceuticals in strict terms, probiotics can modify the gut microbiome, thereby altering the bioavailability of dietary compounds and affecting the entire energy metabolism. For these reasons, the impact of probiotics and the gut microbiome on metabolic changes associated with obesity has been the focus of contemporary research.

Several mechanisms have been proposed to explain the hypocholesterolemic effects of probiotics: decreased absorption of intestinal cholesterol through its precipitation with deconjugated bile salts; assimilation of cholesterol by microbial cells; metabolic transformation to coprostanol; or decreased expression of cholesterol transporter in the enterocyte membrane [122]. In line with this, the beneficial effects of probiotics on LDL-C have been reported [123,124], although not in all studies [125]. A recent study by Michael et al. [126] analyzed the influence of lactobacilli and bifidobacteria supplementation (50 billion CFU/day) for six months in overweight and obese individuals. Apart from a significant decrease in body weight, hypercholesterolemic patients also experienced a reduction in sdLDL-C following supplementation, which is an interesting finding that should be further explored. The use of probiotics is generally considered safe, but one should not neglect that adverse effects have been reported in vulnerable populations (e.g., infants, immunocompromised patients) [127]. Thus, further investigations are needed to fully evaluate the possible benefits of probiotics in controlling lipid profile abnormalities.

5. Conclusions

Even though sdLDL has been long recognized as an essential feature of atherosclerosis development, it is still neither a part of the routine assessment of CVD risk, nor a specific therapeutic target. At present, commercially available electrophoretic systems such as Lipoprint represent the most reliable routinely applicable method for the assessment of sdLDL levels [2]. In addition to sdLDL, this method provides an insight into the entire spectrum of LDL subclasses in plasma and is more economical than other methodologies [2]. Regarding the measurement of sdLDL alone, automated homogenous enzymatic assays for sdLDL-C concentration determination are the most readily available for medical laboratories, and therefore could be recommended as an optimal and feasible methodology for assessing sdLDL in clinical practice. Numerous investigations have demonstrated that both conventional pharmacological treatment and novel therapeutic approaches designed to affect specific aspects of lipid metabolism also target sdLDL particles. In addition, there is a plethora of evidence that nutraceuticals, besides their confirmed effects on LDL-C, can also modify a qualitative aspect of these particles. However, additional large-scale clinical trials are needed to fully evaluate the capabilities of various pharmacological and non-pharmacological approaches to improve LDL quality by reducing the sdLDL content.

Bearing in mind that genetic factors have recently been shown to contribute to the effectiveness of pharmaceutical approaches by targeting LDL, these factors should also be considered in the context of effective cardiovascular prevention. Namely, it is now firmly established that numerous genetic variants may cause inter-individual variations in response to lipid-lowering therapy [128]. So far, ample evidence is available confirming the association between the efficacy of statin therapy and certain single nucleotide polymorphisms of the genes encoding proteins that participate in cholesterol synthesis and removal from plasma such as HMG-CoA reductase, LDL-receptor, and PCSK9, but also apolipoprotein E. Investigators of the Prospective Study of Pravastatin in the Elderly at Risk (PROSPER) reported that polymorphism in the 3′-untranslated region (UTR) of the LDL-receptor gene contributed to different therapeutic response to pravastatin [129], while researchers of the Cholesterol and Pharmacogenetics (CAP) trial showed that a common haplotype within 3′-UTR of the LDL-receptor gene is associated with reduced response to simvastatin [130]. In the same study, the presence of both LDL-receptor and HMG-CoA reductase gene polymorphisms was associated with an additionally attenuated lipid-lowering effect of simvastatin [130]. The results of the Justification for the Use of Statins in Prevention: an Intervention Trial Evaluating Rosuvastatin (JUPITER) trial suggested that certain genetic variants of PCSK9 are also able to modulate response to statin therapy [131]. In line with the previous, Feng et al. [132] recently demonstrated a more favorable response to statins in the carriers of loss-of-function variants of the *PCSK9* gene. Regarding apolipoprotein E gene polymorphism, it was shown that the carriers of ε_2 allele have more favorable response to atorvastatin [133], in contrast to the carriers of the ε_4 allele [134]. Genetic variations of

PCSK9 have also been proposed to affect the response to PCSK9 inhibitor therapy observed in clinical trials [135], but currently there is no available data to confirm this assumption. Overall, genetic testing could be useful for the identification of high-risk patients that cannot achieve therapeutic LDL-C goals. According to available evidence, the presence of mutations responsible for severe defects in the LDL-receptor and/or gain-of-function mutations of the *PCSK9* gene might suggest an unsatisfactory response to statin therapy. Given the fact that the latest guidelines recommend the addition of emerging lipid-lowering agents to statin therapy in patients requiring further LDL-C lowering, pharmacogenomic studies with combined therapy are highly welcomed. These data would hopefully pave the way for a personalized approach toward more efficient targeting of sdLDL.

Funding: No funding was received for the preparation of the present article.

Institutional Review Board Statement: Not applicable.

Informed Consent Statement: Not applicable.

Data Availability Statement: Not applicable.

Acknowledgments: The authors from the University of Belgrade-Faculty of Pharmacy appreciate the support from the Ministry of Education, Science and Technological Development, Republic of Serbia (grant no. 451-03-68/2022-14/200161).

Conflicts of Interest: The authors declare no conflict of interest.

Disclosures: The authors declare that the present article was written independently, without any industry role.

References

1. Mach, F.; Baigent, C.; Catapano, A.L.; Koskinas, K.C.; Casula, M.; Badimon, L.; Chapman, M.J.; De Backer, G.G.; Delgado, V.; Ference, B.A.; et al. 2019 ESC/EAS Guidelines for the management of dyslipidaemias: Lipid modification to reduce cardiovascular risk. *Eur. Heart J.* **2020**, *41*, 111–188. [CrossRef] [PubMed]
2. Mikhailidis, D.P.; Elisaf, M.; Rizzo, M.; Berneis, K.; Griffin, B.; Zambon, A.; Athyros, V.; de Graaf, J.; Marz, W.; Parhofer, K.G.; et al. "European panel on low density lipoprotein (LDL) subclasses": A statement on the pathophysiology, atherogenicity and clinical significance of LDL subclasses. *Curr. Vasc. Pharmacol.* **2011**, *9*, 533–571. [CrossRef] [PubMed]
3. Rizzo, M.; Berneis, K.; Zeljkovic, A.; Vekic, J. Should we routinely measure low-density and high-density lipoprotein subclasses? *Clin. Lab.* **2009**, *55*, 421–429. [PubMed]
4. Giglio, R.V.; Pantea Stoian, A.; Al-Rasadi, K.; Banach, M.; Patti, A.M.; Ciaccio, M.; Rizvi, A.A.; Rizzo, M. Novel Therapeutical Approaches to Managing Atherosclerotic Risk. *Int. J. Mol. Sci.* **2021**, *22*, 4633. [CrossRef] [PubMed]
5. Cicero, A.F.G.; Fogacci, F.; Stoian, A.P.; Vrablik, M.; Al Rasadi, K.; Banach, M.; Toth, P.P.; Rizzo, M. Nutraceuticals in the Management of Dyslipidemia: Which, When, and for Whom? Could Nutraceuticals Help Low-Risk Individuals with Non-optimal Lipid Levels? *Curr. Atheroscler. Rep.* **2021**, *23*, 57. [CrossRef] [PubMed]
6. Diffenderfer, M.R.; Schaefer, E.J. The composition and metabolism of large and small LDL. *Curr. Opin. Lipidol.* **2014**, *25*, 221–226. [CrossRef]
7. Rizzo, M.; Berneis, K. Low-density lipoprotein size and cardiovascular risk assessment. *QJM* **2006**, *99*, 1–14. [CrossRef]
8. Zeljkovic, A.; Spasojevic-Kalimanovska, V.; Vekic, J.; Jelic-Ivanovic, Z.; Topic, A.; Bogavac-Stanojevic, N.; Spasic, S.; Vujovic, A.; Kalimanovska-Ostric, D. Does simultaneous determination of LDL and HDL particle size improve prediction of coronary artery disease risk? *Clin. Exp. Med.* **2008**, *8*, 109–116. [CrossRef]
9. Zeljkovic, A.; Vekic, J.; Spasojevic-Kalimanovska, V.; Jelic-Ivanovic, Z.; Bogavac-Stanojevic, N.; Gulan, B.; Spasic, S. LDL and HDL subclasses in acute ischemic stroke: Prediction of risk and short-term mortality. *Atherosclerosis* **2010**, *210*, 548–554. [CrossRef]
10. Chen, C.H.; Jiang, T.; Yang, J.H.; Jiang, W.; Lu, J.; Marathe, G.K.; Pownall, H.J.; Ballantyne, C.M.; McIntyre, T.M.; Henry, P.D.; et al. Low-density lipoprotein in hypercholesterolemic human plasma induces vascular endothelial cell apoptosis by inhibiting fibroblast growth factor 2 transcription. *Circulation* **2003**, *107*, 2102–2108. [CrossRef]
11. Tang, D.; Lu, J.; Walterscheid, J.P.; Chen, H.H.; Engler, D.A.; Sawamura, T.; Chang, P.Y.; Safi, H.J.; Yang, C.Y.; Chen, C.H. Electronegative LDL circulating in smokers impairs endothelial progenitor cell differentiation by inhibiting Akt phosphorylation via LOX-1. *J. Lipid Res.* **2008**, *49*, 33–47. [CrossRef] [PubMed]
12. Puig, N.; Montolio, L.; Camps-Renom, P.; Navarra, L.; Jimenez-Altayo, F.; Jimenez-Xarrie, E.; Sanchez-Quesada, J.L.; Benitez, S. Electronegative LDL Promotes Inflammation and Triglyceride Accumulation in Macrophages. *Cells* **2020**, *9*, 583. [CrossRef] [PubMed]
13. Rivas-Urbina, A.; Rull, A.; Ordonez-Llanos, J.; Sanchez-Quesada, J.L. Electronegative LDL: An Active Player in Atherogenesis or a By-Product of Atherosclerosis? *Curr. Med. Chem.* **2019**, *26*, 1665–1679. [CrossRef] [PubMed]

14. Noda, K.; Zhang, B.; Uehara, Y.; Miura, S.; Matsunaga, A.; Saku, K. Potent capillary isotachophoresis (cITP) for analyzing a marker of coronary heart disease risk and electronegative low-density lipoprotein (LDL) in small dense LDL fraction. *Circ. J.* **2005**, *69*, 1568–1570. [CrossRef]
15. Zhang, B.; Matsunaga, A.; Rainwater, D.L.; Miura, S.; Noda, K.; Nishikawa, H.; Uehara, Y.; Shirai, K.; Ogawa, M.; Saku, K. Effects of rosuvastatin on electronegative LDL as characterized by capillary isotachophoresis: The ROSARY Study. *J. Lipid Res.* **2009**, *50*, 1832–1841. [CrossRef]
16. Vekic, J.; Zeljkovic, A.; Stefanovic, A.; Jelic-Ivanovic, Z.; Spasojevic-Kalimanovska, V. Obesity and dyslipidemia. *Metabolism* **2019**, *92*, 71–81. [CrossRef]
17. Berneis, K.K.; Krauss, R.M. Metabolic origins and clinical significance of LDL heterogeneity. *J. Lipid Res.* **2002**, *43*, 1363–1379. [CrossRef]
18. Rizzo, M.; Kotur-Stevuljevic, J.; Berneis, K.; Spinas, G.; Rini, G.B.; Jelic-Ivanovic, Z.; Spasojevic-Kalimanovska, V.; Vekic, J. Atherogenic dyslipidemia and oxidative stress: A new look. *Transl. Res.* **2009**, *153*, 217–223. [CrossRef]
19. Ivanova, E.A.; Myasoedova, V.A.; Melnichenko, A.A.; Grechko, A.V.; Orekhov, A.N. Small Dense Low-Density Lipoprotein as Biomarker for Atherosclerotic Diseases. *Oxidative Med. Cell. Longev.* **2017**, *2017*, 1273042. [CrossRef]
20. Poznyak, A.V.; Nikiforov, N.G.; Markin, A.M.; Kashirskikh, D.A.; Myasoedova, V.A.; Gerasimova, E.V.; Orekhov, A.N. Overview of OxLDL and Its Impact on Cardiovascular Health: Focus on Atherosclerosis. *Front. Pharmacol.* **2020**, *11*, 613780. [CrossRef]
21. Kanonidou, C. Small dense low-density lipoprotein: Analytical review. *Clin. Chim. Acta* **2021**, *520*, 172–178. [CrossRef] [PubMed]
22. Seidah, N.G. The PCSK9 discovery, an inactive protease with varied functions in hypercholesterolemia, viral infections, and cancer. *J. Lipid Res.* **2021**, *62*, 100130. [CrossRef] [PubMed]
23. Sabatine, M.S.; Giugliano, R.P.; Keech, A.C.; Honarpour, N.; Wiviott, S.D.; Murphy, S.A.; Kuder, J.F.; Wang, H.; Liu, T.; Wasserman, S.M.; et al. Evolocumab and Clinical Outcomes in Patients with Cardiovascular Disease. *N. Engl. J. Med.* **2017**, *376*, 1713–1722. [CrossRef] [PubMed]
24. Schwartz, G.G.; Steg, P.G.; Szarek, M.; Bhatt, D.L.; Bittner, V.A.; Diaz, R.; Edelberg, J.M.; Goodman, S.G.; Hanotin, C.; Harrington, R.A.; et al. Alirocumab and Cardiovascular Outcomes after Acute Coronary Syndrome. *N. Engl. J. Med.* **2018**, *379*, 2097–2107. [CrossRef]
25. Ray, K.K.; Wright, R.S.; Kallend, D.; Koenig, W.; Leiter, L.A.; Raal, F.J.; Bisch, J.A.; Richardson, T.; Jaros, M.; Wijngaard, P.L.J.; et al. Two Phase 3 Trials of Inclisiran in Patients with Elevated LDL Cholesterol. *N. Engl. J. Med.* **2020**, *382*, 1507–1519. [CrossRef]
26. Wright, R.S.; Ray, K.K.; Raal, F.J.; Kallend, D.G.; Jaros, M.; Koenig, W.; Leiter, L.A.; Landmesser, U.; Schwartz, G.G.; Friedman, A.; et al. Pooled Patient-Level Analysis of Inclisiran Trials in Patients With Familial Hypercholesterolemia or Atherosclerosis. *J. Am. Coll. Cardiol.* **2021**, *77*, 1182–1193. [CrossRef]
27. Lamb, Y.N. Inclisiran: First Approval. *Drugs* **2021**, *81*, 389–395. [CrossRef]
28. Zhang, Y.; Xu, R.X.; Li, S.; Zhu, C.G.; Guo, Y.L.; Sun, J.; Li, J.J. Association of plasma small dense LDL cholesterol with PCSK9 levels in patients with angiographically proven coronary artery disease. *Nutr. Metab. Cardiovasc. Dis.* **2015**, *25*, 426–433. [CrossRef]
29. Nozue, T.; Hattori, H.; Ogawa, K.; Kujiraoka, T.; Iwasaki, T.; Hirano, T.; Michishita, I. Correlation between serum levels of proprotein convertase subtilisin/kexin type 9 (PCSK9) and atherogenic lipoproteins in patients with coronary artery disease. *Lipids Health Dis.* **2016**, *15*, 165. [CrossRef]
30. Toth, P.P.; Hamon, S.C.; Jones, S.R.; Martin, S.S.; Joshi, P.H.; Kulkarni, K.R.; Banerjee, P.; Hanotin, C.; Roth, E.M.; McKenney, J.M. Effect of alirocumab on specific lipoprotein non-high-density lipoprotein cholesterol and subfractions as measured by the vertical auto profile method: Analysis of 3 randomized trials versus placebo. *Lipids Health Dis.* **2016**, *15*, 28. [CrossRef]
31. Di Minno, A.; Gentile, M.; Iannuzzo, G.; Calcaterra, I.; Tripaldella, M.; Porro, B.; Cavalca, V.; Di Taranto, M.D.; Tremoli, E.; Fortunato, G.; et al. Endothelial function improvement in patients with familial hypercholesterolemia receiving PCSK-9 inhibitors on top of maximally tolerated lipid lowering therapy. *Thromb. Res.* **2020**, *194*, 229–236. [CrossRef] [PubMed]
32. Di Minno, M.N.D.; Gentile, M.; Di Minno, A.; Iannuzzo, G.; Calcaterra, I.; Buonaiuto, A.; Di Taranto, M.D.; Giacobbe, C.; Fortunato, G.; Rubba, P.O.F. Changes in carotid stiffness in patients with familial hypercholesterolemia treated with Evolocumab(R): A prospective cohort study. *Nutr. Metab. Cardiovasc. Dis.* **2020**, *30*, 996–1004. [CrossRef] [PubMed]
33. Ray, K.K.; Stoekenbroek, R.M.; Kallend, D.; Leiter, L.A.; Landmesser, U.; Wright, R.S.; Wijngaard, P.; Kastelein, J.J.P. Effect of an siRNA Therapeutic Targeting PCSK9 on Atherogenic Lipoproteins: Prespecified Secondary End Points in ORION 1. *Circulation* **2018**, *138*, 1304–1316. [CrossRef] [PubMed]
34. Banach, M.; Rizzo, M.; Obradovic, M.; Montalto, G.; Rysz, J.; Mikhailidis, D.P.; Isenovic, E.R. PCSK9 inhibition—A novel mechanism to treat lipid disorders? *Curr. Pharm. Des.* **2013**, *19*, 3869–3877. [CrossRef]
35. Brandts, J.; Ray, K.K. Bempedoic acid, an inhibitor of ATP citrate lyase for the treatment of hypercholesterolemia: Early indications and potential. *Expert Opin. Investig. Drugs* **2020**, *29*, 763–770. [CrossRef]
36. Kelly, M.S.; Sulaica, E.M.; Beavers, C.J. Role of Bempedoic Acid in Dyslipidemia Management. *J. Cardiovasc. Pharmacol.* **2020**, *76*, 376–388. [CrossRef]
37. Ballantyne, C.M.; Bays, H.; Catapano, A.L.; Goldberg, A.; Ray, K.K.; Saseen, J.J. Role of Bempedoic Acid in Clinical Practice. *Cardiovasc. Drugs Ther.* **2021**, *35*, 853–864. [CrossRef]
38. Banach, M.; Duell, P.B.; Gotto, A.M., Jr.; Laufs, U.; Leiter, L.A.; Mancini, G.B.J.; Ray, K.K.; Flaim, J.; Ye, Z.; Catapano, A.L. Association of Bempedoic Acid Administration With Atherogenic Lipid Levels in Phase 3 Randomized Clinical Trials of Patients With Hypercholesterolemia. *JAMA Cardiol.* **2020**, *5*, 1124–1135. [CrossRef]

39. Cicero, A.F.G.; Fogacci, F.; Hernandez, A.V.; Banach, M.; on behalf of the Lipid and Blood Pressure Meta-Analysis Collaboration (LBPMC) Group; the International Lipid Expert Panel (ILEP). Efficacy and safety of bempedoic acid for the treatment of hypercholesterolemia: A systematic review and meta-analysis. *PLoS Med.* **2020**, *17*, e1003121. [CrossRef]
40. Pinkosky, S.L.; Filippov, S.; Srivastava, R.A.; Hanselman, J.C.; Bradshaw, C.D.; Hurley, T.R.; Cramer, C.T.; Spahr, M.A.; Brant, A.F.; Houghton, J.L.; et al. AMP-activated protein kinase and ATP-citrate lyase are two distinct molecular targets for ETC-1002, a novel small molecule regulator of lipid and carbohydrate metabolism. *J. Lipid Res.* **2013**, *54*, 134–151. [CrossRef]
41. Leiter, L.A.; Banach, M.; Catapano, A.L.; Duell, P.B.; Gotto, A.M., Jr.; Laufs, U.; Mancini, G.B.J.; Ray, K.K.; Hanselman, J.C.; Ye, Z.; et al. Bempedoic acid in patients with type 2 diabetes mellitus, prediabetes, and normoglycaemia: A post hoc analysis of efficacy and glycaemic control using pooled data from phase 3 clinical trials. *Diabetes Obes. Metab.* **2022**, *24*, 868–880. [CrossRef] [PubMed]
42. Iqbal, J.; Jahangir, Z.; Al-Qarni, A.A. Microsomal Triglyceride Transfer Protein: From Lipid Metabolism to Metabolic Diseases. *Adv. Exp. Med. Biol.* **2020**, *1276*, 37–52. [CrossRef] [PubMed]
43. Wetterau, J.R.; Gregg, R.E.; Harrity, T.W.; Arbeeny, C.; Cap, M.; Connolly, F.; Chu, C.H.; George, R.J.; Gordon, D.A.; Jamil, H.; et al. An MTP inhibitor that normalizes atherogenic lipoprotein levels in WHHL rabbits. *Science* **1998**, *282*, 751–754. [CrossRef]
44. Hebbachi, A.M.; Brown, A.M.; Gibbons, G.F. Suppression of cytosolic triacylglycerol recruitment for very low density lipoprotein assembly by inactivation of microsomal triglyceride transfer protein results in a delayed removal of apoB-48 and apoB-100 from microsomal and Golgi membranes of primary rat hepatocytes. *J. Lipid Res.* **1999**, *40*, 1758–1768. [PubMed]
45. Cuchel, M.; Meagher, E.A.; du Toit Theron, H.; Blom, D.J.; Marais, A.D.; Hegele, R.A.; Averna, M.R.; Sirtori, C.R.; Shah, P.K.; Gaudet, D.; et al. Efficacy and safety of a microsomal triglyceride transfer protein inhibitor in patients with homozygous familial hypercholesterolaemia: A single-arm, open-label, phase 3 study. *Lancet* **2013**, *381*, 40–46. [CrossRef]
46. Blom, D.J.; Averna, M.R.; Meagher, E.A.; du Toit Theron, H.; Sirtori, C.R.; Hegele, R.A.; Shah, P.K.; Gaudet, D.; Stefanutti, C.; Vigna, G.B.; et al. Long-Term Efficacy and Safety of the Microsomal Triglyceride Transfer Protein Inhibitor Lomitapide in Patients With Homozygous Familial Hypercholesterolemia. *Circulation* **2017**, *136*, 332–335. [CrossRef]
47. Nohara, A.; Otsubo, Y.; Yanagi, K.; Yoshida, M.; Ikewaki, K.; Harada-Shiba, M.; Jurecka, A. Safety and Efficacy of Lomitapide in Japanese Patients with Homozygous Familial Hypercholesterolemia (HoFH): Results from the AEGR-733-301 Long-Term Extension Study. *J. Atheroscler. Thromb.* **2019**, *26*, 368–377. [CrossRef] [PubMed]
48. D'Erasmo, L.; Cefalu, A.B.; Noto, D.; Giammanco, A.; Averna, M.; Pintus, P.; Medde, P.; Vigna, G.B.; Sirtori, C.; Calabresi, L.; et al. Efficacy of Lomitapide in the Treatment of Familial Homozygous Hypercholesterolemia: Results of a Real-World Clinical Experience in Italy. *Adv. Ther.* **2017**, *34*, 1200–1210. [CrossRef]
49. Agabiti Rosei, E.; Salvetti, M. Management of Hypercholesterolemia, Appropriateness of Therapeutic Approaches and New Drugs in Patients with High Cardiovascular Risk. *High Blood Press. Cardiovasc. Prev.* **2016**, *23*, 217–230. [CrossRef]
50. Yahya, R.; Favari, E.; Calabresi, L.; Verhoeven, A.J.M.; Zimetti, F.; Adorni, M.P.; Gomaraschi, M.; Averna, M.; Cefalu, A.B.; Bernini, F.; et al. Lomitapide affects HDL composition and function. *Atherosclerosis* **2016**, *251*, 15–18. [CrossRef]
51. Couture, P.; Otvos, J.D.; Cupples, L.A.; Wilson, P.W.; Schaefer, E.J.; Ordovas, J.M. Absence of association between genetic variation in the promoter of the microsomal triglyceride transfer protein gene and plasma lipoproteins in the Framingham Offspring Study. *Atherosclerosis* **2000**, *148*, 337–343. [CrossRef]
52. Christopoulou, E.; Elisaf, M.; Filippatos, T. Effects of Angiopoietin-Like 3 on Triglyceride Regulation, Glucose Homeostasis, and Diabetes. *Dis. Markers* **2019**, *2019*, 6578327. [CrossRef] [PubMed]
53. Koishi, R.; Ando, Y.; Ono, M.; Shimamura, M.; Yasumo, H.; Fujiwara, T.; Horikoshi, H.; Furukawa, H. Angptl3 regulates lipid metabolism in mice. *Nat. Genet.* **2002**, *30*, 151–157. [CrossRef] [PubMed]
54. Stitziel, N.O.; Khera, A.V.; Wang, X.; Bierhals, A.J.; Vourakis, A.C.; Sperry, A.E.; Natarajan, P.; Klarin, D.; Emdin, C.A.; Zekavat, S.M.; et al. ANGPTL3 Deficiency and Protection Against Coronary Artery Disease. *J. Am. Coll. Cardiol.* **2017**, *69*, 2054–2063. [CrossRef]
55. Surma, S.; Romanczyk, M.; Filipiak, K.J. Evinacumab-The new kid on the block. Is it important for cardiovascular prevention? *Int. J. Cardiol. Cardiovasc. Risk Prev.* **2021**, *11*, 200107. [CrossRef]
56. Harada-Shiba, M.; Ali, S.; Gipe, D.A.; Gasparino, E.; Son, V.; Zhang, Y.; Pordy, R.; Catapano, A.L. A randomized study investigating the safety, tolerability, and pharmacokinetics of evinacumab, an ANGPTL3 inhibitor, in healthy Japanese and Caucasian subjects. *Atherosclerosis* **2020**, *314*, 33–40. [CrossRef]
57. Raal, F.J.; Rosenson, R.S.; Reeskamp, L.F.; Hovingh, G.K.; Kastelein, J.J.P.; Rubba, P.; Ali, S.; Banerjee, P.; Chan, K.C.; Gipe, D.A.; et al. Evinacumab for Homozygous Familial Hypercholesterolemia. *N. Engl. J. Med.* **2020**, *383*, 711–720. [CrossRef]
58. Gaudet, D.; Gipe, D.A.; Pordy, R.; Ahmad, Z.; Cuchel, M.; Shah, P.K.; Chyu, K.Y.; Sasiela, W.J.; Chan, K.C.; Brisson, D.; et al. ANGPTL3 Inhibition in Homozygous Familial Hypercholesterolemia. *N. Engl. J. Med.* **2017**, *377*, 296–297. [CrossRef]
59. Reeskamp, L.F.; Millar, J.S.; Wu, L.; Jansen, H.; van Harskamp, D.; Schierbeek, H.; Gipe, D.A.; Rader, D.J.; Dallinga-Thie, G.M.; Hovingh, G.K.; et al. ANGPTL3 Inhibition With Evinacumab Results in Faster Clearance of IDL and LDL apoB in Patients With Homozygous Familial Hypercholesterolemia-Brief Report. *Arterioscler. Thromb. Vasc. Biol.* **2021**, *41*, 1753–1759. [CrossRef]
60. Markham, A. Evinacumab: First Approval. *Drugs* **2021**, *81*, 1101–1105. [CrossRef]
61. Murawska, K.; Krintus, M.; Kuligowska-Prusinska, M.; Szternel, L.; Stefanska, A.; Sypniewska, G. Relationship between Serum Angiopoietin-like Proteins 3 and 8 and Atherogenic Lipid Biomarkers in Non-Diabetic Adults Depends on Gender and Obesity. *Nutrients* **2021**, *13*, 4339. [CrossRef] [PubMed]

62. Harada, M.; Yamakawa, T.; Kashiwagi, R.; Ohira, A.; Sugiyama, M.; Sugiura, Y.; Kondo, Y.; Terauchi, Y. Association between ANGPTL3, 4, and 8 and lipid and glucose metabolism markers in patients with diabetes. *PLoS ONE* **2021**, *16*, e0255147. [CrossRef] [PubMed]
63. Fukami, H.; Morinaga, J.; Nakagami, H.; Hayashi, H.; Okadome, Y.; Matsunaga, E.; Kadomatsu, T.; Horiguchi, H.; Sato, M.; Sugizaki, T.; et al. Vaccine targeting ANGPTL3 ameliorates dyslipidemia and associated diseases in mouse models of obese dyslipidemia and familial hypercholesterolemia. *Cell Rep. Med.* **2021**, *2*, 100446. [CrossRef] [PubMed]
64. Gylling, H.; Simonen, P. Phytosterols, Phytostanols, and Lipoprotein Metabolism. *Nutrients* **2015**, *7*, 7965–7977. [CrossRef] [PubMed]
65. Poli, A.; Barbagallo, C.M.; Cicero, A.F.G.; Corsini, A.; Manzato, E.; Trimarco, B.; Bernini, F.; Visioli, F.; Bianchi, A.; Canzone, G.; et al. Nutraceuticals and functional foods for the control of plasma cholesterol levels. An intersociety position paper. *Pharmacol. Res.* **2018**, *134*, 51–60. [CrossRef]
66. Musa-Veloso, K.; Poon, T.H.; Elliot, J.A.; Chung, C. A comparison of the LDL-cholesterol lowering efficacy of plant stanols and plant sterols over a continuous dose range: Results of a meta-analysis of randomized, placebo-controlled trials. *Prostaglandins Leukot. Essent. Fat. Acids* **2011**, *85*, 9–28. [CrossRef]
67. Alizadeh-Fanalou, S.; Nazarizadeh, A.; Alian, F.; Faraji, P.; Sorori, B.; Khosravi, M. Small dense low-density lipoprotein-lowering agents. *Biol. Chem.* **2020**, *401*, 1101–1121. [CrossRef]
68. Talebi, S.; Bagherniya, M.; Atkin, S.L.; Askari, G.; Orafai, H.M.; Sahebkar, A. The beneficial effects of nutraceuticals and natural products on small dense LDL levels, LDL particle number and LDL particle size: A clinical review. *Lipids Health Dis.* **2020**, *19*, 66. [CrossRef]
69. Sialvera, T.E.; Pounis, G.D.; Koutelidakis, A.E.; Richter, D.J.; Yfanti, G.; Kapsokefalou, M.; Goumas, G.; Chiotinis, N.; Diamantopoulos, E.; Zampelas, A. Phytosterols supplementation decreases plasma small and dense LDL levels in metabolic syndrome patients on a westernized type diet. *Nutr. Metab. Cardiovasc. Dis.* **2012**, *22*, 843–848. [CrossRef]
70. Garoufi, A.; Vorre, S.; Soldatou, A.; Tsentidis, C.; Kossiva, L.; Drakatos, A.; Marmarinos, A.; Gourgiotis, D. Plant sterols-enriched diet decreases small, dense LDL-cholesterol levels in children with hypercholesterolemia: A prospective study. *Ital. J. Pediatr.* **2014**, *40*, 42. [CrossRef]
71. Mantovani, L.M.; Pugliese, C. Phytosterol supplementation in the treatment of dyslipidemia in children and adolescents: A systematic review. *Rev. Paul. Pediatr.* **2020**, *39*, e2019389. [CrossRef] [PubMed]
72. Izar, M.C.; Tegani, D.M.; Kasmas, S.H.; Fonseca, F.A. Phytosterols and phytosterolemia: Gene-diet interactions. *Genes Nutr.* **2011**, *6*, 17–26. [CrossRef] [PubMed]
73. Lattimer, J.M.; Haub, M.D. Effects of dietary fiber and its components on metabolic health. *Nutrients* **2010**, *2*, 1266–1289. [CrossRef] [PubMed]
74. Romero, A.L.; West, K.L.; Zern, T.; Fernandez, M.L. The seeds from Plantago ovata lower plasma lipids by altering hepatic and bile acid metabolism in guinea pigs. *J. Nutr.* **2002**, *132*, 1194–1198. [CrossRef]
75. Santini, A.; Novellino, E. To Nutraceuticals and Back: Rethinking a Concept. *Foods* **2017**, *6*, 74. [CrossRef]
76. Ho, H.V.; Sievenpiper, J.L.; Zurbau, A.; Blanco Mejia, S.; Jovanovski, E.; Au-Yeung, F.; Jenkins, A.L.; Vuksan, V. The effect of oat beta-glucan on LDL-cholesterol, non-HDL-cholesterol and apoB for CVD risk reduction: A systematic review and meta-analysis of randomised-controlled trials. *Br. J. Nutr.* **2016**, *116*, 1369–1382. [CrossRef]
77. Shrestha, S.; Volek, J.S.; Udani, J.; Wood, R.J.; Greene, C.M.; Aggarwal, D.; Contois, J.H.; Kavoussi, B.; Fernandez, M.L. A combination therapy including psyllium and plant sterols lowers LDL cholesterol by modifying lipoprotein metabolism in hypercholesterolemic individuals. *J. Nutr.* **2006**, *136*, 2492–2497. [CrossRef]
78. Xiong, Z.; Cao, X.; Wen, Q.; Chen, Z.; Cheng, Z.; Huang, X.; Zhang, Y.; Long, C.; Zhang, Y.; Huang, Z. An overview of the bioactivity of monacolin K/lovastatin. *Food Chem. Toxicol.* **2019**, *131*, 110585. [CrossRef]
79. Galletti, F.; Fazio, V.; Gentile, M.; Schillaci, G.; Pucci, G.; Battista, F.; Mercurio, V.; Bosso, G.; Bonaduce, D.; Brambilla, N.; et al. Efficacy of a nutraceutical combination on lipid metabolism in patients with metabolic syndrome: A multicenter, double blind, randomized, placebo controlled trial. *Lipids Health Dis.* **2019**, *18*, 66. [CrossRef]
80. Gentile, M.; Calcaterra, I.; Strazzullo, A.; Pagano, C.; Pacioni, D.; Speranza, E.; Rubba, P.; Marotta, G. Effects of Armolipid Plus on small dense LDL particles in a sample of patients affected by familial combined hyperlipidemia. *Clin. Lipidol.* **2015**, *10*, 475–480. [CrossRef]
81. Nam, D.E.; Yun, J.M.; Kim, D.; Kim, O.K. Policosanol Attenuates Cholesterol Synthesis via AMPK Activation in Hypercholesterolemic Rats. *J. Med. Food* **2019**, *22*, 1110–1117. [CrossRef] [PubMed]
82. Feng, X.; Sureda, A.; Jafari, S.; Memariani, Z.; Tewari, D.; Annunziata, G.; Barrea, L.; Hassan, S.T.S.; Smejkal, K.; Malanik, M.; et al. Berberine in Cardiovascular and Metabolic Diseases: From Mechanisms to Therapeutics. *Theranostics* **2019**, *9*, 1923–1951. [CrossRef] [PubMed]
83. Adorni, M.P.; Zimetti, F.; Lupo, M.G.; Ruscica, M.; Ferri, N. Naturally Occurring PCSK9 Inhibitors. *Nutrients* **2020**, *12*, 1440. [CrossRef] [PubMed]
84. Fogacci, F.; Banach, M.; Mikhailidis, D.P.; Bruckert, E.; Toth, P.P.; Watts, G.F.; Reiner, Z.; Mancini, J.; Rizzo, M.; Mitchenko, O.; et al. Safety of red yeast rice supplementation: A systematic review and meta-analysis of randomized controlled trials. *Pharmacol. Res.* **2019**, *143*, 1–16. [CrossRef] [PubMed]

85. Bok, S.H.; Lee, S.H.; Park, Y.B.; Bae, K.H.; Son, K.H.; Jeong, T.S.; Choi, M.S. Plasma and hepatic cholesterol and hepatic activities of 3-hydroxy-3-methyl-glutaryl-CoA reductase and acyl CoA: Cholesterol transferase are lower in rats fed citrus peel extract or a mixture of citrus bioflavonoids. *J. Nutr.* **1999**, *129*, 1182–1185. [CrossRef] [PubMed]
86. Toth, P.P.; Patti, A.M.; Nikolic, D.; Giglio, R.V.; Castellino, G.; Biancucci, T.; Geraci, F.; David, S.; Montalto, G.; Rizvi, A.; et al. Bergamot Reduces Plasma Lipids, Atherogenic Small Dense LDL, and Subclinical Atherosclerosis in Subjects with Moderate Hypercholesterolemia: A 6 Months Prospective Study. *Front. Pharmacol.* **2015**, *6*, 299. [CrossRef]
87. Miwa, Y.; Mitsuzumi, H.; Sunayama, T.; Yamada, M.; Okada, K.; Kubota, M.; Chaen, H.; Mishima, Y.; Kibata, M. Glucosyl hesperidin lowers serum triglyceride level in hypertriglyceridemic subjects through the improvement of very low-density lipoprotein metabolic abnormality. *J. Nutr. Sci. Vitaminol. (Tokyo)* **2005**, *51*, 460–470. [CrossRef]
88. Giglio, R.V.; Patti, A.M.; Cicero, A.F.G.; Lippi, G.; Rizzo, M.; Toth, P.P.; Banach, M. Polyphenols: Potential Use in the Prevention and Treatment of Cardiovascular Diseases. *Curr. Pharm. Des.* **2018**, *24*, 239–258. [CrossRef]
89. Duncan, R.E.; El-Sohemy, A.; Archer, M.C. Regulation of HMG-CoA reductase in MCF-7 cells by genistein, EPA, and DHA, alone and in combination with mevastatin. *Cancer Lett.* **2005**, *224*, 221–228. [CrossRef]
90. Taku, K.; Umegaki, K.; Sato, Y.; Taki, Y.; Endoh, K.; Watanabe, S. Soy isoflavones lower serum total and LDL cholesterol in humans: A meta-analysis of 11 randomized controlled trials. *Am. J. Clin. Nutr.* **2007**, *85*, 1148–1156. [CrossRef]
91. Hall, W.L.; Vafeiadou, K.; Hallund, J.; Bugel, S.; Reimann, M.; Koebnick, C.; Zunft, H.J.; Ferrari, M.; Branca, F.; Dadd, T.; et al. Soy-isoflavone-enriched foods and markers of lipid and glucose metabolism in postmenopausal women: Interactions with genotype and equol production. *Am. J. Clin. Nutr.* **2006**, *83*, 592–600. [CrossRef] [PubMed]
92. Ross, J.A.; Kasum, C.M. Dietary flavonoids: Bioavailability, metabolic effects, and safety. *Annu. Rev. Nutr.* **2002**, *22*, 19–34. [CrossRef] [PubMed]
93. Panahi, Y.; Ahmadi, Y.; Teymouri, M.; Johnston, T.P.; Sahebkar, A. Curcumin as a potential candidate for treating hyperlipidemia: A review of cellular and metabolic mechanisms. *J. Cell. Physiol.* **2018**, *233*, 141–152. [CrossRef] [PubMed]
94. Zingg, J.M.; Meydani, M. Curcumin–from tradition to science. *Biofactors* **2013**, *39*, 1. [CrossRef]
95. Hewlings, S.J.; Kalman, D.S. Curcumin: A Review of Its Effects on Human Health. *Foods* **2017**, *6*, 92. [CrossRef]
96. Moohebati, M.; Yazdandoust, S.; Sahebkar, A.; Mazidi, M.; Sharghi-Shahri, Z.; Ferns, G.; Ghayour-Mobarhan, M. Investigation of the effect of short-term supplementation with curcuminoids on circulating small dense low-density lipoprotein concentrations in obese dyslipidemic subjects: A randomized double-blind placebo-controlled cross-over trial. *ARYA Atheroscler.* **2014**, *10*, 280–286.
97. Panahi, Y.; Khalili, N.; Hosseini, M.S.; Abbasinazari, M.; Sahebkar, A. Lipid-modifying effects of adjunctive therapy with curcuminoids-piperine combination in patients with metabolic syndrome: Results of a randomized controlled trial. *Complementary Ther. Med.* **2014**, *22*, 851–857. [CrossRef]
98. Kelley, D.S.; Siegel, D.; Vemuri, M.; Mackey, B.E. Docosahexaenoic acid supplementation improves fasting and postprandial lipid profiles in hypertriglyceridemic men. *Am. J. Clin. Nutr.* **2007**, *86*, 324–333. [CrossRef]
99. Maki, K.C.; Van Elswyk, M.E.; McCarthy, D.; Hess, S.P.; Veith, P.E.; Bell, M.; Subbaiah, P.; Davidson, M.H. Lipid responses to a dietary docosahexaenoic acid supplement in men and women with below average levels of high density lipoprotein cholesterol. *J. Am. Coll. Nutr.* **2005**, *24*, 189–199. [CrossRef]
100. Satoh, N.; Shimatsu, A.; Kotani, K.; Sakane, N.; Yamada, K.; Suganami, T.; Kuzuya, H.; Ogawa, Y. Purified eicosapentaenoic acid reduces small dense LDL, remnant lipoprotein particles, and C-reactive protein in metabolic syndrome. *Diabetes Care* **2007**, *30*, 144–146. [CrossRef]
101. Sherratt, S.C.R.; Juliano, R.A.; Mason, R.P. Eicosapentaenoic acid (EPA) has optimal chain length and degree of unsaturation to inhibit oxidation of small dense LDL and membrane cholesterol domains as compared to related fatty acids in vitro. *Biochim. Biophys. Acta–Biomembr.* **2020**, *1862*, 183254. [CrossRef] [PubMed]
102. Ide, K.; Koshizaka, M.; Tokuyama, H.; Tokuyama, T.; Ishikawa, T.; Maezawa, Y.; Takemoto, M.; Yokote, K. N-3 polyunsaturated fatty acids improve lipoprotein particle size and concentration in Japanese patients with type 2 diabetes and hypertriglyceridemia: A pilot study. *Lipids Health Dis.* **2018**, *17*, 51. [CrossRef] [PubMed]
103. Agouridis, A.P.; Kostapanos, M.S.; Tsimihodimos, V.; Kostara, C.; Mikhailidis, D.P.; Bairaktari, E.T.; Tselepis, A.D.; Elisaf, M.S. Effect of rosuvastatin monotherapy or in combination with fenofibrate or omega-3 fatty acids on lipoprotein subfraction profile in patients with mixed dyslipidaemia and metabolic syndrome. *Int. J. Clin. Pract.* **2012**, *66*, 843–853. [CrossRef] [PubMed]
104. Masuda, D.; Miyata, Y.; Matsui, S.; Yamashita, S. Omega-3 fatty acid ethyl esters improve low-density lipoprotein subclasses without increasing low-density lipoprotein-cholesterol levels: A phase 4, randomized study. *Atherosclerosis* **2020**, *292*, 163–170. [CrossRef] [PubMed]
105. Sorensen, G.V.; Svensson, M.; Strandhave, C.; Schmidt, E.B.; Jorgensen, K.A.; Christensen, J.H. The Effect of n-3 Fatty Acids on Small Dense Low-Density Lipoproteins in Patients With End-Stage Renal Disease: A Randomized Placebo-Controlled Intervention Study. *J. Ren. Nutr.* **2015**, *25*, 376–380. [CrossRef]
106. Kawakami, Y.; Yamanaka-Okumura, H.; Naniwa-Kuroki, Y.; Sakuma, M.; Taketani, Y.; Takeda, E. Flaxseed oil intake reduces serum small dense low-density lipoprotein concentrations in Japanese men: A randomized, double blind, crossover study. *Nutr. J.* **2015**, *14*, 39. [CrossRef]
107. Wilkinson, P.; Leach, C.; Ah-Sing, E.E.; Hussain, N.; Miller, G.J.; Millward, D.J.; Griffin, B.A. Influence of alpha-linolenic acid and fish-oil on markers of cardiovascular risk in subjects with an atherogenic lipoprotein phenotype. *Atherosclerosis* **2005**, *181*, 115–124. [CrossRef]

108. Tuccinardi, D.; Farr, O.M.; Upadhyay, J.; Oussaada, S.M.; Klapa, M.I.; Candela, M.; Rampelli, S.; Lehoux, S.; Lazaro, I.; Sala-Vila, A.; et al. Mechanisms underlying the cardiometabolic protective effect of walnut consumption in obese people: A cross-over, randomized, double-blind, controlled inpatient physiology study. *Diabetes Obes. Metab.* **2019**, *21*, 2086–2095. [CrossRef]
109. Chang, C.H.; Tseng, P.T.; Chen, N.Y.; Lin, P.C.; Lin, P.Y.; Chang, J.P.; Kuo, F.Y.; Lin, J.; Wu, M.C.; Su, K.P. Safety and tolerability of prescription omega-3 fatty acids: A systematic review and meta-analysis of randomized controlled trials. *Prostaglandins Leukot. Essent. Fat. Acids* **2018**, *129*, 1–12. [CrossRef]
110. Franck, M.; de Toro-Martin, J.; Guenard, F.; Rudkowska, I.; Lemieux, S.; Lamarche, B.; Couture, P.; Vohl, M.C. Prevention of Potential Adverse Metabolic Effects of a Supplementation with Omega-3 Fatty Acids Using a Genetic Score Approach. *Lifestyle Genom.* **2020**, *13*, 32–42. [CrossRef]
111. Silva, M.A.; Albuquerque, T.G.; Pereira, P.; Ramalho, R.; Vicente, F.; Oliveira, M.; Costa, H.S. Opuntia ficus-indica (L.) Mill.: A Multi-Benefit Potential to Be Exploited. *Molecules* **2021**, *26*, 951. [CrossRef] [PubMed]
112. Giglio, R.V.; Carruba, G.; Cicero, A.F.G.; Banach, M.; Patti, A.M.; Nikolic, D.; Cocciadiferro, L.; Zarcone, M.; Montalto, G.; Stoian, A.P.; et al. Pasta Supplemented with Opuntia ficus-indica Extract Improves Metabolic Parameters and Reduces Atherogenic Small Dense Low-Density Lipoproteins in Patients with Risk Factors for the Metabolic Syndrome: A Four-Week Intervention Study. *Metabolites* **2020**, *10*, 428. [CrossRef] [PubMed]
113. Khan, N.; Mukhtar, H. Tea polyphenols for health promotion. *Life Sci.* **2007**, *81*, 519–533. [CrossRef] [PubMed]
114. Ng, K.W.; Cao, Z.J.; Chen, H.B.; Zhao, Z.Z.; Zhu, L.; Yi, T. Oolong tea: A critical review of processing methods, chemical composition, health effects, and risk. *Crit. Rev. Food Sci. Nutr.* **2018**, *58*, 2957–2980. [CrossRef] [PubMed]
115. Shishikura, Y.; Khokhar, S.; Murray, B.S. Effects of tea polyphenols on emulsification of olive oil in a small intestine model system. *J. Agric. Food Chem.* **2006**, *54*, 1906–1913. [CrossRef]
116. Shimada, K.; Kawarabayashi, T.; Tanaka, A.; Fukuda, D.; Nakamura, Y.; Yoshiyama, M.; Takeuchi, K.; Sawaki, T.; Hosoda, K.; Yoshikawa, J. Oolong tea increases plasma adiponectin levels and low-density lipoprotein particle size in patients with coronary artery disease. *Diabetes Res. Clin. Pract.* **2004**, *65*, 227–234. [CrossRef]
117. Lovati, M.R.; Manzoni, C.; Gianazza, E.; Arnoldi, A.; Kurowska, E.; Carroll, K.K.; Sirtori, C.R. Soy protein peptides regulate cholesterol homeostasis in Hep G2 cells. *J. Nutr.* **2000**, *130*, 2543–2549. [CrossRef]
118. Choi, S.K.; Adachi, M.; Utsumi, S. Identification of the bile acid-binding region in the soy glycinin A1aB1b subunit. *Biosci. Biotechnol. Biochem.* **2002**, *66*, 2395–2401. [CrossRef]
119. Caponio, G.R.; Wang, D.Q.; Di Ciaula, A.; De Angelis, M.; Portincasa, P. Regulation of Cholesterol Metabolism by Bioactive Components of Soy Proteins: Novel Translational Evidence. *Int. J. Mol. Sci.* **2020**, *22*, 227. [CrossRef]
120. Blanco Mejia, S.; Messina, M.; Li, S.S.; Viguiliouk, E.; Chiavaroli, L.; Khan, T.A.; Srichaikul, K.; Mirrahimi, A.; Sievenpiper, J.L.; Kris-Etherton, P.; et al. A Meta-Analysis of 46 Studies Identified by the FDA Demonstrates that Soy Protein Decreases Circulating LDL and Total Cholesterol Concentrations in Adults. *J. Nutr.* **2019**, *149*, 968–981. [CrossRef]
121. Desroches, S.; Mauger, J.F.; Ausman, L.M.; Lichtenstein, A.H.; Lamarche, B. Soy protein favorably affects LDL size independently of isoflavones in hypercholesterolemic men and women. *J. Nutr.* **2004**, *134*, 574–579. [CrossRef] [PubMed]
122. Reis, S.A.; Conceicao, L.L.; Rosa, D.D.; Siqueira, N.P.; Peluzio, M.C.G. Mechanisms responsible for the hypocholesterolaemic effect of regular consumption of probiotics. *Nutr. Res. Rev.* **2017**, *30*, 36–49. [CrossRef] [PubMed]
123. Gadelha, C.; Bezerra, A.N. Effects of probiotics on the lipid profile: Systematic review. *J. Vasc. Bras.* **2019**, *18*, e20180124. [CrossRef] [PubMed]
124. Barengolts, E. Gut Microbiota, Prebiotics, Probiotics, and Synbiotics in Management of Obesity and Prediabetes: Review of Randomized Controlled Trials. *Endocr. Pract.* **2016**, *22*, 1224–1234. [CrossRef]
125. Taylor, B.L.; Woodfall, G.E.; Sheedy, K.E.; O'Riley, M.L.; Rainbow, K.A.; Bramwell, E.L.; Kellow, N.J. Effect of Probiotics on Metabolic Outcomes in Pregnant Women with Gestational Diabetes: A Systematic Review and Meta-Analysis of Randomized Controlled Trials. *Nutrients* **2017**, *9*, 461. [CrossRef]
126. Michael, D.R.; Jack, A.A.; Masetti, G.; Davies, T.S.; Loxley, K.E.; Kerry-Smith, J.; Plummer, J.F.; Marchesi, J.R.; Mullish, B.H.; McDonald, J.A.K.; et al. A randomised controlled study shows supplementation of overweight and obese adults with lactobacilli and bifidobacteria reduces bodyweight and improves well-being. *Sci. Rep.* **2020**, *10*, 4183. [CrossRef]
127. Suez, J.; Zmora, N.; Segal, E.; Elinav, E. The pros, cons, and many unknowns of probiotics. *Nat. Med.* **2019**, *25*, 716–729. [CrossRef]
128. Ahangari, N.; Doosti, M.; Ghayour Mobarhan, M.; Sahebkar, A.; Ferns, G.A.; Pasdar, A. Personalised medicine in hypercholesterolaemia: The role of pharmacogenetics in statin therapy. *Ann. Med.* **2020**, *52*, 462–470. [CrossRef]
129. Polisecki, E.; Muallem, H.; Maeda, N.; Peter, I.; Robertson, M.; McMahon, A.D.; Ford, I.; Packard, C.; Shepherd, J.; Jukema, J.W.; et al. Genetic variation at the LDL receptor and HMG-CoA reductase gene loci, lipid levels, statin response, and cardiovascular disease incidence in PROSPER. *Atherosclerosis* **2008**, *200*, 109–114. [CrossRef]
130. Mangravite, L.M.; Medina, M.W.; Cui, J.; Pressman, S.; Smith, J.D.; Rieder, M.J.; Guo, X.; Nickerson, D.A.; Rotter, J.I.; Krauss, R.M. Combined influence of LDLR and HMGCR sequence variation on lipid-lowering response to simvastatin. *Arterioscler. Thromb. Vasc. Biol.* **2010**, *30*, 1485–1492. [CrossRef]
131. Chasman, D.I.; Giulianini, F.; MacFadyen, J.; Barratt, B.J.; Nyberg, F.; Ridker, P.M. Genetic determinants of statin-induced low-density lipoprotein cholesterol reduction: The Justification for the Use of Statins in Prevention: An Intervention Trial Evaluating Rosuvastatin (JUPITER) trial. *Circ. Cardiovasc. Genet.* **2012**, *5*, 257–264. [CrossRef] [PubMed]

132. Feng, Q.; Wei, W.Q.; Chung, C.P.; Levinson, R.T.; Bastarache, L.; Denny, J.C.; Stein, C.M. The effect of genetic variation in PCSK9 on the LDL-cholesterol response to statin therapy. *Pharm. J.* **2017**, *17*, 204–208. [CrossRef] [PubMed]
133. Kirac, D.; Bayam, E.; Dagdelen, M.; Gezmis, H.; Sarikaya, S.; Pala, S.; Altunok, E.C.; Genc, E. HMGCR and ApoE mutations may cause different responses to lipid lowering statin therapy. *Cell. Mol. Biol.* **2017**, *63*, 43–48. [CrossRef] [PubMed]
134. O'Neill, F.H.; Patel, D.D.; Knight, B.L.; Neuwirth, C.K.; Bourbon, M.; Soutar, A.K.; Taylor, G.W.; Thompson, G.R.; Naoumova, R.P. Determinants of variable response to statin treatment in patients with refractory familial hypercholesterolemia. *Arterioscler. Thromb. Vasc. Biol.* **2001**, *21*, 832–837. [CrossRef] [PubMed]
135. Krittanawong, C.; Khawaja, M.; Rosenson, R.S.; Amos, C.I.; Nambi, V.; Lavie, C.J.; Virani, S.S. Association of PCSK9 Variants With the Risk of Atherosclerotic Cardiovascular Disease and Variable Responses to PCSK9 Inhibitor Therapy. *Curr. Probl. Cardiol.* **2021**, 101043. [CrossRef] [PubMed]

Article

Efficacy and Safety of Novel Aspirin Formulations: A Randomized, Double-Blind, Placebo-Controlled Study

Rocco Mollace [1,2,†], Micaela Gliozzi [1,†], Roberta Macrì [1], Annamaria Tavernese [1], Vincenzo Musolino [1], Cristina Carresi [1], Jessica Maiuolo [1], Carolina Muscoli [1,2], Carlo Tomino [2], Giuseppe Maria Rosano [2], Massimo Fini [2], Maurizio Volterrani [2], Bruno Silvestrini [1] and Vincenzo Mollace [1,2,*]

1. Department of Health Science, Institute of Research for Food Safety & Health IRC-FSH, University Magna Graecia, 88100 Catanzaro, Italy; rocco.mollace@gmail.com (R.M.); micaela.gliozzi@gmail.com (M.G.); robertamacri85@gmail.com (R.M.); an.tavernese@gmail.com (A.T.); xabaras3@hotmail.com (V.M.); carresi@unicz.it (C.C.); jessicamaiuolo@virgilio.it (J.M.); muscoli@unicz.it (C.M.); bruno.silvestrini@alice.it (B.S.)
2. IRCCS San Raffaele Pisana, Via di Valcannuta, 00163 Rome, Italy; carlo.tomino@uniroma5.it (C.T.); giuseppe.rosano@sanraffaele.it (G.M.R.); massimo.fini@sanraffaele.it (M.F.); maurizio.volterrani@sanraffaele.it (M.V.)
* Correspondence: mollace@libero.it
† Both authors equally contributed to the manuscript.

Abstract: Low-dose aspirin represents the best option in the secondary prevention of coronary artery disease, but its extensive use in primary prevention is limited by the occurrence of gastric mucosal lesions and increased risk of bleeding. We investigated the safety profile of a novel sublingual aspirin formulation in 200 healthy volunteers, randomly assigned to ten (n = 20 each) different 7-day once-daily treatment regimens. Gastric mucosal injury based on the modified Lanza score (MLS), the histopathology of gastric mucosa and the serum determination of thromboxane B_2 (TXB_2) and urinary 11-dehydro-TXB_2 levels were evaluated at basal as well as after 7 days of each placebo or aspirin treatment regimen. In Groups A and B (placebo—oral and sublingual, respectively), no changes in MLS and in gastric mucosal micro-vessel diameter were found at day 7. In contrast, in Groups C and D (oral standard aspirin—100 and 50 mg daily, respectively), the median MLS was significantly increased. Very few changes were found in Groups E and F (standard sublingual aspirin—100 and 50 mg, respectively). Groups G and H (oral administration of micronized collagen-cogrinded aspirin) showed gastric protection compared to Groups C and D. Moreover, Groups I and L (sublingual collagen-cogrinded aspirin—100 and 50 mg, respectively) showed a significant reduction (Group I) or total abolition (Group L) of gastric mucosal lesions and no difference compared to the standard one in serum TXB_2 and urinary 11-dehydro-TXB_2 levels. In conclusion, our data show that the new formulation leads to a better safety profile compared to standard aspirin, representing a better therapeutic option for extended use in primary and secondary prevention of cardiovascular diseases.

Keywords: aspirin; coronary artery disease prevention; gastric protection; micronization; collagen cogrinding

1. Introduction

Aspirin is the most successful drug in history. It was discovered over a hundred years ago, and, now, one billion tablets are consumed every year worldwide. In particular, evidence has been collected showing that low-dose aspirin may play a crucial role in the secondary prevention of both cardiovascular and cerebrovascular diseases [1–3]. Moreover, due to its direct, as well as indirect, damaging effect on gastric mucosa, the occurrence of aspirin-related peptic ulcers is increasing [4–6], and upper intestine bleeding still represents a major issue in patients chronically using aspirin.

The effect of aspirin has been assessed in the last forty years. In particular, it is known that aspirin inhibits cyclooxygenase-1 (COX-1) in platelets, leading to a reduction in platelet thromboxane A_2 (TXA_2) and the subsequent inhibition of platelet adhesion and aggregation, which are major steps that contribute to preventing cardiovascular complications [6,7]. However, the activity of aspirin is accompanied by a reduction in the protective activity exerted by the biosynthesis of gastric mucosal prostaglandin E_2 (PGE_2), an effect that increases the risk of gastric lesions and bleeding [8]. However, the inhibition of COX-1 as a result of taking aspirin is accompanied by the enhanced production of another class of COX-related products, namely, leukotrienes, mostly leukotriene B_4, which leads to vasoconstriction and inflammation in gastric tissues, an effect associated with aspirin-induced gastric injury [9]. Finally, direct gastric mucosal lesion has been found to occur in patients undergoing long-term low-dose aspirin treatment, mostly due to its direct entry into gastric mucosal cells via non-ionic mechanisms, an effect associated with the back diffusion of hydrogen ions into mucosal cells [10].

The occurrence of damage of the gastric mucosa and the bleeding found in patients undergoing chronic oral treatment with low-dose aspirin have recently been confirmed in the ASCEND study [11], which elucidated that gastric injury counteracts the benefit derived from a more extended use of low-dose aspirin in the primary prevention in patients with diabetes, though further studies are required in this area. This, however, represents the basis for assessing therapeutic strategies aimed at combining gastro-protective drugs with aspirin in order to attenuate its potential damaging effect at the gastric level [11,12]. In fact, the use of protonic pump inhibitors (PPIs), as well as H_2 histamine receptor antagonists, has been proven to be effective in protecting the gastric mucosa in patients undergoing low-dose aspirin treatment; this strategy, however, is associated with an increase in sanitary cost and is drug metabolism dependent [13,14]. Moreover, the use of aspirin formulations, in which the drug is combined with compounds that increase gastric pH, is associated with impaired aspirin absorption, as its entry into the cells is influenced by changes in its solubility, which decreases at higher pH levels [15–17]. Thus, the development of a better aspirin formulation still represents a challenge for researchers working in this area.

Recently, we developed and tested a new aspirin formulation based on an original process, which includes micronization and cogrinding with collagen of its crystalline form, thereby achieving a better drug absorption associated with significant protection of gastric mucosa [18].

In particular, both oral and sublingual administration of the novel aspirin formulation showed an early occurrence of serum concentration peak response compared to the standard crystalline drug formulation. This effect was associated with a decrease in both TXB_2 serum concentration (the metabolite of platelet TXA_2) and urinary 6-keto-PGF1α, which represents another reliable bio-marker of aspirin efficacy at the COX level [18].

Finally, experiments in rats have been performed in order to verify the attenuated impact of the novel aspirin formulation on the gastric mucosa. In particular, aspirin, either standard or collagen-cogrinded aspirin, at doses previously proven to produce gastric lesions, was given orally to rats to compare their damaging effects. Under these experimental conditions, we found that the severity of the aspirin-induced ulceration of the gastric mucosa was reduced when aspirin was cogrinded with collagen, an effect confirmed by histopathological studies [18]. Thus, the novel aspirin formulation seems to possess non-inferiority efficacy compared to standard aspirin and a better safety profile as evaluated in the experimental models of aspirin-related gastric damage.

The present randomized, double-blind, placebo-controlled study was performed in healthy volunteers in order to assess the safety profile of the novel formulation based on micronization and the cogrinding of aspirin with collagen.

2. Materials and Methods

2.1. Materials

Type I bovine collagen hydrolysate was purchased from LapiGelatin (Pistoia, Italy). Aspirin (acetylsalicylic acid), maltodextrin, microcrystalline cellulose, sodium carboxymethyl starch, sucralose and magnesium stearate were purchased from Sigma-Aldrich (Milan, Italy).

2.2. Preparation of Aspirin Formulations

A mixture of hydrolyzed bovine collagen and crystalline aspirin was micronized and cogrinded in a ratio of 1 to 1 by means of a pin rotor mortar, which leads to micronization of powder particles at <40 µm (Pulverisette 14, Fisher, Idar Oberstein, Germany). Optical microscopy showed, after 20 min, the disappearance of micro-crystals of aspirin, replaced by amorphous particles surrounded by collagen. The amorphization of aspirin was confirmed by means of differential scanning calorimetry (DSC), performed with Perkin Elmer apparatus DSC7 and calibrated with Indium. The samples were examined with a scanning speed of 5.0 C/min. Granular aspirin was tested, highlighting the melting peak in the range of 133.9–136.8, which characterizes the crystalline building. In contrast, when evaluating aspirin micronized and cogrinded with bovine collagen hydrolysate via DSC, the melting peak between 135 °C and 138 °C disappeared. The aspirin amorphization after cogrinding with collagen was also confirmed by Raman microspectroscopy, as previously described [18].

In the second step, standard crystalline aspirin and aspirin micronized and cogrinded with collagen powders were used to obtain oral and sublingual formulations (tablets) by means of mechanical compression (Ronchi, Italy) under good manufacturing procedure (GMP-Institute of Research for Food Safety & Health, University of Catanzaro, Catanzaro, Italy) conditions. Microcrystalline cellulose, sodium carboxy-methyl starch, sucralose and magnesium stearate were thus used as excipients. When required, maltodextrin was used to obtain a homogeneous final weight for each tablet, as well as in the formulations for placebo. Placebo was obtained by substitution of aspirin and/or collagen in tablets with maltodextrin.

2.3. Study Design

A randomized, double-blind, placebo-controlled study was performed to evaluate the effect of oral, as well as sublingual, standard aspirin and micronized and collagen-cogrinded aspirin on gastric mucosal lesions and on serum TXB_2 and 11-dehydro-TXB_2 urinary levels. The study was carried out in 200 healthy volunteers, and data were compared with a placebo-treated group. The study complied with the principles of the Good Clinical Practice International Conference on Harmonization rules, was performed according to the CONSORT Statement and its checklist (http://www.consort-statement.org/, accessed on 9 January 2022; see Supplementary Materials) and was approved by the Regional Ethics Committee (extension study of EudraCT N. 2013-002980-24, 1 July 2013). Each study participant provided written informed consent. Inclusion and exclusion criteria are listed in the Supplementary Materials.

A total of 200 healthy volunteers were randomized using computerized random number generation by an independent investigator (CIRM, Milan, Italy) on a double-blind basis and randomly assigned to 10 groups (20 subjects each) according to the type and dose of aspirin or placebo (Table 1 summarizes subjects' demographics). In particular, healthy volunteers received 7-day, once-daily treatment regimens: Groups A and B received oral and sublingual placebo, respectively; Groups C and D received standard oral aspirin of 100 mg or 50 mg, respectively; Groups E and F received sublingual aspirin of 100 mg or 50 mg, respectively; Groups G and H received oral micronized and collagen-cogrinded aspirin of 100 mg or 50 mg, respectively; and, finally, Groups I and L received sublingual micronized and collagen-cogrinded aspirin of 100 mg or 50 mg, respectively. On day 7, healthy volunteers entering the study received two low-fat meals (lunch and dinner at 12 and 18 h, respectively). Only mineral water was allowed.

Table 1. Demographics of healthy volunteers enrolled in the study. Values are expressed as mean ± SD.

Group	N.	Age (Years)	Gender (Male/Female)	Body Weight (Kg)	Body Mass Index (Kg/m^2)	Smoking	Concomitant Treatment
A—placebo oral	20	32 ± 6	10 M and 10 F	68 ± 8	23 ± 2	0	0
B—placebo sublingual	20	35 ± 4	10 M and 10 F	66 ± 7	25 ± 4	0	0
C—oral standard aspirin 100 mg	20	34 ± 4	9 M and 11 F	66 ± 6	24 ± 4	0	0
D—oral standard aspirin 50 mg	20	34 ± 5	11 M and 9 F	68 ± 7	23 ± 5	0	0
E—sublingual standard aspirin 100 mg	20	34 ± 5	11 M and 9 F	65 ± 8	23 ± 3	0	0
F—sublingual standard aspirin 50 mg	20	35 ± 5	9 M and 11 F	68 ± 8	24 ± 3	0	0
G—oral micronized collagen-cogrinded aspirin 100 mg	20	33 ± 4	10 M and 10 F	67 ± 6	24 ± 4	0	0
H—oral micronized collagen-cogrinded aspirin 50 mg	20	34 ± 5	11 M and 9 F	66 ± 6	25 ± 3	0	0
I—sublingual micronized collagen-cogrinded aspirin 100 mg	20	35 ± 4	10 M and 10 F	66 ± 8	25 ± 4	0	0
L—sublingual micronized collagen-cogrinded aspirin 50 mg	20	34 ± 4	9 M and 11 F	68 ± 8	23 ± 5	0	0

Gastroscopy and blood and urine sample collection for analytical tests were performed in fasted volunteers on days 1 and 7 alongside the administration of the first and last doses of the drugs or the placebo. All of the procedures required the supervision of an investigator, who also instructed the healthy volunteers on the correct procedures for taking the aspirin or placebo at their home. A pill count was performed on day 7 in order to verify the compliance and adherence of subjects to the assigned treatment, which was 100%. This was also confirmed by contacting healthy volunteers by telephone on days 2–6. All subjects were instructed to not eat any meal for at least 6 h after taking the aspirin or placebo. Finally, drinking water was not allowed for at least 1 h before and after taking the aspirin or placebo.

Before administration of aspirin formulations or placebo and after the sixth dose, all subjects performed a 24 h urine collection in order to study the effect of aspirin on urinary levels of 11-dehydro-TXB$_2$ (by means of ELISA immunoassay; BioRad, Milan, Italy).

Plasma TXB$_2$ and urinary 11-dehydro-TXB$_2$ were validated for precision and accuracy according to EMA guidelines. The mean serum levels of TXB$_2$ and urinary 11-dehydro-TXB$_2$ in healthy volunteers were 306 ± 45 ng/mL and 465 ± 58 pg/mg creatinine, respectively. Changes in these parameters were assumed to calculate the % response after aspirin treatment.

2.4. Endoscopy and Collection of Gastric Mucosal Samples for Histopathology

Gastroduodenal endoscopy was performed in healthy volunteers enrolled in the study after they fasted overnight, with an Olympus GIF-XQ 240 flexible gastroscope

(Olympus Corporation, Tokyo, Japan). A blinded endoscopist collected the pictures and video sequences necessary for assessing the status of gastric mucosa during gastroscopy in both placebo- and aspirin-treated patients. The extent of gastric lesions was scored via the so-called modified Lanza score (MLS) system (Grade 0 = no erosion/hemorrhage, Grade 1 = 1–2 lesions of erosion and/or hemorrhage found in one area of the stomach, Grade 2 = 3–5 lesions of erosion and/or hemorrhage localized in one area of the stomach, Grade 3 = 6–9 lesions of erosion and/or hemorrhage detected in one area of the stomach or no more than 10 lesions in two areas in the stomach, Grade 4 = erosion and/or hemorrhage detected in three areas in the stomach or no less than 10 lesions in the whole stomach, and Grade 5 = gastric ulcer). The MLS was assessed as a means of three evaluations made by three independent endoscopists unaware of the group composition of the subjects undergoing gastroduodenal endoscopy. Gastric mucosa biopsy was collected from three different areas representative of the total gastric surface. Gastric specimens were stained with hematoxylin–eosin, and the sub-epithelial microvessels were measured according to their short-axis section. A mean of thirty vessels for each subject was taken as representative for assessing microvascular impairment in the subepithelial vessels.

2.5. Statistical Analysis

For the evaluation of data in our comparison between the groups, we used the statistical software SPSS version 22. The data were expressed as mean ± SD, and statistical comparisons were made by parametric tests (Student's t-test or repeated measures analysis of variance, followed by the Student–Newman–Keuls test). The Shapiro–Wilk test was used to evaluate the distribution of the normality data. A probability value of $p < 0.05$ was considered to be statistically significant.

3. Results

3.1. Dissolution Studies

We investigated the in vitro dissolution of standard aspirin, as well as micronized collagen-cogrinded aspirin, in 50 and 100 mg tablets. The procedures defined by the USP/NF monograph dissolution procedure for aspirin tablets were followed for dissolution studies. In particular, the dissolution profiles of the products were defined in samples determined at times 1, 3, 6 and 15 min with a Q point at 30 min. A modified test procedure was also performed by using dissolution media prepared in accordance with the USP reagents section on the preparation of buffers at pH 1.2 and 6.8, respectively.

For calibration procedures, solutions contained aspirin at a concentration of 1 mg/mL under the same pH conditions as those of the dissolution buffer. Solutions of 1mg/mL were also used to obtain the isosbestic point for aspirin. Measurements were performed via a Cary Model 50 spectrophotometer (Agilent Technologies, Santa Clara, CA, USA), which were carried out after the collection and filtering of each sample. The procedures were performed according to GMP requirements.

At the two pH values, the aspirin tablet formulations were dissolved to an extent of 92.5 ± 2 and 99.2 ± 3%, respectively, at 15 min, while at the same time, the standard aspirin tablet was dissolved to an extent of 47.6 ± 3 and 82.8 ± 3%, at the two pH values, respectively. The dissolution studies carried out in vitro showed that the tablet containing aspirin micronized and cogrinded with collagen is characterized by a substantially faster dissolution compared to standard aspirin tablets at pH conditions ranging from 1.2 to 6.8 levels. Moreover, a pH-dependent dissolution capacity was found for both forms of aspirin, with lower dissolution rates detected at lower pH levels.

In all of the 200 subjects enrolled, the study was completed according to protocols between January 2018 and December 2019 at the IRC-FSH (Institute of Research for Food Safety & Health, University of Catanzaro, Catanzaro, Italy). There were no significant differences in the demographic or clinical characteristics (e.g., age and sex) at baseline among the different groups (Table 1). None of the subjects experienced any consistent adverse events associated with aspirin, such as gastrointestinal hemorrhage or major abdominal symptoms.

3.2. Gastric Mucosal Injury Induced by Standard Aspirin or Aspirin Micronized and Cogrinded with Collagen

The changes in the MLS in each subject associated with the different treatments are shown in Figure 1. The median (range) MLS in Groups A and B (placebo) was 0 (0–1). A significant increase in the median MLS (3, 0) was observed in Group C, who received oral standard aspirin (100 mg daily for 7 days), in comparison with that in the groups receiving placebo (Groups A and B; Figure 1). This effect was moderately attenuated in Group D, who received 50 mg of oral standard aspirin, and in Groups E and F, who received standard aspirin sublingually at doses of 100 and 50 mg, respectively. The administration of oral aspirin micronized and cogrinded with collagen (Groups G and H), at doses of 100 and 50 mg, respectively, produced a further reduction in the aspirin impact on gastric mucosa. Indeed, the MLS was 2 and 1, respectively, compared to standard aspirin. A better response was found when micronized and collagen-cogrinded aspirin was given sublingually at doses of 100 mg (Group I—MLS 1) and 50 mg (Group L—MLS 0), the latter effect being similar to the one found with the placebo groups (Figure 1). Thus, aspirin micronized and cogrinded with collagen seems to display a better safety profile compared to standard aspirin.

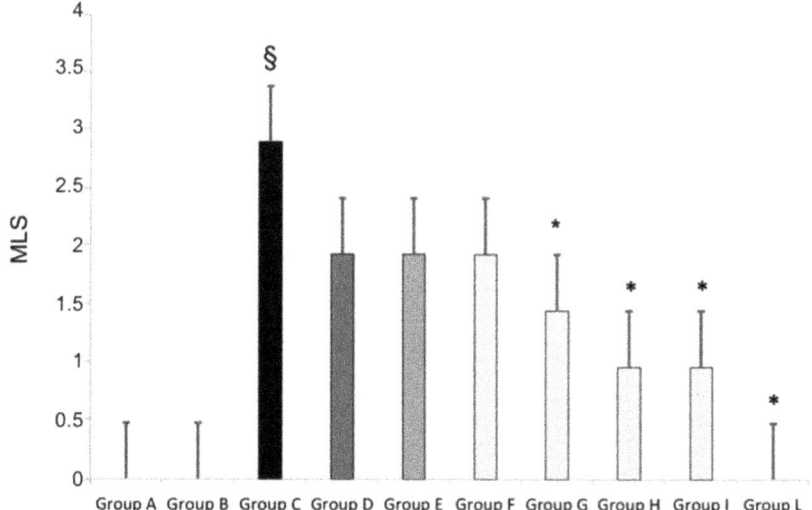

Figure 1. Gastric modified Lanza score (MLS) gastroscopy evaluation in healthy volunteers receiving placebo orally or sublingually (Groups A and B, respectively); receiving 100 or 50 mg of standard aspirin orally (Groups C and D, respectively); receiving 100 or 50 mg of standard aspirin sublingually (Groups E and F, respectively); receiving aspirin micronized and cogrinded with collagen orally (Groups G and H) or sublingually (Groups I and L). § $p < 0.05$ standard aspirin vs. placebo; * $p < 0.05$ collagen cogrinded aspirin vs. standard aspirin.

3.3. Gastric Micro-Vessel Vasodilatation Induced by Standard as Well as Micronized and Collagen-Cogrinded Aspirin

Treatment with oral standard aspirin (Groups C and D; 100 and 50 mg/daily, respectively) for 7 days significantly increased the median diameter of the sub-epithelial micro-vessels as compared with that of the groups receiving placebo (Groups A and B; Figure 2). A similar response was seen when standard aspirin, 100 and 50 mg/day, was given to healthy volunteers (Groups E and F, respectively; Figure 2). In contrast, this effect was found to be attenuated when micronized and collagen-cogrinded aspirin was given to the study population. In particular, in healthy volunteers taking aspirin micronized and cogrinded with collagen orally (Groups G and I) or sublingually (Groups H and L), a significant decrease in the diameter was found as compared with that of the standard aspirin regimen; in fact, the median diameter of the micro-vessels in the sublingual aspirin group was almost the same as the one found in the placebo group (Figure 2).

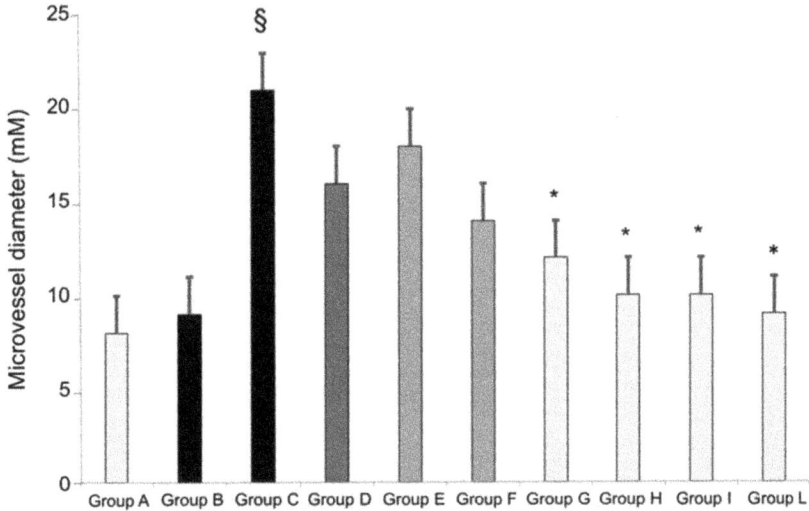

Figure 2. Gastric sub-epithelial micro-vessel diameter in healthy volunteers receiving placebo orally or sublingually (Groups A and B, respectively); receiving 100 or 50 mg of standard aspirin orally (Groups C and D, respectively); receiving 100 or 50 mg of standard aspirin sublingually (Groups E and F, respectively); receiving aspirin micronized and cogrinded with collagen orally (Groups G and H) or sublingually (Groups I and L). § $p < 0.05$ standard aspirin vs. placebo; * $p < 0.05$ collagen cogrinded aspirin vs. standard aspirin.

3.4. TXB$_2$ and Urinary 11-Dehydro-TX B$_2$ Determinations

The administration of oral aspirin, as well as sublingual aspirin (100 and 50 mg), either standard or micronized and cogrinded with collagen, was associated with decreased TXB$_2$ serum levels as detected at day 7 compared to the groups receiving placebo. No significant changes were seen among the different regimens of aspirin treatment. Moreover, urinary measurements of 11-dehydro-TXB$_2$ showed a similar response, thereby confirming that aspirin micronized and cogrinded with collagen showed a non-inferiority response to the COX enzyme compared to the crystalline standard formulation (Table 2).

The administration of standard aspirin and aspirin micronized and cogrinded with collagen given orally or sublingually did not produce any change in routine blood analytical biomarkers. In addition, no side effects or adverse drug reactions were described. Finally, the compliance and adherence were 100% in all groups and all the enrolled subjects in the study.

Table 2. The effect of standard aspirin, collagen-cogrinded aspirin and placebo, given orally or sublingually to healthy volunteers, on serum TXB$_2$ (ng/mL) and urinary 6-dehydro-TXB$_2$ (pg/mg creatinine) at Time 0 before treatment and after 7 days of treatment. Values are expressed as mean ± SD * $p < 0.05$ treatment vs. placebo.

Group	Serum TXB$_2$ Time 0	Serum TXB$_2$ 7 Days	Urinary 11-dehydro-TXB$_2$ Time 0	Urinary 11-dehydro-TXB$_2$ 7 Days
A—placebo oral	302 ± 44	278 ± 48	485 ± 54	490 ± 58
B—placebo sublingual	298 ± 38	281 ± 45	498 ± 50	486 ± 46
C—oral standard aspirin 100 mg	286 ± 40	38 ± 12 *	485 ± 52	86 ± 26 *
D—oral standard aspirin 50 mg	295 ± 38	71 ± 18 *	505 ± 48	108 ± 27 *
E—sublingual standard aspirin 100 mg	304 ± 42	48 ± 14 *	495 ± 50	95 ± 18 *
F—sublingual standard aspirin 50 mg	302 ± 35	70 ± 15 *	502 ± 46	118 ± 22 *
G—oral micronized collagen-cogrinded aspirin 100 mg	300 ± 44	36 ± 12 *	494 ± 54	77 ± 16 *
H—oral micronized collagen-cogrinded aspirin 50 mg	286 ± 40	64 ± 15 *	506 ± 54	106 ± 20 *
I—sublingual micronized collagen-cogrinded aspirin 100 mg	290 ± 44	30 ± 14 *	496 ± 48	66 ± 18 *
L—sublingual micronized collagen-cogrinded aspirin 50 mg	302 ± 38	46 ± 20 *	502 ± 48	88 ± 18 *

4. Discussion

The occurrence of gastric lesions in patients undergoing low-dose aspirin treatment for cardiovascular risk prevention represents a relevant issue, which, in some cases, limits the extensive use of such an antiplatelet drug [19,20].

In particular, data originating from very recent clinical trials and a meta-analysis performed on this topic confirmed that the efficacy of low-dose aspirin in the primary prevention of cardiovascular risk is seriously counteracted by the concomitant increased risk of gastric bleeding [21–24]. Thus, the limitation of aspirin-induced gastric injury and the development of a better aspirin may be considered relevant challenges for the research in this area [18,25,26].

The pathogenesis of aspirin-related gastric injury is complex and involves many players, including a reduced production of the protective gastric mucous associated with changes in gastric pH and direct gastrolesive action [27]. Furthermore, the dysregulation of nitric oxide (NO) production has been shown to contribute to the gastric lesions found in patients undergoing aspirin treatment. This fits with the evidence showing that aspirin induces inflammation in the gastric mucosa [28,29] as expressed by the dilatation of gastric microvessels.

Here, we reported that a better formulation of aspirin may represent an innovative way to maintain consistent antiplatelet activity as found with standard aspirin with a significant reduction in gastric injury and a better safety profile.

In particular, the micronization of aspirin and the cogrinding of the crystalline form of this drug with collagen lead to an innovative formulation that enhances drug absorption, thereby reducing gastric lesions associated with 7-day treatment with this drug. This confirms the previous evidence, in which we measured the serum concentration of aspirin both standard and micronized and cogrinded with collagen. These data are not surprising, as it is known that the micronization of crystalline drugs is clearly accompanied by an enhanced absorption of aspirin. In particular, evidence has been accumulated that micronization, which is able to reduce the size of crystalline aspirin, is associated with better drug absorption throughout both the gastric and sublingual mucosa. This has been confirmed by evidence obtained by means of Raman spectroscopy, which showed that the micronization of aspirin leads to a complete de-structuring of the crystalline form of the drug, an effect that has been demonstrated to increase the speed and rate of the absorption of many drugs, including aspirin. However, cogrinding aspirin with collagen leads to significant gastric protection. Indeed, collagen has been shown to produce both direct and indirect protection of the gastric mucosa, mostly due to its effect on gastric mucous. This effect occurs with no changes in gastric pH, compared to many of the compounds combined with aspirin in recent years, which are associated with an elevation of gastric pH. In particular, this effect is associated with a reduction in aspirin-related gastric injury, with the consequence, however, of poor aspirin absorption and subsequent reduced aspirin activity.

The innovative formulation of aspirin micronized and cogrinded with collagen seems to resolve many of the previous issues found with standard aspirin. Indeed, the extent of gastric erosions subsequent to oral aspirin was reduced when aspirin was micronized and cogrinded with collagen as detected via gastroscopy and measured via the Lanza's score [30]. In particular, the use of the sublingual formulation of the micronized aspirin occurred with no changes in the gastric mucosa compared with standard aspirin. However, this effect was associated with comparable effects of novel aspirin formulation in the biomarkers of antiplatelet activity. Indeed, both the levels of TXB_2 (the footprint of aspirin activity on platelet COX) and the levels of 11-dehydro-TXB_2 (the urinary metabolite of TXA_2) were comparable when using both sublingual and oral aspirin micronized and cogrinded with collagen when compared to standard aspirin, suggesting a non-inferiority profile of the novel formulations in the efficacy of aspirin. The better safety profile of novel aspirin is confirmed by the data from histopathological studies, which showed that the diameter of the microvessels of the gastric mucosa is reduced in subjects undergoing 7-day treatment with novel aspirin compared to the standard one, an effect that may be explained on the basis of the anti-inflammatory role of collagen when combined with aspirin, as expected with the micronized formulation compared to the standard, crystalline drug.

5. Conclusions

In conclusion, the present study demonstrated that low-dose standard aspirin induces gastric mucosal injury in healthy volunteers, an effect associated with the dilatation of the micro-vessels of gastric tissues. This response was attenuated when aspirin was micronized and cogrinded with collagen, with no significant changes in the ability of the new formulations to inhibit thromboxane formation.

Further studies are required in patients to verify the efficacy and safety of better aspirin formulations in both primary and secondary cardiovascular risk prevention in patients.

Supplementary Materials: The following are available online at https://www.mdpi.com/article/10.3390/pharmaceutics14010187/s1, Clinical Study Protocol.

Author Contributions: V.M. (Vincenzo Mollace), M.F., M.V., B.S. and G.M.R.: conceptualization and supervision; R.M. (Rocco Mollace) and M.G.: writing—original draft, investigation and methodology; R.M. (Roberta Macrì), A.T., V.M. (Vincenzo Musolino), C.C., J.M., C.M. and C.T.: investigation, methodology and formal analysis. All authors have read and agreed to the published version of the manuscript.

Funding: The work was supported by the public resources from the Italian Ministry of Research. PON-MIUR 03PE000_78_1 and PONMIUR 03PE000_78_2. POR Calabria FESR FSE 2014–2020 Asse 12-Azioni 10.5.6 e 10.5.12.

Institutional Review Board Statement: The study was conducted in accordance with the Declaration of Helsinki, and approved by the Ethics Committee of IRCCS San Raffaele Pisana, Rome, Italy (protocol ASA-001, EudraCT N. 2013-002980-24, 1 July 2013).

Informed Consent Statement: Informed consent was obtained from all subjects involved in the study.

Data Availability Statement: The data presented in this study are available upon request from the corresponding author.

Acknowledgments: This work was supported by PON-MIUR 03PE000_78_1 and PONMIUR 03PE 000_78_2. POR Calabria FESR FSE 2014–2020 Asse 12-Azioni 10.5.6 e 10.5.12.

Conflicts of Interest: The authors declare no conflict of interest.

References

1. Awtry, E.H.; Loscalzo, J. Aspirin. *Circulation* **2000**, *101*, 1206–1218. [CrossRef]
2. Baigent, C.; Blackwell, L.; Collins, R.; Emberson, J.; Godwin, J.; Peto, R.; Buring, J.; Hennekens, C.; Kearney, P.; Meade, C.; et al. Aspirin in the primary and secondary prevention of vascular disease: Collaborative meta-analysis of individual participant data from randomised trials. *Lancet* **2009**, *373*, 1849–1860. [PubMed]
3. Schrör, K. Aspirin and platelets: The antiplatelet action of aspirin and its role in thrombosis treatment and prophylaxis. *Semin. Thromb. Hemost.* **1997**, *23*, 349–356. [CrossRef] [PubMed]
4. Taha, A.S.; Angerson, W.J.; Knill-Jones, R.P.; Blatchford, O. Upper gastrointestinal haemorrhage associated with low-dose aspirin and anti-thrombotic drugs—A 6-year analysis and comparison with non-steroidal anti-inflammatory drugs. *Aliment. Pharmacol. Ther.* **2005**, *22*, 285–289. [CrossRef] [PubMed]
5. Serrano, P.; Lanas, A.; Arroyo, M.T.; Ferreira, I.J. Risk of upper gastrointestinal bleeding in patients taking low-dose aspirin for the prevention of cardiovascular diseases. *Aliment. Pharmacol. Ther.* **2002**, *16*, 1945–1953. [CrossRef]
6. Antiplatelet Trialists' Collaboration. Collaborative overview of randomised trials of antiplatelet therapy–I: Prevention of death, myocardial infarction, and stroke by prolonged antiplatelet therapy in various categories of patients. *BMJ* **1994**, *308*, 81–106. [CrossRef]
7. Warner, T.D.; Nylander, S.; Whatling, C. Anti-platelet therapy: Cyclo-oxygenase inhibition and the use of aspirin with particular regard to dual anti-platelet therapy. *Br. J. Clin. Pharmacol.* **2011**, *72*, 619–633. [CrossRef]
8. Schoen, R.T.; Vender, R.J. Mechanisms of nonsteroidal anti- inflammatory drug-induced gastric damage. *Am. J. Med.* **1989**, *86*, 449–458. [CrossRef]
9. Halter, F. Mechanism of gastrointestinal toxicity of NSAIDs. *Scand. J. Rheumatol. Suppl.* **1988**, *73*, 16–21. [CrossRef]
10. Yeomans, N.D.; Lanas, A.I.; Talley, N.J.; Thomson, A.B.R.; Daneshjoo, R.; Eriksson, B.; Appelman-Eszczuk, S.; Långström, G.; Naesdal, J.; Serrano, P.; et al. Prevalence and incidence of gastroduodenal ulcers during treatment with vascular protective doses of aspirin. *Aliment. Pharmacol. Ther.* **2005**, *22*, 795–801. [CrossRef]
11. Bowman, L.; Mafham, M.; Stevens, W.; Haynes, R.; Aung, T.; Chen, F.; Buck, G.; Collins, R.; Armitage, J.; The ASCEND Study Collaborative Group. ASCEND: A Study of Cardiovascular Events iN Diabetes: Characteristics of a randomized trial of aspirin and of omega-3 fatty acid supplementation in 15,480 people with diabetes. *Am. Heart J.* **2018**, *198*, 135–144. [CrossRef]
12. Derry, S.; Loke, Y.K. Risk of gastrointestinal haemorrhage with long term use of aspirin: Meta-analysis. *BMJ* **2000**, *321*, 1183–1187. [CrossRef] [PubMed]
13. Pilotto, A.; Franceschi, M.; Leandro, G.; Paris, F.; Cascavilla, L.; Longo, M.G.; Niro, V.; Andriulli, A.; Scarcelli, C.; Di Mario, F. Proton-pump inhibitors reduce the risk of uncomplicated peptic ulcer in elderly either acute or chronic users of aspirin/non-steroidal anti-inflammatory drugs. *Aliment. Pharmacol. Ther.* **2004**, *20*, 1091–1097. [CrossRef]
14. Huang, M.; Han, M.; Han, W.; Kuang, L. Proton pump inhibitors versus histamine-2 receptor blockers for stress ulcer prophylaxis in patients with sepsis: A retrospective cohort study. *J. Int. Med. Res.* **2021**, *49*, 03000605211025130. [CrossRef] [PubMed]
15. Dotevall, G.; Ekenved, G. The absorption of acetylsalicylic acid from the stomach in relation to intragastric pH. *Scand. J. Gastroenterol.* **1976**, *11*, 801–805. [CrossRef] [PubMed]
16. Cooke, A.R.; Hunt, J.N. Relationship between pH and absorption of acetylsalicylic acid from the stomach. *Gut* **1969**, *10*, 77–78.
17. Mitra, A.; Kesisoglou, F. Impaired drug absorption due to high stomach pH: A review of strategies for mitigation of such effect to enable pharmaceutical product development. *Mol. Pharm.* **2013**, *10*, 3970–3979. [CrossRef] [PubMed]
18. Mollace, V.; Rosano, G.; Malara, N.; Di Fabrizio, E.; Vitale, C.; Coluccio, M.; Maiuolo, J.; Wasti, A.A.; Muscoli, C.; Gliozzi, M.; et al. Aspirin wears smart. *Eur. Heart J. Cardiovasc. Pharmacother.* **2017**, *3*, 185–188. [CrossRef]
19. Lavie, C.J.; Howden, C.W.; Scheiman, J.; Tursi, J. Upper Gastrointestinal Toxicity Associated With Long-Term Aspirin Therapy: Consequences and Prevention. *Curr. Probl. Cardiol.* **2017**, *42*, 146–164. [CrossRef]
20. Sostres, C.; Lanas, A. Gastrointestinal effects of aspirin. *Nat. Rev. Gastroenterol. Hepatol.* **2011**, *8*, 385–394. [CrossRef]
21. García Rodríguez, L.A.; Vora, P.; Brobert, G.; Soriano-Gabarrò, M.; Cea Soriano, L. Bleeding associated with low-dose aspirin: Comparison of data from the COMPASS randomized controlled trial and routine clinical practice. *Int. J. Cardiol.* **2020**, *318*, 21–24. [CrossRef]
22. Cea Soriano, L.; Lanas, A.; Soriano-Gabarró, M.; García Rodríguez, L.A. Incidence of Upper and Lower Gastrointestinal Bleeding in New Users of Low-Dose Aspirin. *Clin. Gastroenterol. Hepatol.* **2019**, *17*, 887–895.e6. [CrossRef]
23. Cea Soriano, L.; Gaist, D.; Soriano-Gabarró, M.; García Rodríguez, L.A. Incidence of intracranial bleeds in new users of low-dose aspirin: A cohort study using The Health Improvement Network. *J. Thromb. Haemost.* **2017**, *15*, 1055–1064. [CrossRef] [PubMed]

24. Li, L.; Geraghty, O.C.; Mehta, Z.; Rothwell, P.M.; Oxford Vascular Study. Age-specific risks, severity, time course, and outcome of bleeding on long-term antiplatelet treatment after vascular events: A population-based cohort study. *Lancet* **2017**, *390*, 490–499. [CrossRef]
25. Scheiman, J.M. Strategies to reduce the GI risks of antiplatelet therapy. *Rev. Cardiovasc. Med.* **2005**, *6* (Suppl. 4), S23–S31. [PubMed]
26. Zhao, C.; Wang, J.; Xiao, Q. Efficacy of Teprenone for Prevention of NSAID-Induced Gastrointestinal Injury: A Systematic Review and Meta-Analysis. *Front. Med.* **2021**, *8*, 647494. [CrossRef] [PubMed]
27. Nishino, M.; Sugimoto, M.; Kodaira, C.; Yamade, M.; Shirai, N.; Ikuma, M.; Tanaka, T.; Sugimura, H.; Hishida, A.; Furuta, T. Relationship between low-dose aspirin-induced gastric mucosal injury and intragastric pH in healthy volunteers. *Dig. Dis. Sci.* **2009**, *55*, 1627–1636. [CrossRef]
28. Kitay, A.M.; Ferstl, F.S.; Geibel, J.P. Induction of Secretagogue Independent Gastric Acid Secretion via a Novel Aspirin-Activated Pathway. *Front. Physiol.* **2019**, *10*, 1264. [CrossRef]
29. Lanas, A.; Wu, P.; Medin, J.; Mills, E. Low doses of acetylsalicylic acid increase risk of gastrointestinal bleeding in a meta-analysis. *J. Clin. Gastroenterol. Hepatol.* **2011**, *9*, 762–768.e6. [CrossRef]
30. Lanza, F.L.; Royer, G.L., Jr.; Nelson, R.S.; Chen, T.T.; Seckman, C.E.; Rack, M.F. A comparative endoscopic evaluation of the damaging effects of nonsteroidal anti-inflammatory agents on the gastric and duodenal mucosa. *Am. J. Gastroenterol.* **1981**, *75*, 17–21.

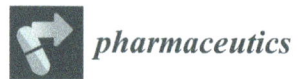 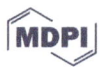

Review

The Impact of Angiotensin-Converting Enzyme-2/Angiotensin 1-7 Axis in Establishing Severe COVID-19 Consequences

Minela Aida Maranduca [1,2,†], Daniela Maria Tanase [1,3,†], Cristian Tudor Cozma [2,*], Nicoleta Dima [1,3], Andreea Clim [2], Alin Constantin Pinzariu [2], Dragomir Nicolae Serban [2] and Ionela Lacramioara Serban [2]

1. Internal Medicine Clinic, "St. Spiridon" County Clinical Emergency Hospital, 700115 Iasi, Romania
2. Department of Morpho-Functional Sciences II, Discipline of Physiology, "Grigore T. Popa" University of Medicine and Pharmacy, 700115 Iasi, Romania
3. Department of Internal Medicine, "Grigore T. Popa" University of Medicine and Pharmacy, 700115 Iasi, Romania
* Correspondence: cozmatudor19@gmail.com
† These authors contributed equally to this work.

Abstract: The COVID-19 pandemic has put a tremendous stress on the medical community over the last two years. Managing the infection proved a lot more difficult after several research communities started to recognize the long-term effects of this disease. The cellular receptor for the virus was identified as angiotensin-converting enzyme-2 (ACE2), a molecule responsible for a wide array of processes, broadly variable amongst different organs. Angiotensin (Ang) 1-7 is the product of Ang II, a decaying reaction catalysed by ACE2. The effects observed after altering the level of ACE2 are essentially related to the variation of Ang 1-7. The renin-angiotensin-aldosterone system (RAAS) is comprised of two main branches, with ACE2 representing a crucial component of the protective part of the complex. The ACE2/Ang (1-7) axis is well represented in the testis, heart, brain, kidney, and intestine. Infection with the novel SARS-CoV-2 virus determines downregulation of ACE2 and interrupts the equilibrium between ACE and ACE2 in these organs. In this review, we highlight the link between the local effects of RAAS and the consequences of COVID-19 infection as they arise from observational studies.

Keywords: renin-angiotensin-aldosterone system; RAAS; angiotensin-converting enzyme-2; ACE2; angiotensin 1-7; Ang (1-7); COVID-19; long-term effects

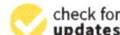

Citation: Maranduca, M.A.; Tanase, D.M.; Cozma, C.T.; Dima, N.; Clim, A.; Pinzariu, A.C.; Serban, D.N.; Serban, I.L. The Impact of Angiotensin-Converting Enzyme-2/Angiotensin 1-7 Axis in Establishing Severe COVID-19 Consequences. *Pharmaceutics* 2022, 14, 1906. https://doi.org/10.3390/pharmaceutics14091906

Academic Editors: Jesus Perez-Gil, Maria Nowakowska, Radu Iliescu and Ionut Tudorancea

Received: 31 July 2022
Accepted: 3 September 2022
Published: 8 September 2022

Publisher's Note: MDPI stays neutral with regard to jurisdictional claims in published maps and institutional affiliations.

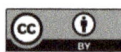

Copyright: © 2022 by the authors. Licensee MDPI, Basel, Switzerland. This article is an open access article distributed under the terms and conditions of the Creative Commons Attribution (CC BY) license (https://creativecommons.org/licenses/by/4.0/).

1. Introduction

Angiotensin-converting enzyme-2 (ACE2), a type I transmembrane protein expressed in many organs such as the heart, kidneys, lungs (type II alveolar cell), and intestine, plays a central role in the pathology of COVID-19 infection [1]. As it was in the case of SARS-CoV, the coupling of the virus molecule to the ACE2 receptor leads to fusion and downregulation [2,3]. Angiotensin-converting enzyme (ACE) and ACE2 are involved in the function regulation of several organs, metabolic condition, and, ultimately, the renin-angiotensin-aldosterone system (RAAS). Currently, this axis is described as two closely interlocking components: a deleterious arm—ACE—and a protective arm—ACE2 [4]. Despite the beneficial side of ACE2, a higher propensity for severe forms of infection has been previously assigned to higher levels of circulating ACE2 [5]. The vast majority of the effects precipitated by COVID-19 infection on key peripheral organs are linked to derangement of the ACE2/ACE axis. There is an ever-growing number of studies focused on observing the impact of the infection outside the lung. Additionally, the considerable amount of medical records allows for a thorough analysis of risk factors.

In this review, we aim to shed light on the molecular mechanisms underlying the tremendous consequences of COVID-19 infection, while keeping the RAAS at the heart of the discussion.

2. RAAS—The Classical View

The classical view of the renin-angiotensin-aldosterone system considers three peptides whose names comprise the acronym RAA axis. Angiotensinogen is converted to angiotensin I by renin, then further to Ang II by ACE.

Conventionally, the receptors angiotensin II binds to are only angiotensin receptor (AT) type-1 (AT1-R) and AT2-R. There have been other subtypes reported, such as AT3-R and AT4-R; however, the former has not been assigned a gene, so its existence is uncertain, while the latter is part of the AT4-R/Ang IV yet poses no affinity towards Ang II or its analogues (Figure 1) [6].

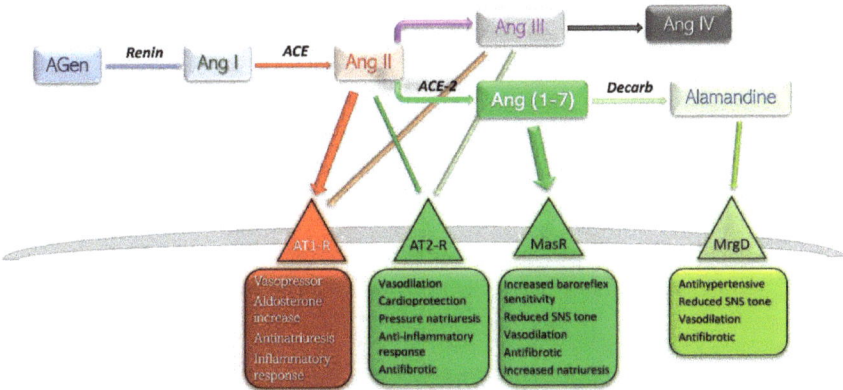

Figure 1. Schematic representation of RAAS components, their main receptors, and main actions. Deleterious side is shown in red-rimmed boxes; protective side is shown in green-rimmed boxes. Abbreviations: Agen, angiotensinogen; Ang, angiotensin; ACE, angiotensin-converting enzyme; Decarb, unspecified decarboxylases; MasR, Mas receptor pathway; MrgD, Mas-related G protein coupled receptor; AT, angiotensin receptor.

Currently, RAAS is viewed as a balance between, on one side, the detrimental actions of Ang II—AT1-R, and, on the other side, the protective effects of Ang II—AT2-R, Ang (1-7)—Mas receptor pathway, and Alamandine—Mas-related G protein receptor pathway. Stimulation of AT1-R subtype by the main peptide driver of RAAS—Ang II—leads to vasoconstriction, antinatriuresis, aldosterone level increase, sympathetic nervous system upregulation, and inflammation-mediated organ damage. Stimulation of AT2-R is generally considered to yield opposite effects, and is therefore protective [6]. The effects mediated by Ang (1-7)—MasR and Alamandine—MrgD are thoroughly discussed further in this text.

The degree of independence between the AT1 and AT2 receptors is highlighted by in vivo consequences after angiotensin-receptor blockers (ARB) administration [7]. Selective blockade of AT1-R would lead to a proportionally higher quantity of substrate binding to the remaining substrate, AT2-R. Furthermore, blockade of AT1-R at renal level results in increased levels of circulating renin and therefore higher levels of circulating Ang II, which would exhibit its protective effects on the only free receptors, AT2. Several studies have reported dramatically increased effects of AT2-R selective stimulation in the presence of small-dose ARB, which may be explained by a higher constitutive expression of AT1-R compared to AT2-R [8–10].

Metabolism end-products of Ang are Ang III and Ang IV. The former has a half-life five times lower in plasma than Ang II, and the latter exhibits its effects largely at the central level, with very low influence on peripheral AT1/2 subtypes [11]. For these reasons, Ang III and Ang IV contribute only slightly to the whole array of effects of Ang II.

3. RAAS—The Alternative Pathway

A new involvement in blood pressure control was unveiled in the early 2000s [12,13]. In this axis, Ang II is converted to Ang (1-7) by the catalytic activity of the then novel discovery, ACE2. The ACE–Ang II–AT1-R axis hyperactivation commonly leads to deleterious effects such as vasoconstriction, inflammation, endothelial dysfunction, thrombosis, and the well-established pro-hypertensive profile; the other, ACE2–Ang (1-7)–MasR typically reverts the forementioned effects. Ang (1-7) is found at a rather pseudo-stationary concentration state. There are at least three enzymes which aid in synthesis of Ang (1-7), and the reaction with the highest rate is different among the peripheral organs [14] (Figure 2).

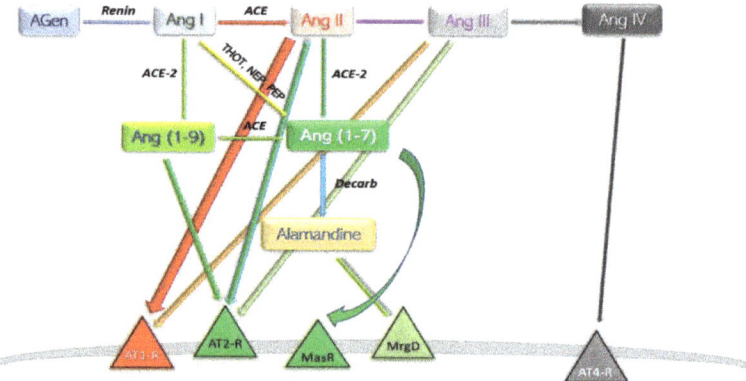

Figure 2. Schematic depiction of the modern view ACE2 axis and its products. AGen, angiotensinogen; Ang, angiotensin; ACE, angiotensin-converting enzyme; Decarb, unspecified aspartate decarboxylases; THOT, thimet oligopeptidase; NEP, neutral endopeptidase; PEP, prolyl endopeptidase; MasR, Mas axis; MrgD, Mas-related G protein receptor; AT–R, angiotensin receptor subtype.

3.1. ACE2 Enzyme

Following the efforts of discovering "ACE-like enzymes" in Drosophila melanogaster, mammalian homologue of ACE has been cloned and named "angiotensin-converting enzyme 2" (ACE2) [12,13,15]. ACE2 is an extracellular transmembrane protein expressed more restrictively to the surface of specific tissues including heart, kidney, endothelium, and testis [13]. Like ACE, it can be cleaved from the cell surface, resulting in the soluble form sACE2 [16]. Despite exhibiting considerable similarity and identity to human ACE, ACE2 functions exclusively as a carboxypeptidase, cleaving only the C-terminal residue from Ang I, yielding Ang (1-9) and from Ang II, likewise yielding Ang (1-7). Regardless, both the structures of ACE2 and ACE display a zinc-binding motif; typical angiotensin-converting enzyme inhibitors (ACEI) do not return any inhibition on ACE2 activity [12]. Arguably, inhibitors designed to act on C-terminal dipeptide-releasing enzymes—ACE—do not bind efficiently to C-terminal cleaving enzymes—ACE2.

3.2. SARS-CoV-2 and Its Receptor, ACE2

A full-fledged crisis emerged as the severe acute respiratory syndrome virus 2 (SARS-CoV-2) pandemics took over in late 2019. Most coronaviruses determine moderate enteric and pulmonary distress through the establishment of a proinflammatory profile [17]. SARS-Cov-2 belongs to the genus Betacoronavirus, but unlike the common coronaviruses, precipitates serious respiratory dysfunction [18,19]. ACE2 behaves as a receptor for SARS-CoV-2, and once the complex is formed, it is immediately internalized [20,21]. Surface expression of ACE2 is therefore diminished through consumption; circulating serum levels—sACE2—may also decrease, accounting for an absolute decrease in shedding. A decline in ACE2 levels will most probably be denoted by an alteration in synthesis of both Ang (1-9) and

Ang (1-7). Furthermore, degradation of the hypertensive components of RAAS may be impeded by the low levels of enzyme ACE2. Therefore, a disequilibrium throughout the entire RAA axis is expected. While Ang (1-9) exhibits only few of the characteristics SARS-CoV-2 interferes with, Ang (1-7) is the most important substrate to account for the extensive effects of the infection.

3.3. Angiotensin (1-9)

Ang (1-9) is considered an intermediate product. The production step is catalysed by ACE-2, while consumption is catalysed by ACE. Ang (1-9) should exhibit in vivo a pseudo-stationary concentration; the absolute value of concentration at a specific time is directly determined by—amongst other factors—the ratio of the enzymatic activities of ACE-2 and ACE. Any alteration in ACE-2 activity would therefore yield significant effects on a systemic scale. The first direct receptor-mediated effect turned out to be the antihypertrophic effect mediated by AT2-R, independent of MasR pathway manipulation [22].

Infusion of Ang (1-9) in hypertensive elevated Ang II level rats resulted in significant blood pressure drop and circulating Ang II level reduction. A co-infusion experiment aimed to disclose the receptor for Ang (1-9) proved that MasR antagonist did not affect the beneficial properties of Ang (1-9), while AT2-R antagonist completely reversed the effects [22]. Controversial claims regarding either a possible interaction of Ang (1-9) with AT1-R, or in vivo transformation of this peptide to Ang II, were advanced in an attempt to explain the in vivo arterial pro-thrombotic activity exhibited by Ang (1-9) in rats [23,24]. To date, there are no reports of an enzyme to aid in conversion of Ang (1-9) to Ang II, nor a quantified affinity towards receptor subtypes other than AT2-R angiotensin. Extracellular signal-regulated kinase (ERK)1/2 pathway downregulation seems to be the key mechanism involved in the antifibrotic and antihypertrophic properties exhibited through AT2-R stimulation [25].

3.4. Angiotensin (1-7)

Angiotensin (1-7) is the most potent product of the protective arm of RAAS. Synthesis can take place three ways: (a) directly and most efficient, from Ang II by catalytic action of ACE2 [26]; (b) directly, from Ang I, catalysed by thimet oligopeptidase (THOT), neutral endopeptidase (NEP), and prolyl endopeptidase (PEP) [27,28]; and (c) through an intermediary product Ang (1-9), and therefore with a slow reaction speed, by means of ACE2 then ACE [29]. Degradation of Ang (1-7) takes place by parallel first-order kinetic reactions; decarboxylation yields a novel compound—Alamandine—by a not currently individualised enzyme. Interaction of alamandine with Mas-related G protein-coupled receptor (MrgD) explained some of the previously noted effects of Ang (1-7) which could not be assigned to Mas axis [30].

3.4.1. Intracellular Signalling Pathways Employed by Angiotensin (1-7)

The majority of the effects generated by this heptapeptide are mediated by the MasR pathway. Downstream activation leads to Akt phosphorylation, upregulation of inducible nitric oxide synthases, and intracellular cyclic guanosine monophosphate (GMP) increase.

Besides the classical MasR pathway, Ang (1-7) mediates some of its cardioprotective effects by behaving as a beta-arrestin recruiter. Agonistic action at the active site of AT1-R leads to recruitment of beta1/2 arrestins, intracellular molecules which effectively block the active site in an irreversible manner. AT1-R engagement by Ang (1-7) leads ultimately to a transient activation of ERK1/2 axis, displaying a cardioprotective profile [31]. The affinity towards receptors other than MasR was also independently demonstrated by using human kidney (HK-2) cells [32]. Effects of low-concentration MasR agonist were not influenced by subsequent MasR blockade, but reversed by AT2 and AT1-R blockade, which owes a degree of affinity of Ang (1-7) to both receptors (Figure 3).

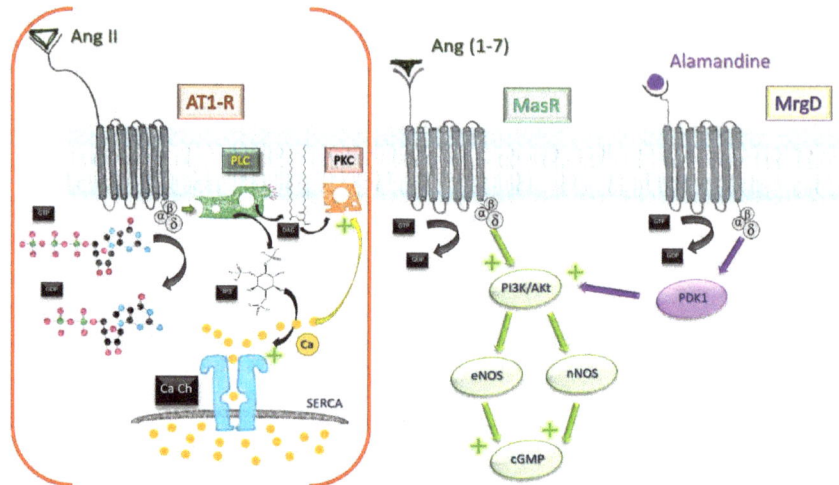

Figure 3. Comparative mechanisms of Ang II and Ang (1-7). Ang, angiotensin; MrgD, Mas-related G protein receptor D; AT1-R, angiotensin receptor type I; GTP, guanosine triphosphate; GDP, guanosine diphosphate; PLC, phospholipase C; PKC, protein kinase C; DAG, diacylglycerol; IP3, triphosphate inositol; Ca Ch, Calcium channel of smooth endoplasmic reticulum; eNOS, endothelial nitric oxide synthase; nNOS, neuronal; PI3K/Akt pathway; PDK1, phosphoinositide-dependent protein kinase 1.

Influence on Metabolism

Activation of Glycogen Synthase Kinase-3 beta (GSK3β), a crucial insulin mediator, may be Akt-dependent or direct; nevertheless, metabolic effects should be expected after manipulation of Ang (1-7), and indeed, oral administration of coated peptide attenuates hyperglycaemia in type 2 diabetes mellitus rodents showing impaired insulin sensitivity [33,34]. While GSK3β further downstream controls glycogen synthesis, phosphorylation of Akt Substrate-160 (AS160) by Akt is required for Glucose Transporter Type-4 translocation to occur. GSK3β and AS160 synergically inhibit phosphorylation of the inhibitory site at Insulin Receptor Substrate 1.

ACE2 knockout mice showed reduced concentration of tryptophan and other large amino acids in blood (valine, threonine, and tyrosine) [35]. Histologically, the mice displayed diffuse mucosal inflammation and altered intestinal microbiota. Inflammatory susceptibility in ACE2-deficient subjects was remedied by supplying only tryptophan, which may indicate a benefit in a tryptophan rich diet in COVID patients. Along with the current knowledge regarding blood sugar levels and microbiota, insulin resistance and impaired glucose homeostasis can be partially explained by an imbalance of ACE forms [36].

Oxidative Stress

Nicotinamide adenine dinucleotide phosphate (NADPH) inhibition leads to reduced oxidative stress by inhibiting the detrimental activity of inducible nitric oxide (NO) synthase [37]. ACE2 knockout display hypertensive phenotypes aggravated by endothelial dysfunction, proved by the worse outcome induced by diabetes- and shock-induced kidney injury, viral lung injury, and chronic liver injury [38]. The unifying characteristic among these models is an increase in oxidative stress in ACE2 knockout male mice [39,40].

Arterial Blood Pressure

Vascular smooth muscle tone may be modulated either directly—as determined by upregulation of endothelial and neuronal NO synthase, subsequent cyclic GMP rise and vasodilation—or indirectly. Ang 1-7 treatment leads to normalisation of surface expression of the proteins Tumor Necrosis Factor (TNF)-Alpha Converting Enzyme (TACE) and Sodium Hydrogen Exchanger-3 (NHE3) in proximal renal tubule cells [41]. TACE is responsible for surface ACE-2 shedding; the high levels expressed in hypertension only compound the problem regarding low activity of Ang 1-7 [42]. NHE3 is a key transporter in proximal renal tubule cells; upregulation leads to increased reabsorption and drop in diuresis [43]. The reactive oxidative species (ROS) and NO generation in genetic deletion of ACE2 enabled researchers to observe the direct effect of Ang (1-7), and only slight but consistent elevation of blood pressure was noted [39]. Results are, however, discordant among different genetic mouse strains [44]. Vascular dysfunction—loss of the vessel ability to modulate local tone—only reinforces the previously noted consistently increased vascular tone [41].

Apoptosis

Mitogen-activated protein kinase pathway and nuclear factor kappa-light-chain-enhancer of activated B cells (NF-kB) transcription factor are both toned down in vascular smooth muscle cells, endothelium, and proximal tubule in kidney after infusion of the heptapeptide [45,46], resulting in a lesser inflammatory response, reduced cell death, reduced fibrosis, and satisfactory preservation of organ function. Finally, stimulation of MrgD by alamandine may account for the effects observed in triple blockade (MasR, AT1, AT2-R). Through phosphoinositide-dependent protein kinase 1 (PDK1), it mediates phosphorylation and activation of Akt, which downstream will activate inducible NO synthases. Figure 4 sums up the most important paths Ang (1-7) acts.

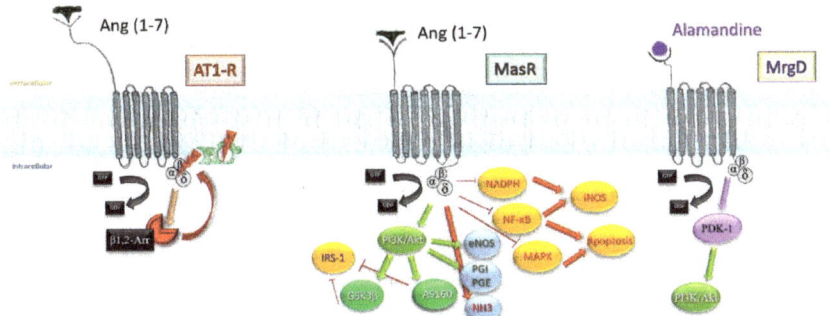

Figure 4. An extensive scheme displaying the mechanisms Ang (1-7) influences on an intracellular level. β-arr1/2, β-arrestins; GSK3β, glycogen synthase kinase 3β; AS160, Akt substrate 160; IRS-1, insulin receptor substrate 1; PGI, PGE, prostaglandins; NHE3, sodium hydrogen exchanger 3; NF-KB, nuclear transcription factor; iNOS, inducible nitrous oxide synthase; MAPK, mithogen-activated protein kinase; NADPH, nicotin-amide-diphospho-hydrogenase.

3.4.2. Effects Mediated by Angiotensin (1-7) in Specific Organs

In order to assess the effects mediated by Ang (1-7) in an individual setting, several strategies have been employed to manipulate either the substrate or the receptor activities: pharmacological concentration alterations of circulating Ang (1-7), genetically modified expression of ACE2, and MasR. Significantly involved in the Ang (1-7)/MasR axis due to the high local Mas expression, the brain exhibits both local and systemic effects in response to manipulation of this axis.

Brain

Metabolism of the heptapeptide closely resembles the description in Figure 2. All components of RAS described above have been determined in brain tissue; however, not every compartment exhibits all of them, nor has any neuron type been identified to produce all those substances [47]. Despite that, Ang (1-7) presence has only been selectively demonstrated; ACE2 is present through every single brain compartment, mainly in neurons rather than glia cells [48]. MasR was identified in certain compartments mostly—but not exclusively—related to cardiovascular control: nucleus tract solitary (NTS), rostral and caudal ventrolateral medulla (RVLM, CVLM), paraventricular nucleus (PVN), and supraoptic nucleus (SON) [49].

Improved modulation of baroreflex by enhancing the bradycardic component, cardiac autonomic balance regaining, and renal sympathetic tone control restoration stand as explanation for the experiment in which long-term stimulation of Ang (1-7) axis leads to significant drop in hypertensive response to Aldosterone-NaCl artificial infusions or high-salt regime [50,51]. Aldosterone-NaCl treatment mimics the effect of Ang II systemically, while also downregulating any intrinsic renin or Ang II secretion. Deoxycorticosterone acetate (DOCA)-salt hypertension is predominantly characterized by upregulated sympathetic activity. Mas knockout mice (equivalent to ACE imbalanced profile) displayed—besides impaired baroreflex and aberrant renal sympathetic tone activity rise—blunted Jarisch-Bezold and chemoreceptor reflexes, with the entire neural network for blood pressure control being influenced [52].

The baroreflex response is the most intricate of all previously mentioned cardiovascular mechanisms. ACE inhibition led to improvement of bradycardic component in normotensive and spontaneous hypertensive rats (SHR). Inhibition of ACE2 axis by infusion of A-779 (an antagonist of Ang (1-7)) led to a significantly depressed sensitivity in normotensive, yet to a mild, almost insignificant attenuation of baroreflex in SHR, which comes to emphasize the imbalance between the two Angiotensin axis in the hypertensive subjects [53]. Infusion of A-779 in ACE inhibitor-treated SHR subjects promptly reverted the beneficial effects [54]. The favourable outcome met by ACEI treatment was most likely exhibited through Ang (1-7). Increased levels of Ang (1-7) at NTS—a key cardiovascular reflex command centre—and signalling through Phosphoinositide 3-kinase (PI3K) pathway may be responsible [55].

Fructose-fed rats treated with intracerebroventricular high-dose Ang (1-7) displayed protective (High-density lipoprotein) HDL-Cholesterol values, normal glucose tolerance, and normal levels of insulin. The peripheral cardioprotective and metabolic effects of central administration of Ang (1-7) were mediated via shifting Ang II/ACE2 equilibrium and further consequences on NO production rise (neuronal NOS activation via Mas axis) [56,57].

Emotional stress and anxiety-like syndromes were noted in Mas-deficient animals [58]. Chronic intracerebroventricular infusion of Ang (1-7) proved effective in reducing both anxiety- and depression-like syndromes [59]. Increase in ACE2 activity by use of ACEI showed a mood improvement in depression-suffering hypertensive patients [60]. The emotional response to stress can therefore be improved by administering ACEI class drugs, discontinuation of which would be deeply unwise from perspectives of both cardiovascular risk and cerebral involvement. Further benefit comes from the modulation of cardiovascular response evoked by acute emotional stress. Microinjections of Ang (1-7) into the basolateral amygdala—an area of the limbic system—lead to attenuation of pressor reflex in response to acute psychic stress [61].

Cardiac Direct Involvement

Coronary vessels seem to be favourably responsive at nanomolar order of concentration, with higher concentrations exhibiting no or constrictive effect [62].

Cardiomyocytes acutely exposed to Ang (1-7) only display a slight elevation in NO release by activation of endothelial and neuronal nitric oxide synthase (eNOS, nNOS) [63]; chronic exposure leads to significant effects on calcium-handling proteins, with increased expression of Sarcoendoplasmic Reticulum Calcium ATPase-2 (SERCA2), higher Calcium (Ca) transient amplitude and faster Ca uptake. This may explain the beneficial effects of ACE2 axis stimulation in chronic heart failure subjects [64].

Identification of Ang (1-7) and Mas axis in sinoatrial node provides the morphopathological fundamentals for the observed biphasic effect (an excessively high local peptide concentration worsened the prognosis) in administration of different concentration of Ang (1-7), only one order of magnitude apart [65,66]. Long-term overproduction of Ang (1-7) has proved to reduce cardiac fibrosis in many studies, reducing oxidative stress, autophagy prevention, and reducing mitogen-activated fibroblast proliferation [67,68]. The main axis involved are Mas-R, Insulin-like Growth Factor-1 Receptor (IGF1R)/PI3K/Akt, and alteration of mitogenic prostaglandin profile [69].

Contradicting its expected cardioprotective effects, overexpression of human ACE2 in mouse heart lead to ventricular tachycardia and sudden death [70]. An explanation may arise from the role of apelin, a peptide involved in a variety of cardiovascular pathological processes. Apelin serves as substrate for ACE2 and as a biomarker in cardiovascular diseases including coronary artery disease, stroke, ischemic heart disease, and infarction [71]. The lower the level of apelin, the worse the prognosis in those subjects. Manipulation of ACE axis towards a deep imbalance in favour of ACE2/Ang (1-7)/MasR may, therefore, prove detrimental in already fragile COVID patients.

Kidney

Inside the kidney water regulation network, Ang (1-7) and antidiuretic hormone (AVP) are involved in a very delicate balance. The effects of Ang 1-7 at central level may not parallel the ones on a peripheral level.

Ang (1-7) effects are distinct among different brain areas. Even in the same cerebral structure, there may be a whole range of distinctive effects owing to certain physiopathological conditions. As such, infusions in the PVN in rodents exhibit different effects according to the state of the subject involved. Following Ang (1-7) microinjection in a healthy subject, an increase in AVP was demonstrated [72]. However, an inverse relationship was noted between Ang (1-7) concentration and AVP release in haemorrhagic conditions of an ethanol-intoxicated model [57]. The underlying mechanism is the already consistent NO-induced release by Ang (1-7), which in the second study displayed an inhibitory effect on AVP secretion.

Ang (1-7) presents a wide array of effects on kidney function, which are way beyond our target. In almost all instances, perfusion/injection of Ang (1-7) in the microenvironment of the studied kidney (or glomerular portion) resulted either in no effect, or natriuresis/diuresis, antiproteinuric, or rarely Ang II antagonism [27]. Antidiuretic effects were noted in only two instances. Worth mentioning is the possible involvement of receptors other than Mas pathway; antidiuretic effects noticed in healthy normotensive rats could be blocked by pre-treatment with Angiotensin Receptor Blockers (ARB) Losartan—Ang (1-7) may display some affinity towards AT1R [73]. Additionally, antidiuretic effect in inner medullary-collecting tubule cells of water-loaded rats seems to involve V2-AVP receptor [74]. Administering A-779 prior to AVP blunted the water reabsorption; similarly, AVP antagonist forskolin prior to Ang (1-7) resulted in no increase in cyclic Adenosine Monophosphate (cAMP) and in no effect in the collecting tubule cell. Cross-antagonist administration following the inspected substance returned no inhibition; the mechanism underlying AVP/Ang (1-7) and their interconnecting substrate-receptor affinity may rely upon binding with subsequent cross-internalization of complex.

Renal vasculature in vitro exhibited afferent arteriole vasodilation in response to Ang (1-7) [75]. Recent in vivo studies prove the vasodilatory effect, yet also the inverse dependence on the degree of RAAS activation [76]; thus, low sodium intake and co-infusion of Ang II lead to hyperactivity of RAAS in the hypertensive human, which diminishes the beneficial effect of intrarenal infusion of Ang (1-7).

Vascular Actions

Ang (1-7) is endogenously produced by vascular endothelium, and therefore induces endothelium-dependent vasorelaxation. Furthermore, it enhances the vasodilator effect of bradykinin in several vascular beds [77].

Besides the well-known effect of vasodilation, Ang (1-7) exhibits antiproliferative and antithrombotic actions [78,79]. The antiproliferative side is mediated through an increase in prostacyclin (PGI2), which in turn reduced activity of mitogen-activated protein kinase (MAPK) Ang II-stimulated pathway. Neointimal thickness and stenosis reduction in rat stenting model, slowing of the osteogenic transition of vascular smooth muscle cells in calcified specimens, and cardiac fibroblast antiproliferative potential were noted [68,80,81]. The antithrombotic side is mediated by the increase in prostacyclin PGI2 and enhanced release of NO from platelets, both part of the Mas axis [82].

Most of the work around Ang (1-7) has been aimed at understanding its effect on vessels and blood pressure. While Ang II/AT1R is widely distributed in all vascular beds, Ang (1-7)/Mas is specific to certain vascular beds—kidney, lungs, adrenals, brain. In normotensive rats, either short or long-term infusion of Ang (1-7) resulted in increased conductance in the previously mentioned vascular beds. However, a proportional cardiac output increase allowed these subjects to not display any significant blood pressure changes [83].

Many of the vascular effects Ang (1-7) exhibits in vivo are mediated through Mas-R activation, which in turn activates eNOS and enhances NO release. Previously, we noted also the nNO inducting activity of the same Mas-R. Ang (1-7) is also involved in a fine-tuned network involving PI3K/Akt pathway, as demonstrated by the NO levels in Mas-transfected cells and in vivo transcription activation of Forkhead box protein O1 (FOXO1), a well-known negative regulator of Akt cascade [84,85]. The same PI3K/Akt pathway is—peripherally—involved in improvement of insulin sensitivity in fructose-fed rats [33].

In human endothelium, Ang (1-7) counteracts effects mediated by Ang II through a common enzyme, Src homology-2 domain-containing protein tyrosine phosphatase-2 (SHP-2). Antioxidant action occurs by opposing the activation of NADPH oxidase by AT1-R, while anti-inflammatory activity occurs through inhibition of NFκB nuclear factor translocation in nuclear cells and attenuation of Vascular Cell Adhesion Molecule-1 (VCAM-1) expression, otherwise an early marker of endothelial dysfunction [86,87].

Restoration of ACE2 function in stroke-prone spontaneously hypertensive rats (which constitutively present a low ACE2 level) leads to significant stroke risk decrease, lower blood pressure profiles, and improved endothelial function [88–90]. Function restoration and perhaps overshooting the imbalance of ACE axis towards the protective side may yield strongly beneficial therapeutic results.

4. Medium and Long-Term Complications Determined by Infection with SARS-CoV-2

4.1. Brain

Neurological involvement has been recognized in more than 80% of severe cases of SARS-CoV-2 infection [91]. The choroid plexus cells proved to be the sense and relay station for neuroinflammation in the context of SARS-CoV-2 infection [92]. Additionally, persistence of the virus for several months in various anatomic sites other than the lungs has brought the brain into focus [93]. There is a wide range of central nervous system (CNS) severe complications in infected patients, generating five pathological profiles: encephalopathies, inflammatory conditions, ischemic strokes, peripheral disorders, and other miscellaneous neurological impairments [94].

A constant clinical finding which emerges even before the onset of respiratory symptoms is the distress in smell and taste sensations in patients infected with SARS-CoV-2 [95]. A decrease of the sensory input leads to a corresponding decrease in the grey matter of the relay and final cerebral stations [96]. The olfactory system encompasses connections to and from the piriform cortex, hippocampus, parahippocampal gyrus, entorhinal cortex, and orbitofrontal cortex [97]. Therefore, it is sensible to put more effort into analysing the previously mentioned regions from whole brain slices. Significant alteration of any of those components (piriform cortex, hippocampus, parahippocampal gyrus, and orbitofrontal cortex) may indicate a direct effect of the infection while simultaneously reducing the error arising from cerebral degeneration owing to pre-existing conditions.

Computer Tomography (CT) and Magnetic Resonance Imaging (MRI) are the most useful imaging techniques for cerebral tissue. A longitudinal analysis employing images both prior and after infection would reinforce the direct correlation between brain slice aspect and long-term disease consequences [98].

Multimodal brain imaging of 401 patients both before and after infection with SARS-CoV-2 allowed researchers to gain more insight into the long-term effects of mild-to-moderate infection [97]. Case-versus-control analysis of brain slices returned significant longitudinal changes in several olfactory-related areas; among the 10 most significantly altered areas were the amygdala, the hippocampus, and the piriform cortex. An imbalance in the ACE2/ACE axis in the context of SARS-CoV-2 infection, along with important staining in the same mentioned areas for the Mas receptor, may explain the observed longitudinal alteration (persistent relative decrease of function) of the hippocampus, piriform region of the frontal lobe, and the amygdala [49,99].

A critical role of the RAAS is represented by the involvement in learning and memory control; long-term potentiation of limbic structures, particularly the hippocampus and amygdala, is mediated through the Mas axis [100]; the imbalance in the ACE axis will therefore disturb the stress response, learning, and memory through a dual coupled mechanism—organic volume density and function. Indeed, studies have already been advanced regarding COVID-19 infection and mental health [101,102]. Neurocognitive symptoms have been consistently mentioned, such as delirium, chronic attention span worsening, and decreased memory capacity. A key aspect regarding mental health is represented by the social burden the pandemic has brought along [101]; the social aspect in a patient with already altered mental health may be more significant than previously expected.

A worsened stress management, owing to the transformations occurred in the amygdala and hippocampus, will also have peripheral consequences, which will most probably parallel the direct effects of the Ang (1-7) level decrease on specific organs. Cardiovascular response to acute stress has been linked to local concentration of Ang (1-7) in amygdala [61].

Cognitive impairment is a characteristic for post-COVID patients, the older ages exhibiting the most significant difference when compared to uninfected subjects [98]. Recently, a correlation has been established between an increase in the protective arm of the RAA axis and cognitive function and depression attenuation [103,104]. An imbalance of the ACE axis, with the prevalence of the deleterious arm, may account for the overwhelming reports of depression in post-COVID patients [102,105–107].

4.2. Heart

Acute cardiac injury was commonly reported as a complication, and was 13 times more often in Intensive Care Unit (ICU) patients than in non-critical cases [108]. Several studies reported a direct correlation between cardiac Troponin T (TnT)—mirroring acute cardiac injury—and inflammatory profile markers (C-reactive protein CRP, leucocytosis, dimer, and procalcitonin) [109,110]. Anatomopathological analysis of tissue in non-survivors returned macrophage as the key cell owing to the local inflammation [111]. The category of patients with underlying cardiovascular disease (CVD) displayed a higher frequency of elevated TnT levels compared to patients with no history of CVD [109]. The same group of patients recorded a higher risk ratio of major complications—including arrythmias—and a higher infection severity. As such, TnT level could stand as the link between acute cardiac injury and life-threatening arrythmias, two major cardiac complications of COVID-19 infection.

The propensity for cardiac injury in severe forms of SARS-CoV-2 infection has been positively correlated to elevated Troponin I (TnI) levels immediately after hospital admission [112]. In addition, normal TnI levels in the first 24 h after admission are significantly linked to lower mortality [113].

Heart failure—quantified by N-Terminal pro B-type Natriuretic Peptide BNP (NT-proBNP)—was also in a direct relationship with inflammation and injury markers [109,110]. It is not yet clear whether this manifestation is due to pre-existing left ventricular dysfunction or is an acute phenomenon in the context of myocarditis. Apart from ACE2 involvement, lung injury may explain heart failure; drop in functional residual volume results in pulmonary hypertension and acute right heart failure.

Arrhythmias were observed significantly more frequently in patients presenting acute cardiac injury, and the incidence of the two complications were statistically correlated. Up to 44% of patients transferred to ICU displayed cardiac arrhythmia at some point during admission [114]. Although both ventricular and atrial arrhythmias were noted, the former may be the first apparent [115].

4.3. Renal

The pooled incidence of Acute Kidney Injury (AKI) in USA and Europe was 28.6%, and only 5.5% in China, the difference being represented by the definitions used [116]. With increasing severity of the disease, the proportion of AKI cases increases too. Physiopathology of AKI is an interlocking blend of local and systemic inflammation, endothelial injury, activation of coagulation pathways, and RAAS imbalance.

Anatomopathological findings reveal a more severe decline in renal function compared to actual necrotic process in the nephron tubule—characteristic decoupling for septic shock related AKI [117]. Other analysis returned thrombotic microangiopathy besides acute tubular injury and collapsing glomerulopathy [118]. The latter is the first clue in favour of endothelial activation and pro-thrombotic local status. Collapsing glomerulopathy, named, COVID-19 associated nephropathy (COVAN), is most likely explained by the same mechanism underlying HIV-associated nephropathy. The mechanism involved is represented by podocyte injury—reinforced by presence of viral particles inside cells—and filtration membrane disruption with subsequent proteinuria [119].

Endothelial dysfunction plays, again, a key role in pathology. Worth remembering is the association of elevated inflammatory markers with the poor prognosis of COVID-19-infected patients. Micro- and macro-vascular thrombosis in the context of endotheliitis have been thoroughly reported, including in the kidney vascular system [120,121]. Platelet activation, microvascular vasodilation, enhancement of immune cell adhesion (assembly of Neutrophil Extracellular Traps (NETs)), and increased vascular permeability all come to reinforce the pro-thrombotic status of a COVID-19 patient [122]. Patients at high risk of severe COVID-19 present with hypertension or diabetes, which themselves depict chronic endothelial dysfunction; reduction in bioavailability of NO may be a central element in explaining the severe course in these patients.

Sepsis-like injury may be explained by the direct action of inflammatory mediators such as TNF at renal endothelial and tubule cell level [123]. Interferon upregulation by the viral infection may represent the (or one of the) cytokines involved in podocyte injury-related proteinuria [124]. Complement activation also plays a pivotal role in endothelial dysfunction and AKI persistence and progression to fibrosis/chronic kidney disease. Higher levels of anaphylatoxins have been constantly recognized in COVID-19 patients, which led to a greater binding of C5a to its receptor on both endothelial (EC) and tubule epithelial cell [125].

4.4. Vascular

Reports from hospitalized patients revealed an imbalanced and exhausted immune profile, an apparent hyperactivation consistent with "cytokine storm", macrophage activating syndrome, most severe in sickest patients. In these cases, immunoparalysis is characterized by significant drop in Human Leukocyte Antigen (HLA)-DR molecule expression on CD14 monocytes, and CD4 and Natural Killer (NK) cell cytopenia inversely correlated with IL-6 and CRP levels. IL-1β levels were lower than expected for such a tremendous inflammatory response [126].

EC activation occurs as response to IL-6, IL-1 (secondary to IL-6), damage- and pathogen- associated molecular pattern (result of viral-mediated cell death). Activated

ECs exhibit pro-inflammatory gene expression, immune cell adhesion and chemotaxis, increased vascular permeability, and alteration of local thrombotic potential.

Kawasaki-like diseases (KD) coexisting with multisystem inflammatory syndrome in children (MIS-C) were reported in several instances of COVID-19 infection [127,128]. It seems that acute vasculitis in children may progress towards giant coronary artery aneurysms significantly more frequent in COVID-19 affected patients than in the KD patient, pre-COVID-19 era [129].

Pulmonary ECs dysfunction surely represents part of the picture of severe hypoxia and acute distress syndrome by altering the air–blood barrier thickness and permeability. Thrombosis in ECs activation is mediated both by EC secretion of Plasminogen Activator Inhibitor-1, Tissue Factor, von Willebrand factor, and NETs formation. Several reports returned up to 25% incidence of venous thromboembolism, with correlation between thrombotic events and lack of prophylactic anticoagulation [130,131]. Macrovascular thrombosis evidence is brought by a case series of ST-segment elevation myocardial infarction patients, but with no sign of plaque rupture at angiography [132]. EC dysfunction may contribute along the EC activation to the potential for thrombosis; knockout ACE2 rodents demonstrated EC dysfunction, and this has been recently linked to the thrombotic events susceptibility [39,133] (Figure 5).

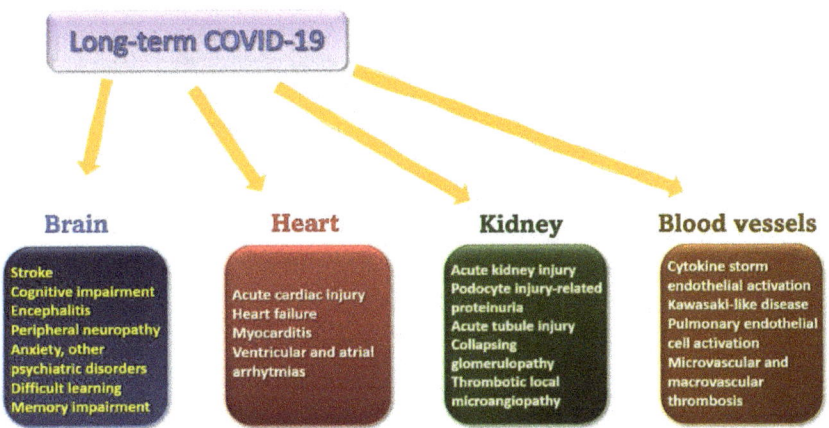

Figure 5. A summary of the previously described consequences of COVID-19 infection.

5. COVID-19 Infection Severity: Proven Risk Factors and Their Link to ACE2 Expression

5.1. Age

COVID-19 infection plot for percentage of critical care cases (out of seropositive individuals) vs age displayed intriguing and oddly inconsistent behaviour. While infection was most mild in children, its severity escalated with age, particularly in the above-80-year-olds group.

It is currently known that children infected with COVID-19 have either no or mild symptoms. Depending on the study design and therapy reporting, asymptomatic patients represented from 16% to 36% [134–136]. Again, these rates are fairly underestimated due to the low detection in the asymptomatic category. No significant sex difference was noted, and no statistically relevant age distribution profile was noted after examining several studies [134–139]. There is conflicting evidence regarding risk factors for contracting the infection: obesity, chronic respiratory conditions, viral co-infection, and immunodepression [140]. Interestingly, though, the highest rate of patients to require critical care was consistently found in the lowest age groups [134,141–143]. Evidence was, however, difficult to find, due to most authors not linking cases which required invasive treatment to age groups. However, rates of both contracting the infection and requiring ICU were systematically reported as lower than in adults [138].

Several articles released in 2020 reporting COVID-19 cases in <19-year-olds have highlighted that young frail patients are at risk for developing severe form of infection [134,142,143]. In all cases, most patients demanding ICU or assisted ventilation were under 1 year-old. Furthermore, the category of patients 1 month-old or less were reported to be most vulnerable [134]. Independent risks under multivariable analysis were age, male sex, respiratory symptoms at presentation, and pre-existing medical conditions. Median interquartile range (IQR) age in patients requiring intensive care versus all admitted cases showed a shift towards lower values, presumably due to the high proportion of under 1 year-old subjects considered in this study.

A sensible theory to explain the peak in severity profile in infants advances the higher serum expression of ACE2 receptors in children owing to the higher predisposition of this age category to infection. Serum concentration of ACE2 in infants <1 year-old were reported to be significantly higher than any other children and adult age group [5]. This was, however, the only statistically significant finding of the authors, other age groups reporting similar quantities of sACE2. Availability of the pathogen's receptor in the bloodstream may explain the higher symptomatic rate and mortality in the <1 year-old age group. It is worth noting the inverse relationship between ACE2 expression and infection intensity, which is particular only to infants. The biphasic role of ACE2 expression in tissues vs plasma has been noted in previous outbursts of SARS infections [144]. Nevertheless, recent work has produced conflicting evidence regarding sACE2 levels and patient prognostic [145,146].

Age-stratified mortality and ICU necessity rates reveal a steep profile with increasing age; considering that most of the infections in children and young adults go unnoticed, the steepness increases even more dramatically towards the elderly group. Many countries unfortunately became understaffed during the first peak of the pandemic in May 2020, so an in-hospital death rate drop in the highest age categories may observed.

Several studies have separately discussed risk factors for contracting the infection, while others have focused on disease progression. However, it was essential to establish a strong link between risk factors for development of disease, and severity or progression of infection once it was attained [140].

5.2. Demographic Factors

Age and male sex proved to be independent risk factors both for contracting the disease and admission to ICU [147]. Intriguingly, though, a study from the same year (2020) highlights a more in-depth method of assessing a patient and predicting individual risk of developing a more severe form of infection [148]. A correlation was advanced between biological aging—which in turn takes into consideration up to 9 biological markers—and severity of disease. Ethnicity as an independent risk factor returned inconclusive results; the lower socioeconomic status may be responsible in this analysis.

5.3. Arterial Hypertension

Hypertension was a constant risk factor for severity and mortality for in-hospital patients. It was determined that hypertension along with high average systolic blood pressure and high systole-diastolic variability (not individually) in COVID-19 patients lead to a darker prognosis compared to patients with low and stable blood pressure [149]. Hypertension alone may not be at fault. Advancing in age results in an imbalance between ACE/Angiotensin II and ACE2/Angiotensin (1-7) enzymes. Indeed, curvilinear association between ACE2 levels and age was noted until 55 years old, beyond which the circulating level of enzyme moderately dropped with advancing age [150]. The imbalance between the Ang II and Ang (1-7) axis is easily reinforced by the baseline pro-inflammatory status consistently present in older ages [151].

Shortly after the beginning of the pandemic, ACE2 was proven to be the principal receptor through which the virus gets inside the cell and then the bloodstream. Antihypertensive drugs belonging to the class of RAA axis inhibitors are commonly known to upregulate levels of ACE2, although evidence is scarce and disparate [152,153]. It may seem counterintuitive to continue medication and enhance the virus's natural ability to penetrate in the body by over-expressing the virus receptor.

Still, patient management revealed that poor blood pressure control, both previously and during admission, lead to high mortality. Adequate hypertension management was still necessary. To support this hypothesis, evidence shows that previous hypertension treatment in COVID-19 patients may indeed lower the in-hospital mortality [154]; this surprising result was recognized after observing the outcome of hypertensive patients with a history of at least 6 months of treatment with ACEI/ARB inhibitors. Their conclusion was not, however, supported by similar subsequent studies, yet practitioners were reassured there was no reason to switch to other medication class or discontinue their patients' current hypertension treatment [155].

5.4. Diabetes

Poor blood sugar control (HbA1C) comprised a significant risk factor for worse infection progression, but not for contracting it. It is demonstrated that diabetes patients present an inadequate immune response to infections: impaired cytokine signalling (impaired IFN-alpha synthesis) and high cellular response to molecular signals (highly sensitised monocytes) [156,157]. Concisely, the diabetes patient is vulnerable to fungi and bacterial infections, and shows an unbalanced response to viral agents. Moreover, as a response to ACE upregulation in different tissues, ACE2 enzyme is overexpressed in serum, liver, and pancreas of the diabetic patient, and may partially explain the higher vulnerability to COVID-19 infection [158].

5.5. Obesity

Poor weight management was the third most incriminated risk factor for mortality. Increased plasma ACE2 were positively correlated with body mass index (BMI) and glycosylated haemoglobin (HbA1C), thus predicting the high risk. A typical obese patient presents with the following cohort of diseases: hypertension, insulin-resistant diabetes, and dyslipidaemia [150]. All these factors considered, weight-related ACE2 level may represent too small a fraction of the whole risk to an obese patient.

5.6. Pregnancy

Out of the infected female patients, a significantly higher percentage of pregnant women required hospitalization compared to non-pregnant subjects [159]. The most likely mechanism for the higher susceptibility is represented by the relative immune suppression characteristic to pregnancy state. Increased infection severity in pregnant subjects positively correlated with higher age, greater weight, diabetes, and hypertension [160,161]. Mortality cases were ascribed to respiratory failure and multiple organ failure [162]. The increased susceptibility for acute respiratory distress syndrome may be linked to the alteration of forced vital capacity during pregnancy [160]. Moreover, a synergistic yet deleterious effect may be caused by the pro-thrombotic state common in COVID-19 patients and the hypercoagulable state in pregnancy; the resulting coagulopathy could represent the foundation of multiple organ failure [163].

6. Long-COVID Organ-Specific Management

In spite of the highly assertive vaccination campaigns, there were tremendous numbers of cases, increasingly higher with each wave of the pandemic. The last wave of the pandemic proved to be the most challenging, owing to the new category of "long-haul" COVID-19 subjects [164]. In some individuals, following the acute phase, the virus resides in specific tissues. Reactivation of the virus, accelerated by a prolonged immune dysfunction and a whole range of other systems degradation, may explain the diversity of long-lasting symptoms [165]. Specific follow-up for COVID-19 patients who developed at least one acute complication should be mandatory. This strategy may allow healthcare providers to identify certain long-term complications—found under the term "long-COVID"—in the early phases, and therefore the patients to benefit sooner from adequate treatment.

6.1. CNS Complications Evaluation

Depression-like syndrome, anxiety, and post-traumatic stress disorder (PTSD) are some of the most encountered psychiatric findings in COVID-19 survivors [107,166]. Severity of long-COVID syndrome is unlikely to be related to severity of the infection [167]. Precise identification of COVID-19 survivors who are prone to psychiatric sequels becomes extremely challenging, owing to the wide array of mechanisms through which COVID-19 affects the CNS and the neurological burden a pre-existing illness may exhibit [168]. Independent risk factors for long-COVID "brain fog" were female sex, severity of respiratory symptoms, and admission to ICU during hospitalization [169]. Indeed, acute lung injury has been demonstrated to yield significant long-term neurological impairment, hypoxemia representing a major mechanism [170]. There is important inconsistency regarding the time interval between when the screening for newly onset psychiatric disorders should take place and the infection symptom onset [166,169,171].

Magnetic resonance imaging of the brain proved a very powerful tool in assessing brain damage associated with COVID-19 infection [98,172]. The longitudinal effects were thoroughly documented, allowing for a deeper understanding of the link between olfactory sense loss and brain impact. It is worth remembering that psychiatric disorders may or may not be mirrored by an organic dysfunction. PTSD, as one of the most severe forms of psychiatric sequels in COVID-19 survivors, proves a model for difficult neurological assessment [168]. Differentiating cognitive complaint as belonging to psychological trauma or neurological insult is key to diagnosis of PTSD; however, the healthcare provider must always be aware that the patient they are examining may be displaying a combination of the forementioned. In addition, patients found in high-risk categories for infection may already display a varying degree of neurological impairment secondary to underlying disease. Even COVID-19 survivors who do not exhibit the whole myriad of symptoms characteristic to PTSD—the condition known as post-traumatic stress-disorder—may display subjective and objective cognitive deficits [173].

Therefore, assessment of psychiatric damage in the context of COVID-19 should occur earlier during treatment, target vulnerable categories of patients, and comprise a wider variety of symptoms, and must lower the threshold for diagnosis [168]. Further management of patients is limited only to pre-existing guidelines, but further COVID-19-related pathology should be suspected and the treatment tailored accordingly.

6.2. Cardiovascular Complications Evaluation and Guidance

Onset or persistence of cardiovascular symptoms weeks after the acute infection phase requires the patient to undergo an extensive battery of tests tailored to the main presumed diagnosis. Physical examination should be focused on the patient's symptoms and signs, and the common cardiovascular parameters (heart rhythm evaluation, respiratory sounds, peripheral oxygen saturation, and check for peripheral oedema) [174]. A detailed clinical history must include the full cardiovascular profile obtained in the acute COVID-19 phase, the infection severity as indicated by any newly arising short-term complications, and the treatments the patients has undergone since first symptom onset. Echocardiogram serves as a very useful tool in assessing any wall motion anomalies, indirectly indicating the status of the coronary vessel network.

New or persistent infectious myocardial involvement can be assessed through transthoracic echocardiography (TTE) or more advanced techniques such as cardiac magnetic resonance imaging (CMR) and positron emission tomography (PET) [175,176]. COVID-19 myocarditis treatment strategies involving steroid drugs, purified immunoglobulins, or antiviral therapy have yielded inconclusive results; newer protocols only recommend adapting previous strategies of treatment for viral myocarditis [177,178].

Life-threatening arrhythmias have been significantly correlated to age, basal heart rate, and antiviral therapy [179]. Atrial fibrillation is considered a significant occurrence in the acute phase of infections; new-onset arrhythmias are less encountered in the medium and long-term phases [180]. Drug–drug interactions explain the necessity of a thorough history regarding treatment directly targeted at COVID-19 infection [181]. Prolongation of QT corrected interval (QTc) through repeated electrocardiographic (ECG) recordings may help in identifying patients at risk for developing life-threatening arrhythmias [171,174,179].

Elevated concentration of N-terminal pro-B-type natriuretic peptide in a dyspnoeic post-acute COVID-19 patient may justify the requirement for TTE imaging [182,183]. A diagnosis of heart failure should be further managed according to the already existing guidelines [171]. Despite previous concerns regarding use of ACEI and possibly increased susceptibility of virus cell entry, current protocols encourage continuation of pre-existing treatment [184]. Echocardiography may view any abnormality in pulmonary hemodynamic, therefore predicting the course of acquired lung disease; integration of pulmonary status, right ventricle size and function, left ventricle function, and any valvular abnormality provide a more accurate image of cardiovascular and lung condition [185].

The increased risk for thrombotic events in the context of recent COVID-19 infection may be reversed by administering standard prophylactic anticoagulation: 40 mg enoxaparin daily [186]. Any higher dose did not yield a significant benefit regarding thrombotic versus haemorrhagic event occurrence in an inpatient setting. Outpatient pharmacological prophylaxis has been proposed, and guidelines provide consistent recommendations; severe cases of COVID-19 without any thromboembolic risk factor may benefit from extended anticoagulation, up to 6 months [174,187].

6.3. COVID-19-Related Chronic Kidney Disease Predictors

Acute kidney injury and chronic kidney disease have previously demonstrated a reciprocal correlation, one serving as a major risk factor for the development of the other [188]. Similarly, the relationship between COVID-19 severity and CKD course is, most probably, bidirectional [189]. At the cellular level, CKD is characterized by chronic inflammation, fibrosis, abnormal apoptosis rates, hypoxia, and vascular dysfunction, all processes which have been linked to medium-term consequences of COVID-19 [117,118,120,123,125]. The extent of decline in renal function directly determined by the amplitude of glomerular filtration rate drop during the AKI episode, the balance of regenerative and destructive processes, and, nonetheless, the pre-existing grade of CKD [190,191]. The risk for progression of CKD was evident even in COVID-19 patients who did not require hospitalization; expectedly, risk was highest among the admissions to critical care unit [192]. Oxygen therapy requirement in ICU is not, however, an entirely accurate predictor for rapidly worsening kidney function [193].

Inconsistency in reports regarding long-term kidney damage due to COVID-19 infection may be linked to an inconsistent protocol for CKD staging [194]. Overestimation of kidney damage was presumably attributed to an inadequate diagnostic procedure in the context of late-phase COVID-19 survivors [166,194]. Renal outcome in long-COVID patients should be compared with similar age-group kidney function, but also with CKD prevalence in general population. Proteinuria should be a key diagnostic criterion for COVID-19-related CKD, owing to the age-adapted definition of CKD, and the high frequency proteinuria is reported in COVID-19 patients [195]. These would allow for better identification of subjects at high-risk of rapid worsening renal function and could facilitate adequate medical care in the likelihood of increasing demand for intermittent dialysis [196].

7. Conclusions

SARS-CoV-2 is a currently running search for optimal management both for sick patients and for subjects who have contracted the disease. Renin-angiotensin-aldosterone system control an overwhelming range of processes at the cellular level. RAAS equilibrium disturbance is determined by the downregulation of ACE2 expression in the context of

COVID-19 infection. The diversity and multitude of local effects controlled by this same axis comes to reinforce the strong connection between ACE2 alteration and organ-specific consequences of the disease. The brain, a central compartment exhibiting significant expression of the ACE2/Ang 1-7 axis, displays both local and central relay-controlled mechanisms. The cardiovascular and renal late manifestations of the disease are therefore also determined by a local and the central relay mechanism. There is an intricate network between these organs, and disruption of one will surely produce an echo in all others. Furthermore, there is rapidly emerging evidence concerning persistent or new-onset symptoms several months after COVID-19 infection was diagnosed. Knowledge regarding SARS-CoV-2 target organs and specific damage related to the infection, should enable healthcare providers to assess medical profile of long-COVID patients more precisely and promptly.

More refined protocols for diagnosis of long-COVID target-organ sequels should be elaborated. Brain damage secondary to pre-existing chronic diseases may sharply interfere with cerebral sequels related to long-COVID. Renal damage assessment should include at least one criterion to differentiate from function collapse related to aging—that is, proteinuria. Cardiovascular state evaluation should be thoroughly performed in high-risk categories of patients, in order to easily identify the mechanism for a potentially serious complication. The physician should obtain an anamnesis regarding in-hospital disease course, current and previously administered medication, should pay attention to subjective complaints of the patient, and shall promptly perform an electrocardiogram and echocardiogram.

The protective arm of RAAS influences a myriad of molecular level mechanisms: NO balance influencing, oxidative stress shielding, Na transmembrane transport, inflammation inhibition, apoptosis control and many more. These statements should encourage the scientists into developing more targeted treatments for COVID-19 survivors; we hope that new strategies of upregulating the levels of ACE2/Ang 1-7/MasR axis could prevent instalment of severe long-term consequences of the virus, or at least improve the quality of life for the already diagnosed patients several months post-infection. More research is required in order to clarify whether the ACE2 axis is the only fundamental cornerstone of long-term COVID-19 effects, yet it is nevertheless representative of the pathophysiology of the infection.

Author Contributions: Conceptualization, M.A.M., N.D. and D.N.S.; methodology, A.C. and A.C.P.; software, C.T.C.; validation, N.D., I.L.S. and M.A.M.; formal analysis, D.N.S.; investigation, N.D., D.M.T., A.C.P. and I.L.S.; resources, C.T.C.; data curation, M.A.M.; writing—original draft preparation, M.A.M., D.M.T. and I.L.S.; writing—review and editing, C.T.C.; visualization, A.C.; supervision, D.N.S.; project administration, M.A.M.; funding acquisition, N.D. All authors have read and agreed to the published version of the manuscript.

Funding: This research received no external funding.

Institutional Review Board Statement: Not applicable.

Informed Consent Statement: Not applicable.

Data Availability Statement: Not applicable.

Conflicts of Interest: The authors declare no conflict of interest.

References

1. Hikmet, F.; Mear, L.; Edvinsson, A.; Micke, P.; Uhlen, M.; Lindskog, C. The protein expression profile of ACE2 in human tissues. *Mol. Syst. Biol.* **2020**, *16*, e9610. [CrossRef] [PubMed]
2. Freitas, F.C.; Ferreira, P.H.B.; Favaro, D.C.; Oliveira, R.J. Shedding Light on the Inhibitory Mechanisms of SARS-CoV-1/CoV-2 Spike Proteins by ACE2-Designed Peptides. *J. Chem. Inf. Model.* **2021**, *61*, 1226–1243. [CrossRef] [PubMed]
3. Mehrabadi, M.E.; Hemmati, R.; Tashakor, A.; Homaei, A.; Yousefzadeh, M.; Hemati, K.; Hosseinkhani, S. Induced dysregulation of ACE2 by SARS-CoV-2 plays a key role in COVID-19 severity. *Biomed. Pharmacoter.* **2021**, *137*. [CrossRef]
4. Ahmadi Badi, S.; Tarashi, S.; Fateh, A.; Rohani, P.; Masotti, A.; Siadat, S.D. From the Role of Microbiota in Gut-Lung Axis to SARS-CoV-2 Pathogenesis. *Mediators Inflamm.* **2021**, *2021*, 6611222. [CrossRef]

5. Gu, J.; Yin, J.; Zhang, M.; Li, J.; Wu, Y.; Chen, J.; Miao, H. Study on the Clinical Significance of ACE2 and Its Age-Related Expression. *J. Inflamm. Res.* **2021**, *14*, 2873–2882. [CrossRef] [PubMed]
6. Singh, K.D.; Karnik, S.S. Angiotensin Receptors: Structure, Function, Signaling and Clinical Applications. *J. Cell. Sign.* **2016**, *1*. [CrossRef]
7. Carey, R.M. AT2 Receptors: Potential Therapeutic Targets for Hypertension. *Am. J. Hypertens.* **2017**, *30*, 339–347. [CrossRef]
8. Li, X.C.; Widdop, R.E. AT2 receptor-mediated vasodilatation is unmasked by AT1 receptor blockade in conscious SHR. *Br. J. Pharmacol.* **2004**, *142*, 821–830. [CrossRef]
9. Widdop, R.E.; Matrougui, K.; Levy, B.I.; Henrion, D. AT2 receptor-mediated relaxation is preserved after long-term AT1 receptor blockade. *Hypertension* **2002**, *40*, 516–520. [CrossRef]
10. Siragy, H.M.; de Gasparo, M.; Carey, R.M. Angiotensin type 2 receptor mediates valsartan-induced hypotension in conscious rats. *Hypertension* **2002**, *35*, 1074–1077. [CrossRef]
11. Gammelgaard, I.; Wamberg, S.; Bie, P. Systemic effects of angiotensin III in conscious dogs during acute double blockade of the renin-angiotensin-aldosterone-system. *Acta Physiol.* **2006**, *188*, 129–138. [CrossRef] [PubMed]
12. Tipnis, S.R.; Hooper, N.M.; Hyde, R.; Karran, E.; Christie, G.; Turner, A.J. A human homolog of angiotensin-converting enzyme. Cloning and functional expression as a captopril-insensitive carboxypeptidase. *J. Biol. Chem.* **2000**, *275*, 33238–33243. [CrossRef] [PubMed]
13. Donoghue, M.; Hsieh, F.; Baronas, E.; Godbout, K.; Gosselin, M.; Stagliano, N.; Donovan, M.; Woolf, B.; Robison, K.; Jeyaseelan, R.; et al. A novel angiotensin-converting enzyme-related carboxypeptidase (ACE2) converts angiotensin I to angiotensin 1-9. *Circ. Res.* **2000**, *87*, E1–E9. [CrossRef] [PubMed]
14. Campbell, D.J.; Zeitz, C.J.; Esler, M.D.; Horowitz, J.D. Evidence against a major role for angiotensin converting enzyme-related carboxypeptidase (ACE2) in angiotensin peptide metabolism in the human coronary circulation. *J. Hypertens.* **2004**, *22*, 1971–1976. [CrossRef]
15. Cornell, M.J.; Williams, T.A.; Lamango, N.S.; Coates, D.; Corvol, P.; Soubrier, F.; Hoheisel, J.; Lehrach, H.; Isaac, R.E. Cloning and Expression of an Evolutionary Conserved Single-domain Angiotensin Converting Enzyme from Drosophila melanogaster. *J. Biol. Chem.* **1995**, *270*, 13613–13619. [CrossRef]
16. Lambert, D.W.; Yarski, M.; Warner, F.J.; Thornhill, P.; Parkin, E.T.; Smith, A.I.; Hooper, N.M.; Turner, A.J. Tumor necrosis factor-alpha convertase (ADAM17) mediates regulated ectodomain shedding of the severe-acute respiratory syndrome-coronavirus (SARS-CoV) receptor, angiotensin-converting enzyme-2 (ACE2). *J. Biol. Chem.* **2005**, *280*, 30113–30119. [CrossRef]
17. Glass, W.G.; Subbarao, K.; Murphy, B.; Murphy, P.M. Mechanisms of host defense following severe acute respiratory syndrome-coronavirus (SARS-CoV) pulmonary infection of mice. *J. Immunol.* **2004**, *173*, 4030–4039. [CrossRef]
18. Kadam, S.B.; Sukhramani, G.S.; Bishnoi, P.; Pable, A.A.; Barvkar, V.T. SARS-CoV-2, the pandemic coronavirus: Molecular and structural insights. *J. Basic Microbiol.* **2021**, *61*, 180–202. [CrossRef]
19. Grasselli, G.; Pesenti, A.; Cecconi, M. Critical Care Utilization for the COVID-19 Outbreak in Lombardy, Italy: Early Experience and Forecast During an Emergency Response. *JAMA* **2020**, *323*, 1545–1546. [CrossRef]
20. Lu, R.; Zhao, X.; Li, J.; Niu, P.; Yang, B.; Wu, H.; Wang, W.; Song, H.; Huang, B.; Zhu, N.; et al. Genomic characterisation and epidemiology of 2019 novel coronavirus: Implications for virus origins and receptor binding. *Lancet* **2020**, *395*, 565–574. [CrossRef]
21. Wan, Y.; Shang, J.; Graham, R.; Baric, R.S.; Li, F. Receptor Recognition by the Novel Coronavirus from Wuhan: An Analysis Based on Decade-Long Structural Studies of SARS Coronavirus. *J. Virol.* **2020**, *94*, e00127-20. [CrossRef] [PubMed]
22. Ocaranza, M.P.; Moya, J.; Barrientos, V.; Alzamora, R.; Hevia, D.; Morales, C.; Pinto, M.; Escudero, N.; García, L.; Novoa, U.; et al. Angiotensin-(1-9) reverses experimental hypertension and cardiovascular damage by inhibition of the angiotensin converting enzyme/Ang II axis. *J. Hypertens.* **2014**, *32*, 771–783. [CrossRef] [PubMed]
23. Kramkowski, K.; Mogielnicki, A.; Leszczynska, A.; Buczko, W. Angiotensin-(1-9), the product of angiotensin I conversion in platelets, enhances arterial thrombosis in rats. *J. Physiol. Pharmacol.* **2010**, *61*, 317–324. [PubMed]
24. Mogielnicki, A.; Kramkowski, K.; Hermanowicz, J.M.; Leszczynska, A.; Przyborowski, K.; Buczko, W. Angiotensin-(1-9) enhances stasis-induced venous thrombosis in the rat because of the impairment of fibrinolysis. *J. Renin Angiotensin Aldosterone Syst.* **2014**, *15*, 13–21. [CrossRef] [PubMed]
25. Calò, L.A.; Schiavo, S.; Davis, P.A.; Pagnin, E.; Mormino, P.; D'Angelo, A.; Pessina, A.C. Angiotensin II signaling via type 2 receptors in a human model of vascular hyporeactivity: Implications for hypertension. *J. Hypertens.* **2010**, *28*, 111–118. [CrossRef] [PubMed]
26. Vickers, C.; Hales, P.; Kaushik, V.; Dick, L.; Gavin, J.; Tang, J.; Godbout, K.; Parsons, T.; Baronas, E.; Hsieh, F. Hydrolysis of Biological Peptides by Human Angiotensin-converting Enzyme-related Carboxypeptidase. *J. Biol. Chem.* **2002**, *277*, 14838–14843. [CrossRef] [PubMed]
27. Santos, R.; Sampaio, W.O.; Alzamora, A.C.; Motta-Santos, D.; Alenina, N.; Bader, M.; Campagnole-Santos, M.J. The ACE2/Angiotensin-(1-7)/MAS Axis of the Renin-Angiotensin System: Focus on Angiotensin-(1-7). *Physiol. Rev.* **2018**, *98*, 505–553. [CrossRef]
28. Chappell, M.C.; Allred, A.J.; Ferrario, C.M. Pathways of angiotensin-(1-7) metabolism in the kidney. *Nephrol. Dial. Transplant.* **2001**, *16*, 22–26. [CrossRef]
29. Rice, G.I.; Thomas, D.A.; Grant, P.J.; Turner, A.J.; Hooper, N.M. Evaluation of angiotensin-converting enzyme (ACE), its homologue ACE2 and neprilysin in angiotensin peptide metabolism. *Biochem. J.* **2004**, *383*, 45–51. [CrossRef]

30. Lautner, R.Q.; Villela, D.C.; Fraga-Silva, R.A.; Silva, N.; Verano-Braga, T.; Costa-Fraga, F.; Jankowski, J.; Jankowski, V.; Sousa, F.; Alzamora, A.; et al. Discovery and characterization of alamandine: A novel component of the renin-angiotensin system. *Circ. Res.* **2013**, *112*, 1104–1111. [CrossRef]
31. Teixeira, L.B.; Parreiras-E-Silva, L.T.; Bruder-Nascimento, T.; Duarte, D.A.; Simões, S.C.; Costa, R.M.; Rodríguez, D.Y.; Ferreira, P.; Silva, C.; Abrao, E.P.; et al. Ang-(1-7) is an endogenous β-arrestin-biased agonist of the AT1 receptor with protective action in cardiac hypertrophy. *Sci. Rep.* **2017**, *7*, 11903. [CrossRef] [PubMed]
32. Patel, S.; Hussain, T. Synergism between Angiotensin receptors ligands: Role of Angiotensin-(1-7) in modulating AT2 R agonist response on nitric oxide in kidney cells. *Pharmacol. Res. Perspect.* **2020**, *8*, e00667. [CrossRef] [PubMed]
33. Muñoz, M.C.; Giani, J.F.; Burghi, V.; Mayer, M.A.; Carranza, A.; Taira, C.A.; Dominici, F.P. The Mas receptor mediates modulation of insulin signaling by angiotensin-(1-7). *Regul. Pept.* **2012**, *177*, 1–11. [CrossRef] [PubMed]
34. Santos, S.H.; Giani, J.F.; Burghi, V.; Miquet, J.G.; Qadri, F.; Braga, J.F.; Todiras, M.; Kotnik, K.; Alenina, N.; Dominici, F.P.; et al. Oral administration of angiotensin-(1-7) ameliorates type 2 diabetes in rats. *J. Mol. Med.* **2014**, *92*, 255–265. [CrossRef]
35. Hashimoto, T.; Perlot, T.; Rehman, A.; Trichereau, J.; Ishiguro, H.; Paolino, M.; Sigl, V.; Hanada, T.; Hanada, R.; Lipinski, S. ACE2 links amino acid malnutrition to microbial ecology and intestinal inflammation. *Nature* **2012**, *487*, 477–481. [CrossRef]
36. Niu, M.J.; Yang, J.K.; Lin, S.S.; Ji, X.J.; Guo, L.M. Loss of angiotensin-converting enzyme 2 leads to impaired glucose homeostasis in mice. *Endocrine* **2008**, *34*, 56–61. [CrossRef]
37. Villalobos, L.A.; San Hipólito-Luengo, Á.; Ramos-González, M.; Cercas, E.; Vallejo, S.; Romero, T.; Carraro, R.; Sanchez-Ferrer, C.F.; Peiro, C. The Angiotensin-(1-7)/Mas Axis Counteracts Angiotensin II-Dependent and -Independent Pro-inflammatory Signaling in Human Vascular Smooth Muscle Cells. *Front. Pharmacol.* **2016**, *7*. [CrossRef]
38. Lovren, F.; Pan, Y.; Quan, A.; Teoh, H.; Wang, G.; Shukla, P.C.; Levitt, K.S.; Oudit, G.Y.; Al-Omran, M.; Stewart, D.J. Angiotensin converting enzyme-2 confers endothelial protection and attenuates atherosclerosis. *Am. J. Physiol. Heart Circ. Physiol.* **2008**, *295*, H1377–H1384. [CrossRef]
39. Rabelo, L.A.; Todiras, M.; Nunes-Souza, V.; Qadri, F.; Szijártó, I.A.; Gollasch, M.; Penninger, J.M.; Bader, M.; Santos, R.A.; Alenina, N. Genetic Deletion of ACE2 Induces Vascular Dysfunction in C57BL/6 Mice: Role of Nitric Oxide Imbalance and Oxidative Stress. *PLoS ONE* **2016**, *11*, e0150255. [CrossRef]
40. Wysocki, J.; Ortiz-Melo, D.I.; Mattocks, N.K.; Xu, K.; Prescott, J.; Evora, K.; Ye, M.; Sparks, M.A.; Haque, S.K.; Batlle, D. ACE2 deficiency increases NADPH-mediated oxidative stress in the kidney. *Physiol. Rep.* **2014**, *2*, e00264. [CrossRef]
41. Shi, Y.; Lo, C.S.; Padda, R.; Abdo, S.; Chenier, I.; Filep, J.G.; Ingelfinger, J.R.; Zhang, S.L.; Chan, J.S.D. Angiotensin-(1–7) prevents systemic hypertension, attenuates oxidative stress and tubulointerstitial fibrosis, and normalizes renal angiotensin-converting enzyme 2 and Mas receptor expression in diabetic mice. *Clin. Sci.* **2015**, *128*, 649–663. [CrossRef] [PubMed]
42. Zamilpa, R.; Chilton, R.J.; Lindsey, M.L. Tumor necrosis factor-alpha–converting enzyme roles in hypertension-induced hypertrophy: Look both ways when crossing the street. *Hypertension* **2009**, *54*, 471–472. [CrossRef] [PubMed]
43. Knepper, M.A.; Brooks, H.L. Regulation of the sodium transporters NHE3, NKCC2 and NCC in the kidney. *Curr. Opin. Nephrol.* **2001**, *10*, 655–659. [CrossRef] [PubMed]
44. Moritani, T.; Iwai, M.; Kanno, H.; Nakaoka, H.; Iwanami, J.; Higaki, T.; Ishii, E.; Horiuchi, M. ACE2 deficiency induced perivascular fibrosis and cardiac hypertrophy during postnatal development in mice. *J. Am. Soc. Hypertens.* **2013**, *7*, 259–266. [CrossRef] [PubMed]
45. Zhang, F.; Ren, X.; Zhao, M.; Zhou, B.; Han, Y. Angiotensin-(1-7) abrogates angiotensin II-induced proliferation, migration and inflammation in VSMCs through inactivation of ROS-mediated PI3K/Akt and MAPK/ERK signaling pathways. *Sci. Rep.* **2016**, *6*, 34621. [CrossRef]
46. Gava, E.; Samad-Zadeh, A.; Zimpelmann, J.; Bahramifarid, N.; Kitten, G.T.; Santos, R.A.; Touyz, R.M.; Burns, K.D. Angiotensin-(1-7) activates a tyrosine phosphatase and inhibits glucose-induced signalling in proximal tubular cells. *Nephrol. Dial. Transplant.* **2009**, *24*, 1766–1773. [CrossRef]
47. von Bohlen und Halbach, O.; Albrecht, D. The CNS renin-angiotensin system. *Cell Tissue Res.* **2006**, *326*, 599–616. [CrossRef]
48. Doobay, M.F.; Talman, L.S.; Obr, T.D.; Tian, X.; Davisson, R.L.; Lazartigues, E. Differential expression of neuronal ACE2 in transgenic mice with overexpression of the brain renin-angiotensin system. *Am. J. Physiol. Regul. Integr. Comp. Physiol.* **2007**, *292*, R373–R381. [CrossRef]
49. Becker, L.K.; Etelvino, G.M.; Walther, T.; Santos, R.A.; Campagnole-Santos, M.J. Immunofluorescence localization of the receptor Mas in cardiovascular-related areas of the rat brain. *Am. J. Physiol. Heart Circ. Physiol.* **2007**, *293*, H1416–H1424. [CrossRef]
50. Xue, B.; Zhang, Z.; Johnson, R.F.; Guo, F.; Hay, M.; Johnson, A.K. Central endogenous angiotensin-(1-7) protects against aldosterone/NaCl-induced hypertension in female rats. *Am. J. Physiol. Heart Circ. Physiol.* **2013**, *305*, H699–H705. [CrossRef]
51. Guimaraes, P.S.; Santiago, N.M.; Xavier, C.H.; Velloso, E.P.; Fontes, M.A.; Santos, R.A.; Campagnole-Santos, M.J. Chronic infusion of angiotensin-(1-7) into the lateral ventricle of the brain attenuates hypertension in DOCA-salt rats. *Am. J. Physiol. Heart Circ. Physiol.* **2012**, *303*, H393–H400. [CrossRef] [PubMed]
52. de Moura, M.M.; dos Santos, R.A.; Campagnole-Santos, M.J.; Todiras, M.; Bader, M.; Alenina, N.; Haibara, A.S. Altered cardiovascular reflexes responses in conscious Angiotensin-(1-7) receptor Mas-knockout mice. *Peptides* **2010**, *31*, 1934–1939. [CrossRef] [PubMed]
53. Heringer-Walther, S.; Batista, E.N.; Walther, T.; Khosla, M.C.; Santos, R.A.; Campagnole-Santos, M.J. Baroreflex improvement in shr after ace inhibition involves angiotensin-(1-7). *Hypertension* **2001**, *37*, 1309–1314. [CrossRef] [PubMed]

54. Britto, R.R.; Santos, R.A.; Fagundes-Moura, C.R.; Khosla, M.C.; Campagnole-Santos, M.J. Role of angiotensin-(1-7) in the modulation of the baroreflex in renovascular hypertensive rats. *Hypertension* **1997**, *30*, 549–556. [CrossRef]
55. Wu, Z.T.; Ren, C.Z.; Yang, Y.H.; Zhang, R.W.; Sun, J.C.; Wang, Y.K.; Su, D.F.; Wang, W.Z. The PI3K signaling-mediated nitric oxide contributes to cardiovascular effects of angiotensin-(1-7) in the nucleus tractus solitarii of rats. *Nitric. Oxide* **2016**, *52*, 56–65. [CrossRef]
56. Guimaraes, P.S.; Oliveira, M.F.; Braga, J.F.; Nadu, A.P.; Schreihofer, A.; Santos, R.A.S.; Campagnole-Santos, M.J. Increasing Angiotensin-(1-7) Levels in the Brain Attenuates Metabolic Syndrome-Related Risks in Fructose-Fed Rats. *Hypertension* **2014**, *63*, 1078–1085. [CrossRef]
57. Whitaker, A.M.; Molina, P.E. Angiotensin (1-7) contributes to nitric oxide tonic inhibition of vasopressin release during hemorrhagic shock in acute ethanol intoxicated rodents. *Life Sci.* **2013**, *93*, 623–629. [CrossRef]
58. Walther, T.; Balschun, D.; Voigt, J.P.; Fink, H.; Zuschratter, W.; Birchmeier, C.; Ganten, D.; Bader, M. Sustained long term potentiation and anxiety in mice lacking the Mas protooncogene. *J. Biol. Chem.* **2013**, *273*, 11867–11873. [CrossRef]
59. Almeida-Santos, A.F.; Kangussu, L.M.; Moreira, F.A.; Santos, R.A.; Aguiar, D.C.; Campagnole-Santos, M.J. Anxiolytic- and antidepressant-like effects of angiotensin-(1-7) in hypertensive transgenic (mRen2)27 rats. *Clin. Sci.* **2016**, *130*, 1247–1255. [CrossRef]
60. Braszko, J.J.; Karwowska-Polecka, W.; Halicka, D.; Gard, P.R. Captopril and Enalapril Improve Cognition and Depressed Mood in Hypertensive Patients. *J. Basic Clin. Physiol. Pharmacol.* **2003**, *14*, 323–343. [CrossRef]
61. Oscar, C.G.; de Figueiredo Muller-Ribeiro, F.C.; de Castro, L.G.; Lima, A.M.; Campagnolo-Santos, M.J.; Santos, R.A.S.; Xavier, C.H.; Fontes, M.A.P. Angiotensin-(1–7) in the basolateral amygdala attenuates the cardiovascular response evoked by acute emotional stress. *Brain Res.* **2015**, *1594*, 183–189. [CrossRef] [PubMed]
62. Souza, A.P.S.; Sobrinho, D.B.S.; Almeida, J.F.Q.; Alves, G.M.M.; Macedo, L.M.; Porto, J.E.; Vêncio, E.F.; Colugnati, D.B.; Santos, R.A.S.; Ferreira, A.J.; et al. Angiotensin II Type 1 receptor blockade restores angiotensin-(1-7)-induced coronary vasodilation in hypertrophic rat hearts. *Clin. Sci.* **2013**, *125*, 449–459. [CrossRef] [PubMed]
63. Costa, M.A.; Lopez Verrilli, M.A.; Gomez, K.A.; Nakagawa, P.; Peña, C.; Arranz, C.; Gironacci, M.M. Angiotensin-(1-7) upregulates cardiac nitric oxide synthase in spontaneously hypertensive rats. *Am. J. Physiol. Heart Circ. Physiol.* **2010**, *299*, H1205–H1211. [CrossRef] [PubMed]
64. Gomes, E.R.M.; Santos, R.A.S.; Guatimosim, S. Angiotensin-(1-7)-Mediated Signaling in Cardiomyocytes. *Int. J. Hypertens.* **2012**, *2012*. [CrossRef] [PubMed]
65. Ferreira, A.J.; Moraes, P.L.; Foureaux, G.; Andrade, A.B.; Santos, R.A.; Almeida, A.P. The angiotensin-(1-7)/Mas receptor axis is expressed in sinoatrial node cells of rats. *J. Histochem. Cytochem.* **2011**, *59*, 761–768. [CrossRef]
66. De Mello, W.C.; Ferrario, C.M.; Jessup, J.A. Beneficial versus harmful effects of Angiotensin (1-7) on impulse propagation and cardiac arrhythmias in the failing heart. *J. Renin Angiotensin Aldosterone Syst.* **2007**, *8*, 74–80. [CrossRef]
67. Lin, L.; Liu, X.; Xu, J.; Weng, L.; Ren, J.F.; Ge, J.; Zou, Y. Mas receptor mediates cardioprotection of angiotensin-(1-7) against Angiotensin II-induced cardiomyocyte autophagy and cardiac remodelling through inhibition of oxidative stress. *J. Cell. Mol. Med.* **2016**, *20*, 48–57. [CrossRef]
68. McCollum, L.T.; Gallagher, P.E.; Tallant, E.A. Angiotensin-(1-7) abrogates mitogen-stimulated proliferation of cardiac fibroblasts. *Peptides* **2012**, *34*, 380–388. [CrossRef]
69. Chang, R.L.; Lin, J.W.; Kuo, W.W.; Hsieh, D.J.; Yeh, Y.L.; Shen, C.Y.; Day, C.H.; Ho, T.J.; Viswanadha, V.P.; Huang, C.Y. Angiotensin-(1-7) attenuated long-term hypoxia-stimulated cardiomyocyte apoptosis by inhibiting HIF-1α nuclear translocation via Mas receptor regulation. *Growth Factors* **2016**, *34*, 11–18. [CrossRef]
70. Donoghue, M.; Wakimoto, H.; Maguire, C.T.; Acton, S.; Hales, P.; Stagliano, N.; Fairchild-Huntress, V.; Xu, J.; Lorenz, J.N.; Kadambi, V. Heart block, ventricular tachycardia, and sudden death in ACE2 transgenic mice with downregulated connexins. *J. Mol. Cell. Cardiol.* **2003**, *35*, 1043–1053. [CrossRef]
71. Wysocka, M.B.; Pietraszek-Gremplewicz, K.; Nowak, D. The Role of Apelin in Cardiovascular Diseases, Obesity and Cancer. *Front. Physiol.* **2018**, *9*, 557. [CrossRef] [PubMed]
72. Schiavone, M.T.; Santos, R.A.; Brosnihan, K.B.; Khosla, M.C.; Ferrario, C.M. Release of vasopressin from the rat hypothalamoneurohypophysial system by angiotensin-(1-7) heptapeptide. *Proc. Natl. Acad. Sci. USA* **1988**, *85*, 4095–4098. [CrossRef] [PubMed]
73. Baracho, N.C.; Simões-e-Silva, A.C.; Khosla, M.C.; Santos, R.A. Effect of selective angiotensin antagonists on the antidiuresis produced by angiotensin-(1-7) in water-loaded rats. *Braz. J. Med. Biol. Res.* **1998**, *31*, 1221–1227. [CrossRef] [PubMed]
74. Magaldi, A.J.; Cesar, K.R.; de Araújo, M.; Simões e Silva, A.C.; Santos, R.A. Angiotensin-(1-7) stimulates water transport in rat inner medullary collecting duct: Evidence for involvement of vasopressin V2 receptors. *Pflugers Arch.* **2003**, *447*, 223–230. [CrossRef]
75. Ren, Y.; Garvin, J.L.; Carretero, O.A. Vasodilator action of angiotensin-(1-7) on isolated rabbit afferent arterioles. *Hypertension* **2002**, *39*, 799–802. [CrossRef]
76. van Twist, D.J.; Houben, A.J.; de Haan, M.W.; Mostard, G.J.; Kroon, A.A.; de Leeuw, P.W. Angiotensin-(1-7)-induced renal vasodilation in hypertensive humans is attenuated by low sodium intake and angiotensin II co-infusion. *Hypertension* **2013**, *62*, 789–793. [CrossRef]

77. Li, P.; Chappell, M.C.; Ferrario, C.M.; Brosnihan, K.B. Angiotensin-(1-7) augments bradykinin-induced vasodilation by competing with ACE and releasing nitric oxide. *Hypertension* **1997**, *29*, 394–400. [CrossRef]
78. Tallant, E.A.; Clark, M.A. Molecular mechanisms of inhibition of vascular growth by angiotensin-(1-7). *Hypertension* **2003**, *42*, 574–579. [CrossRef]
79. Fraga-Silva, R.A.; Costa-Fraga, F.P.; De Sousa, F.B.; Alenina, N.; Bader, M.; Sinisterra, R.D.; Santos, R.A. An orally active formulation of angiotensin-(1-7) produces an antithrombotic effect. *Clinics* **2011**, *66*, 837–841. [CrossRef]
80. Langeveld, B.; van Gilst, W.H.; Tio, R.A.; Zijlstra, F.; Roks, A.J. Angiotensin-(1-7) attenuates neointimal formation after stent implantation in the rat. *Hypertension* **2005**, *45*, 138–141. [CrossRef]
81. Sui, Y.B.; Chang, J.R.; Chen, W.J.; Zhao, L.; Zhang, B.H.; Yu, Y.R.; Tang, C.S.; Yin, X.H.; Qi, Y.F. Angiotensin-(1-7) inhibits vascular calcification in rats. *Peptides* **2013**, *42*, 25–34. [CrossRef] [PubMed]
82. Fang, C.; Stavrou, E.; Schmaier, A.A.; Grobe, N.; Morris, M.; Chen, A.; Nieman, M.T.; Adams, G.N.; LaRusch, G.; Zhou, Y.; et al. Angiotensin 1-7 and Mas decrease thrombosis in Bdkrb2-/- mice by increasing NO and prostacyclin to reduce platelet spreading and glycoprotein VI activation. *Blood* **2013**, *121*, 3023–3032. [CrossRef] [PubMed]
83. Sampaio, W.O.; Nascimento, A.A.S.; Santos, R.A.S. Regulation of Cardiovascular Signaling by Kinins and Products of Similar Converting Enzyme Systems. *Am. J. Physiol. Heart Circ. Physiol.* **2003**, *284*, H1985–H1994. [CrossRef]
84. Sampaio, W.O.; Henrique de Castro, C.; Santos, R.A.S.; Schiffrin, E.L.; Touyz, R.M. Angiotensin-(1-7) counterregulates angiotensin II signaling in human endothelial cells. *Hypertension* **2007**, *50*, 1093–1098. [CrossRef] [PubMed]
85. Verano-Braga, T.; Schwämmle, V.; Sylvester, M.; Passos-Silva, D.G.; Peluso, A.A.B.; Etelvino, G.M.; Santos, R.A.S.; Roepstorff, P. Time-resolved quantitative phosphoproteomics: New insights into Angiotensin-(1-7) signaling networks in human endothelial cells. *J. Proteome Res.* **2012**, *11*, 3370–3381. [CrossRef]
86. Pernomian, L.; Gomes, M.S.; Restini, C.B.; de Oliveira, A.M. MAS-mediated antioxidant effects restore the functionality of angiotensin converting enzyme 2-angiotensin-(1-7)-MAS axis in diabetic rat carotid. *BioMed Res. Int.* **2014**, *2014*, 640329. [CrossRef]
87. Zhang, F.; Ren, J.; Chan, K.; Chen, H. Angiotensin-(1-7) regulates Angiotensin II-induced VCAM-1 expression on vascular endothelial cells. *Biochem. Biophys. Res. Commun.* **2013**, *430*, 642–646. [CrossRef]
88. Rentzsch, B.; Todiras, M.; Iliescu, R.; Popova, E.; Campos, L.A.; Oliveira, M.L.; Baltatu, O.C.; Santos, R.A.; Bader, M. Transgenic angiotensin-converting enzyme 2 overexpression in vessels of SHRSP rats reduces blood pressure and improves endothelial function. *Hypertension* **2008**, *52*, 967–973. [CrossRef]
89. Alenina, N.; Xu, P.; Rentzsch, B.; Patkin, E.L.; Bader, M. Genetically altered animal models for Mas and angiotensin-(1-7). *Exp. Physiol.* **2008**, *93*, 528–537. [CrossRef]
90. Regenhardt, R.W.; Mecca, A.P.; Desland, F.; Ritucci-Chinni, P.F.; Ludin, J.A.; Greenstein, D.; Banuelos, C.; Bizon, J.L.; Reinhard, M.K.; Sumners, C. Centrally administered angiotensin-(1-7) increases the survival of stroke-prone spontaneously hypertensive rats. *Exp. Physiol.* **2014**, *99*, 442–453. [CrossRef]
91. Helms, J.; Kremer, S.; Merdji, H.; Clere-Jehl, R.; Schenck, M.; Kummerlen, C.; Collange, O.; Boulay, C.; Fafi-Kremer, S.; Ohana, M.; et al. Neurologic Features in Severe SARS-CoV-2 Infection. *N. Engl. J. Med.* **2020**, *382*, 2268–2270. [CrossRef] [PubMed]
92. Yang, A.C.; Kern, F.; Losada, P.M.; Agam, M.R.; Maat, C.A.; Schmartz, G.P.; Fehlmann, T.; Stein, J.A.; Schaum, N.; Lee, D.P.; et al. Dysregulation of brain and choroid plexus cell types in severe COVID-19. *Nature* **2021**, *595*, 565–571. [CrossRef] [PubMed]
93. Chertow, D.; Stein, S.; Ramelli, S.; Grazioli, A.; Chung, J.Y.; Singh, M.; Yinda, C.K.; Winkler, C.; Dickey, J.; Ylaya, K.; et al. SARS-CoV-2 infection and persistence throughout the human body and brain. *Res. Sq.* 2021, *preprint under review*. [CrossRef]
94. Paterson, R.W.; Brown, R.L.; Benjamin, L.; Nortley, R.; Wiethoff, S.; Bharucha, T.; Jayaseelan, D.L.; Kumar, G.; Raftopoulos, R.E.; Zambreanu, L.; et al. The emerging spectrum of COVID-19 neurology: Clinical, radiological and laboratory findings. *Brain* **2020**, *143*, 3104–3120. [CrossRef] [PubMed]
95. Lechien, J.R.; Chiesa-Estomba, C.M.; De Siati, D.R.; Horoi, M.; Le Bon, S.D.; Rodriguez, A.; Dequanter, D.; Blecic, S.; El Afia, F.; Distinguin, L.; et al. Olfactory and gustatory dysfunctions as a clinical presentation of mild-to-moderate forms of the coronavirus disease (COVID-19): A multicenter European study. *Eur. Arch. Otorhinolaryngol.* **2020**, *277*, 2251–2261. [CrossRef] [PubMed]
96. Postma, E.M.; Smeets, P.A.M.; Boek, W.M.; Boesveldt, S. Investigating morphological changes in the brain in relation to etiology and duration of olfactory dysfunction with voxel-based morphometry. *Sci. Rep.* **2021**, *11*, 12704 . [CrossRef]
97. Carmichael, S.T.; Clugnet, M.C.; Price, J.L. Central olfactory connections in the macaque monkey. *J. Comp. Neurol.* **1994**, *346*, 403–434. [CrossRef]
98. Douaud, G.; Lee, S.; Alfaro-Almagro, F.; Arthofer, C.; Wang, C.; McCarthy, P.; Lange, F.; Andersson, J.; Griffanti, L.; Duff, E.; et al. SARS-CoV-2 is associated with changes in brain structure in UK Biobank. *Nature* **2022**, *604*, 697–707. [CrossRef]
99. Metzger, R.; Bader, M.; Ludwig, T.; Berberich, C.; Bunnemann, B.; Ganten, D. Expression of the mouse and rat mas proto-oncogene in the brain and peripheral tissues. *FEBS lett.* **1995**, *357*, 27–32. [CrossRef]
100. Hellner, K.; Walther, T.; Schubert, M.; Albrecht, D. Angiotensin-(1-7) enhances LTP in the hippocampus through the G-protein-coupled receptor Mas. *Mol. Cell Neurosci.* **2005**, *2*, 427–435. [CrossRef]
101. Valenzano, A.; Scarinci, A.; Monda, V.; Sessa, F.; Messina, A.; Monda, M.; Precenzano, F.; Mollica, M.P.; Carotenuto, M.; Messina, G.; et al. The Social Brain and Emotional Contagion: COVID-19 Effects. *Medicina* **2020**, *56*, 640. [CrossRef] [PubMed]

102. Hellmuth, J.; Barnett, T.A.; Asken, B.M.; Kelly, J.D.; Torres, L.; Stephens, M.L.; Greenhouse, B.; Martin, J.N.; Chow, F.C.; Deeks, E.; et al. Persistent COVID-19-associated neurocognitive symptoms in non-hospitalized patients. *J. Neurovirol.* **2021**, *27*, 191–195. [CrossRef] [PubMed]
103. Chaar, L.J.; Alves, T.P.; Batista Junior, A.M.; Michelini, L.C. Early Training-Induced Reduction of Angiotensinogen in Autonomic Areas-The Main Effect of Exercise on Brain Renin-Angiotensin System in Hypertensive Rats. *PLoS ONE* **2015**, *10*, e0137395. [CrossRef] [PubMed]
104. Kar, S.; Gao, L.; Zucker, I.H. Exercise training normalizes ACE and ACE2 in the brain of rabbits with pacing-induced heart failure. *J. Appl. Physiol.* **2010**, *108*, 923–932. [CrossRef] [PubMed]
105. Renaud-Charest, O.; Lui, L.M.W.; Eskander, S.; Ceban, F.; Ho, R.; Di Vincenzo, J.D.; Rosenblat, J.D.; Lee, Y.; Subramaniapillai, M.; McIntyre, R.S. Onset and frequency of depression in post-COVID-19 syndrome: A systematic review. *Psychiatr. Res.* **2021**, *144*, 129–137. [CrossRef] [PubMed]
106. da Silva Lopes, L.; Silva, R.O.; de Sousa Lima, G.; de Araújo Costa, A.C.; Barros, D.F.; Silva-Néto, R.P. Is there a common pathophysiological mechanism between COVID-19 and depression? *Acta Neurol. Belg.* **2021**, *121*, 1117–1122. [CrossRef]
107. Mazza, M.G.; De Lorenzo, R.; Conte, C.; Poletti, S.; Vai, B.; Bollettini, I.; Melloni, E.; Furlan, R.; Ciceri, F.; Rovere-Querini, P. Anxiety and depression in COVID-19 survivors: Role of inflammatory and clinical predictors. *Brain Behav. Immun.* **2020**, *89*, 594–600. [CrossRef]
108. Li, B.; Yang, J.; Zhao, F.; Zhi, L.; Wang, X.; Liu, L.; Bi, Z.; Zhao, Y. Prevalence and impact of cardiovascular metabolic diseases on COVID-19 in China. *Clin. Res. Cardiol.* **2020**, *109*, 531–538. [CrossRef]
109. Guo, T.; Fan, Y.; Chen, M.; Wu, X.; Zhang, L.; He, T.; Wang, H.; Wan, J.; Wang, X.; Lu, Z. Cardiovascular Implications of Fatal Outcomes of Patients with Coronavirus Disease 2019 (COVID-19). *JAMA Cardiol.* **2020**, *5*, 811–818. [CrossRef]
110. Chen, C.; Zhou, Y.; Wang, D.W. SARS-CoV-2: A potential novel etiology of fulminant myocarditis. *Herz* **2020**, *45*, 230–232. [CrossRef]
111. Immazio, M.; Klingel, K.; Kindermann, I.; Brucato, A.; De Rosa, F.G.; Adler, Y.; De Ferrari, G.M. COVID-19 pandemic and troponin: Indirect myocardial injury, myocardial inflammation or myocarditis? *Heart* **2020**, *106*, 1127–1131. [CrossRef]
112. Lippi, G.; Lavie, C.J.; Sanchis-Gomar, F. Cardiac troponin I in patients with coronavirus disease 2019 (COVID-19): Evidence from a meta-analysis. *Prog. Cardiovasc. Dis.* **2020**, *63*, 390–391. [CrossRef] [PubMed]
113. Abbasi, B.A.; Torres, P.; Ramos-Tuarez, F.; Dewaswala, N.; Abdallah, A.; Chen, K.; Qader, M.A.; Job, R.; Aboulenain, S.; Dziadkwiec, K.; et al. Cardiac Troponin-I and COVID-19: A Prognostic Tool for In-Hospital Mortality. *Cardiol. Res.* **2020**, *11*, 398–404. [CrossRef] [PubMed]
114. Wang, D.; Hu, B.; Hu, C.; Zhu, F.; Liu, X.; Zhang, J.; Wang, B.; Xiang, H.; Cheng, Z.; Xiong, Y.; et al. Clinical Characteristics of 138 Hospitalized Patients With 2019 Novel Coronavirus-Infected Pneumonia in Wuhan, China. *JAMA* **2020**, *323*, 1061–1069. [CrossRef] [PubMed]
115. Kochi, A.N.; Tagliari, A.P.; Forleo, G.B.; Fassini, G.M.; Tondo, C. Cardiac and arrhythmic complications in patients with COVID-19. *J. Cardiovasc. Electrophysiol.* **2020**, *31*, 1003–1008. [CrossRef]
116. Fu, E.L.; Janse, R.J.; de Jong, Y.; van der Endt, V.H.W.; Milders, J.; van der Willik, E.M.; de Rooij, E.N.M.; Dekkers, O.M.; Rotmans, J.I.; van Diepen, M. Acute kidney injury and kidney replacement therapy in COVID-19: A systematic review and meta-analysis. *Clin. Kidney J.* **2020**, *13*, 550–563. [CrossRef]
117. Golmai, P.; Larsen, C.P.; DeVita, M.V.; Wahl, S.J.; Weins, A.; Rennke, H.G.; Bijol, V.; Rosenstock, J.L. Histopathologic and Ultrastructural Findings in Postmortem Kidney Biopsy Material in 12 Patients with AKI and COVID-19. *J. Am. Soc. Nephrol.* **2020**, *31*, 1944–1947. [CrossRef]
118. Akilesh, S.; Nast, C.C.; Yamashita, M.; Henriksen, K.; Charu, V.; Troxell, M.L.; Kambham, N.; Bracamonte, E.; Houghton, D.; Ahmed, N.I.; et al. Multicenter Clinicopathologic Correlation of Kidney Biopsies Performed in COVID-19 Patients Presenting with Acute Kidney Injury or Proteinuria. *Am. J. Kidney Dis.* **2021**, *77*, 82–93. [CrossRef]
119. Sharma, P.; Uppal, N.N.; Wanchoo, R.; Shah, H.H.; Yang, Y.; Parikh, R.; Khanin, Y.; Madireddy, V.; Larsen, C.P.; Jhaveri, K.D.; et al. COVID-19-Associated Kidney Injury: A Case Series of Kidney Biopsy Findings. *J. Am. Soc. Nephrol.* **2020**, *31*, 1948–1958. [CrossRef]
120. Varga, Z.; Flammer, A.J.; Steiger, P.; Haberecker, M.; Andermatt, R.; Zinkernagel, A.S.; Mehra, M.R.; Schuepbach, R.A.; Ruschitzka, F.; Moch, H. Endothelial cell infection and endotheliitis in COVID-19. *Lancet* **2020**, *395*, 1417–1418. [CrossRef]
121. Rapkiewicz, A.V.; Mai, X.; Carsons, S.E.; Pittaluga, S.; Kleiner, D.E.; Berger, J.S. Megakaryocytes and platelet-fibrin thrombi characterize multi-organ thrombosis at autopsy in COVID-19: A case series. *EClinicalMedicine* **2020**, *24*. [CrossRef]
122. Zhang, S.; Liu, Y.; Wang, X.; Yang, L.; Li, H.; Wang, Y.; Liu, M.; Zhao, X.; Xie, Y.; Yang, Y.; et al. SARS-CoV-2 binds platelet ACE2 to enhance thrombosis in COVID-19. *J. Hematol. Oncol.* **2020**, *13*, 120. [CrossRef] [PubMed]
123. Cantaluppi, V.; Quercia, A.D.; Dellepiane, S.; Ferrario, S.; Camussi, G.; Biancone, L. Interaction between systemic inflammation and renal tubular epithelial cells. *Nephrol. Dial. Transplant.* **2014**, *29*, 2004–2011. [CrossRef] [PubMed]
124. Gurkan, S.; Cabinian, A.; Lopez, V.; Bhaumik, M.; Chang, J.M.; Rabson, A.B.; Mundel, P. Inhibition of type I interferon signalling prevents TLR ligand-mediated proteinuria. *J. Pathol.* **2013**, *231*, 248–256. [CrossRef] [PubMed]
125. Cugno, M.; Meroni, P.L.; Gualtierotti, R.; Griffini, S.; Grovetti, E.; Torri, A.; Panigada, M.; Aliberti, S.; Blasi, F.; Tedesco, F. Complement activation in patients with COVID-19: A novel therapeutic. *J. Allergy Clin. Immunol.* **2020**, *146*, 215–217. [CrossRef]

126. Giamarellos-Bourboulis, E.J.; Netea, M.G.; Rovina, N.; Akinosoglou, K.; Antoniadou, A.; Antonakos, N.; Damoraki, G.; Gkavogianni, T.; Adami, M.E.; Katsaounou, P.; et al. Complex Immune Dysregulation in COVID-19 Patients with Severe Respiratory Failure. *Cell Host Microbe* **2020**, *27*, 992–1000. [CrossRef]
127. Richardson, K.L.; Jain, A.; Evans, J.; Uzun, O. Giant coronary artery aneurysm as a feature of coronavirus-related inflammatory syndrome. *BMJ Case Rep.* **2021**, *14*, e238740. [CrossRef]
128. Navaeifar, M.R.; Shahbaznejad, L.; Sadeghi Lotfabadi, A.; Rezai, M.S. COVID-19-Associated Multisystem Inflammatory Syndrome Complicated with Giant Coronary Artery Aneurysm. *Case Rep. Pediatr.* **2021**, *2021*, 8836403. [CrossRef]
129. Pick, J.M.; Wang, S.; Wagner-Lees, S.; Badran, S.; Szmuszkovicz, R.J.; Wong, P.; Votava-Smith, J. Abstract 17092: Coronary Artery Aneurysms Are More Common in Post-COVID-19 Multisystem Inflammatory Syndrome in Children (MIS-C) Than Pre-Pandemic Kawasaki Disease. *Circulation* **2020**, *142*, 17092. [CrossRef]
130. Zhang, C.; Shen, L.; Le, K.J.; Pan, M.M.; Kong, L.C.; Gu, Z.C.; Xu, H.; Zhang, Z.; Ge, W.H.; Lin, H.W. Incidence of Venous Thromboembolism in Hospitalized Coronavirus Disease 2019 Patients: A Systematic Review and Meta-Analysis. *Front. Cardiovasc. Med.* **2020**, *7*, 151. [CrossRef]
131. Birkeland, K.; Zimmer, R.; Kimchi, A.; Kedan, I. Venous Thromboembolism in Hospitalized COVID-19 Patients: Systematic Review. *Interact. J. Med. Res.* **2020**, *9*, e22768. [CrossRef]
132. Bangalore, S.; Sharma, A.; Slotwiner, A.; Yatskar, L.; Harari, R.; Shah, B.; Ibrahim, H.; Friedman, G.H.; Thompson, C.; Alviar, C.L. ST-Segment Elevation in Patients with COVID-19—A Case Series. *N. Engl. J. Med.* **2020**, *382*, 2478–2480. [CrossRef] [PubMed]
133. Nagashima, S.; Mendes, M.C.; Camargo Martins, A.P.; Borges, N.H.; Godoy, T.M.; Miggiolaro, A.; da Silva Dezidério, F.; Machado-Souza, C.; de Noronha, L. Endothelial Dysfunction and Thrombosis in Patients With COVID-19-Brief Report. *Arterioscler. Thromb. Vasc. Biol.* **2020**, *40*, 2404–2407. [CrossRef] [PubMed]
134. Götzinger, F.; Santiago-García, B.; Noguera-Julián, A.; Lanaspa, M.; Lancella, L.; Calò Carducci, F.I.; Gabrovska, N.; Velizarova, S.; Prunk, P.; Osterman, V.; et al. COVID-19 in children and adolescents in Europe: A multinational, multicentre cohort study. *Lancet Child Adolesc. Health* **2020**, *4*, 653–661. [CrossRef]
135. King, J.A.; Whitten, T.A.; Bakal, J.A.; McAlister, F.A. Symptoms associated with a positive result for a swab for SARS-CoV-2 infection among children in Alberta. *CMAJ* **2021**, *193*, E1–E9. [CrossRef]
136. Lu, X.; Zhang, L.; Du, H.; Zhang, J.; Li, Y.Y.; Qu, J.; Zhang, W.; Wang, Y.; Bao, S.; Li, Y.; et al. Chinese Pediatric Novel Coronavirus Study Team (2020). SARS-CoV-2 Infection in Children. *N. Engl. J. Med.* **2020**, *382*, 1663–1665. [CrossRef] [PubMed]
137. Midulla, F.; Cristiani, L.; Mancino, E. Will children reveal their secret? The coronavirus dilemma. *Eur. Respir. J.* **2020**, *55*. [CrossRef]
138. Nikolopoulou, G.B.; Maltezou, H.C. COVID-19 in Children: Where do we Stand? *Arch. Med. Res.* **2022**, *53*, 1–8. [CrossRef]
139. Castagnoli, R.; Votto, M.; Licari, A.; Brambilla, I.; Bruno, R.; Perlini, S.; Rovida, F.; Baldanti, F.; Marseglia, G.L. Severe Acute Respiratory Syndrome Coronavirus 2 (SARS-CoV-2) Infection in Children and Adolescents: A Systematic Review. *JAMA Pediatr.* **2020**, *174*, 882–889. [CrossRef]
140. Siebach, M.K.; Piedimonte, G.; Ley, S.H. COVID-19 in childhood: Transmission, clinical presentation, complications and risk factors. *Pediatr. Pulmonol.* **2021**, *56*, 1342–1356. [CrossRef]
141. Bastolla, U.; Chambers, P.; Abia, D.; Garcia-Bermejo, M.L.; Fresno, M. Is COVID-19 Severity Associated with ACE2 Degradation? *Front. Drug. Discov.* **2022**, *1*, 789710. [CrossRef]
142. Dong, Y.; Mo, X.; Hu, Y.; Qi, X.; Jiang, F.; Jiang, Z.; Tong, S. Epidemiology of COVID-19 Among Children in China. *Pediatrics* **2020**, *145*, e20200702. [CrossRef] [PubMed]
143. Tian, S.; Hu, N.; Lou, J.; Chen, K.; Kang, X.; Xiang, Z.; Chen, H.; Wang, D.; Liu, N.; Liu, D.; et al. Characteristics of COVID-19 infection in Beijing. *J. Infect.* **2020**, *80*, 401–406. [CrossRef] [PubMed]
144. Kuba, K.; Imai, Y.; Rao, S.; Gao, H.; Guo, F.; Guan, B.; Huan, Y.; Yang, P.; Zhang, Y.; Deng, W.; et al. A crucial role of angiotensin converting enzyme 2 (ACE2) in SARS coronavirus-induced lung injury. *Nat. Med.* **2005**, *11*, 875–879. [CrossRef] [PubMed]
145. Kolberg, E.S.; Wickstrøm, K.; Tonby, K.; Dyrhol-Riise, A.M.; Holten, A.R.; Amundsen, E.K. Serum ACE as a prognostic biomarker in COVID-19: A case series. *APMIS* **2021**, *129*, 237–238. [CrossRef]
146. Rieder, M.; Wirth, L.; Pollmeier, L.; Jeserich, M.; Goller, I.; Baldus, N.; Schmid, B.; Busch, H.J.; Hofmann, M.; Kern, W.; et al. Serum ACE2, Angiotensin II, and Aldosterone Levels Are Unchanged in Patients With COVID-19. *Am. J. Hypertens* **2021**, *34*, 278–281. [CrossRef]
147. Gao, Y.D.; Ding, M.; Dong, X.; Zhang, J.J.; Kursat Azkur, A.; Azkur, D.; Gan, H.; Sun, Y.L.; Fu, W.; Li, W.; et al. Risk factors for severe and critically ill COVID-19 patients: A review. *Allergy* **2021**, *76*, 428–455. [CrossRef]
148. Kuo, C.L.; Pilling, L.C.; Atkins, J.C.; Masoli, J.; Delgado, J.; Tignanelli, C.; Kuchel, G.; Melzer, D.; Beckman, K.B.; Levine, M. COVID-19 severity is predicted by earlier evidence of accelerated aging. *medRxiv* **2020**. [CrossRef]
149. Ran, J.; Song, Y.; Zhuang, Z.; Han, L.; Zhao, S.; Cao, P.; Geng, Y.; Xu, L.; Qin, J.; He, D.; et al. Blood pressure control and adverse outcomes of COVID-19 infection in patients with concomitant hypertension in Wuhan, China. *Hypertens Res.* **2020**, *43*, 1267–1276. [CrossRef]
150. AlGhatrif, M.; Tanaka, T.; Moore, A.Z.; Bandinelli, S.; Lakatta, E.G.; Ferrucci, L. Age-associated difference in circulating ACE2, the gateway for SARS-COV-2, in humans: Results from the InCHIANTI study. *GeroScience* **2021**, *43*, 619–627. [CrossRef]
151. Ferrucci, L.; Corsi, A.; Lauretani, F.; Bandinelli, S.; Bartali, B.; Taub, D.D.; Guralnik, J.M.; Longo, D.L. The origins of age-related proinflammatory state. *Blood* **2015**, *105*, 2294–2299. [CrossRef]

152. Akhtar, S.; Benter, I.F.; Danjuma, M.I.; Doi, S.; Hasan, S.S.; Habib, A.M. Pharmacotherapy in COVID-19 patients: A review of ACE2-raising drugs and their clinical safety. *J. Drug. Target.* **2020**, *28*, 683–699. [CrossRef] [PubMed]
153. Emilsson, V.; Gudmundsson, E.F.; Aspelund, T.; Jonsson, B.G.; Gudjonsson, A.; Launer, L.J.; Jennings, L.L.; Gudmundsdottir, V.; Gudnason, V. Antihypertensive medication uses and serum ACE2 levels: ACEIs/ARBs treatment does not raise serum levels of ACE2. *medRxiv* **2020**, *not certified by peer review*. [CrossRef]
154. Gao, C.; Cai, Y.; Zhang, K.; Zhou, L.; Zhang, Y.; Zhang, X.; Li, Q.; Li, W.; Yang, S.; Zhao, X.; et al. Association of hypertension and antihypertensive treatment with COVID-19 mortality: A retrospective observational study. *Eur. Heart J.* **2020**, *41*, 2058–2066. [CrossRef] [PubMed]
155. Fosbøl, E.L.; Butt, J.H.; Østergaard, L.; Andersson, C.; Selmer, C.; Kragholm, K.; Schou, M.; Phelps, M.; Gislason, G.H.; Gerds, T.A.; et al. Association of Angiotensin-Converting Enzyme Inhibitor or Angiotensin Receptor Blocker Use With COVID-19 Diagnosis and Mortality. *JAMA* **2020**, *324*, 168–177. [CrossRef]
156. Summers, K.L.; Marleau, A.M.; Mahon, J.L.; McManus, R.; Hramiak, I.; Singh, B. Reduced IFN-alpha secretion by blood dendritic cells in human diabetes. *Clin. Immunol.* **2020**, *121*, 81–89. [CrossRef]
157. Hu, R.; Xia, C.Q.; Butfiloski, E.; Clare-Salzle, M. Effect of high glucose on cytokine production by human peripheral blood immune cells and type I interferon signaling in monocytes: Implications for the role of hyperglycemia in the diabetes inflammatory process and host defense against infection. *Clin. Immunol.* **2018**, *195*, 139–148. [CrossRef] [PubMed]
158. Roca-Ho, H.; Riera, M.; Palau, V.; Pascual, J.; Soler, M.J. Characterization of ACE and ACE2 Expression within Different Organs of the NOD Mouse. *Int. J. Mol. Sci.* **2017**, *18*, 563. [CrossRef]
159. Qeadan, F.; Mensah, N.A.; Tingey, B.; Stanford, J.B. The risk of clinical complications and death among pregnant women with COVID-19 in the Cerner COVID-19 cohort: A retrospective analysis. *BMC Pregnancy Childbirth* **2021**, *21*, 305. [CrossRef]
160. Harb, J.; Debs, N.; Rima, M.; Wu, Y.; Cao, Z.; Kovacic, H.; Fajloun, Z.; Sabatier, J.M. SARS-CoV-2, COVID-19, and Reproduction: Effects on Fertility, Pregnancy, and Neonatal Life. *Biomedicines* **2022**, *10*, 1775. [CrossRef]
161. Gupta, P.; Kumar, S.; Sharma, S.S. SARS-CoV-2 prevalence and maternal-perinatal outcomes among pregnant women admitted for delivery: Experience from COVID-19-dedicated maternity hospital in Jammu, Jammu and Kashmir (India). *J. Med. Virol.* **2021**, *93*, 5505–5514. [CrossRef]
162. Mirbeyk, M.; Saghazadeh, A.; Rezaei, N. A systematic review of pregnant women with COVID-19 and their neonates. *Arch. Gynecol. Obstet.* **2021**, *304*, 5–38. [CrossRef]
163. Thornton, P.; Douglas, J. Coagulation in pregnancy. *Best Pract. Res. Clin. Obstet. Gynaecol.* **2010**, *24*, 339–352. [CrossRef] [PubMed]
164. Mehandru, S.; Merad, M. Pathological sequelae of long-haul COVID. *Nat. Immunol.* **2022**, *23*, 194–202. [CrossRef]
165. Khazaal, S.; Harb, J.; Rima, M.; Annweiler, C.; Wu, Y.; Cao, Z.; Khattar, Z.A.; Legros, C.; Kovacic, H.; Fajloun, Z.; et al. The Pathophysiology of Long COVID throughout the Renin-Angiotensin System. *Molecules* **2022**, *27*, 2903. [CrossRef] [PubMed]
166. Huang, C.; Huang, L.; Wang, Y.; Li, X.; Ren, L.; Gu, X.; Kang, L.; Guo, L.; Liu, M.; Zhou, X.; et al. 6-month consequences of COVID-19 in patients discharged from hospital: A cohort study. *Lancet* **2021**, *397*, 220–232. [CrossRef]
167. Ledford, H. Can drugs reduce the risk of long COVID? What scientists know so far. *Nature* **2022**, *604*, 21–22. [CrossRef] [PubMed]
168. Kaseda, E.T.; Levine, A.J. Post-traumatic stress disorder: A differential diagnostic consideration for COVID-19 survivors. *Clin. Neuropsychol.* **2020**, *34*, 1498–1514. [CrossRef] [PubMed]
169. Asadi-Pooya, A.A.; Akbari, A.; Emami, A.; Lotfi, M.; Rostamihoseinkhani, M.; Nemati, H.; Barzegar, Z.; Kabiri, M.; Zeraatpisheh, Z.; Farjoud-Kouhanjani, M.; et al. Long COVID syndrome-associated brain fog. *J. Med. Virol.* **2022**, *94*, 979–984. [CrossRef]
170. Mikkelsen, M.E.; Christie, J.D.; Lanken, P.N.; Biester, R.C.; Thompson, B.T.; Bellamy, S.L.; Localio, A.R.; Demissie, E.; Hopkins, R.O.; Angus, D.C. The Adult Respiratory Distress Syndrome Cognitive Outcomes Study Long-Term Neuropsychological Function in Survivors of Acute Lung Injury. *Am. J. Respir. Crit. Care Med.* **2012**, *185*, 1307–1315. [CrossRef]
171. Desai, A.D.; Lavelle, M.; Buorsiquot, B.C.; Wan, E.Y. Long-term complications of COVID-19. *Am. J. Physiol. Cell. Physiol.* **2022**, *322*, 1–11. [CrossRef]
172. Hellgren, L.; Thornberg, U.B.; Samuelsson, K.; Levi, R.; Divanoglou, A.; Blystad, I. Brain MRI and neuropsychological findings at long-term follow-up after COVID-19 hospitalisation: An observational cohort study. *BMJ Open* **2021**, *11*, e055164. [CrossRef]
173. Samuelson, K.W.; Bartel, A.; Valadez, R.; Jordan, J.T. PTSD symptoms and perception of cognitive problems: The roles of posttraumatic cognitions and trauma coping self-efficacy. *Psychol. Trauma* **2017**, *9*, 537–544. [CrossRef] [PubMed]
174. Richter, D.; Guasti, L.; Koehler, F.; Squizzato, A.; Nistri, S.; Christodorescu, R.; Dievart, F.; Gaudio, G.; Asteggiano, R.; Ferrini, M. Late phase of COVID-19 pandemic in General Cardiology. A position paper of the ESC Council for Cardiology Practice. *ESC Heart Fail.* **2021**, *8*, 3483–3494. [CrossRef] [PubMed]
175. Goitein, O.; Matetzky, S.; Beinart, R.; Di Segni, E.; Hod, H.; Bentancur, A.; Konen, E. Acute myocarditis: Noninvasive evaluation with cardiac MRI and transthoracic echocardiography. *AJR Am. J. Roentgenol.* **2009**, *192*, 254–258. [CrossRef]
176. Han, Y.; Chen, T.; Bryant, J.; Bucciarelli-Ducci, C.; Dyke, C.; Eliott, M.D.; Ferrari, V.A.; Friedrich, M.G.; Lawton, C.; Manning, W.J.; et al. Society for Cardiovascular Magnetic Resonance (SCMR) guidance for the practice of cardiovascular magnetic resonance during the COVID-19 pandemic. *J. Cardiovasc. Magn. Reson.* **2020**, *22*, 26. [CrossRef] [PubMed]
177. Mele, D.; Flamigni, F.; Rapezzi, C.; Ferrari, R. Myocarditis in COVID-19 patients: Current problems. *Intern. Emerg. Med.* **2021**, *16*, 1123–1139. [CrossRef] [PubMed]

178. Siripanthong, B.; Nazarian, S.; Muser, D.; Deo, R.; Santangeli, R.; Khanji, M.Y.; Cooper, L.T.; Chahal, C.A.A. Recognizing COVID-19-related myocarditis: The possible pathophysiology and proposed guideline for diagnosis and management. *Heart Rhythm.* **2020**, *17*, 1463–1471. [CrossRef]
179. Santoro, F.; Monitillo, F.; Raimondo, P.; Lopizzo, A.; Brindicci, G.; Gilio, M.; Musaico, F.; Mazzola, M.; Vestito, D.; Di Benedetto, R.; et al. QTc Interval Prolongation and Life-Threatening Arrhythmias During Hospitalization in Patients with Coronavirus Disease 2019 (COVID-19): Results from a Multicenter Prospective Registry. *Clin. Infect. Dis.* **2021**, *73*, 4031–4038. [CrossRef]
180. Giustino, G.; Pinney, S.P.; Lala, A.; Reddy, V.Y.; Johnston-Cox, H.A.; Mechanick, J.I.; Halperin, J.L.; Fuster, V. Coronavirus and Cardiovascular Disease, Myocardial Injury, and Arrhythmia: JACC Focus Seminar. *J. Am. Coll. Cardiol.* **2020**, *76*, 2011–2023. [CrossRef]
181. Dherange, P.; Lang, J.; Qian, P.; Oberfeld, B.; Sauer, W.H.; Koplan, B.; Tedrow, U. Arrhythmias and COVID-19: A Review. *JACC Clin. Electrophysiol.* **2020**, *6*, 1193–1204. [CrossRef]
182. Rudski, L.; Januzzi, J.L.; Rigolin, V.H.; Bohula, E.A.; Blankstein, R.; Patel, A.R.; Bucciarelli-Ducci, C.; Vorovich, E.; Mukheriee, M.; Rao, S.V.; et al. Multimodality Imaging in Evaluation of Cardiovascular Complications in Patients With COVID-19. *J. Am. Coll. Cardiol.* **2020**, *76*, 1345–1357. [CrossRef]
183. Zoghbi, W.A.; DiCarli, M.F.; Blankstein, R.; Choi, A.D.; Dilsizian, V.; Flaschkampf, F.A.; Geske, J.B.; Grayburn, P.A.; Jaffer, F.A.; Kwong, R.Y.; et al. Multimodality Cardiovascular Imaging in the Midst of the COVID-19 Pandemic. *JACC Cardiovasc. Imaging* **2020**, *13*, 1615–1626. [CrossRef] [PubMed]
184. Bozkurt, B.; Kovacs, R.; Harrington, B. Joint HFSA/ACC/AHA Statement Addresses Concerns Re: Using RAAS Antagonists in COVID-19. *J. Card. Fail.* **2020**, *26*, 370. [CrossRef] [PubMed]
185. D'Alto, M.; Romeo, E.; Argiento, P.; Pavelescu, A.; Melot, C.; D'Andrea, A.; Correra, A.; Bossone, E.; Calabro, R.; Russo, M.G.; et al. Echocardiographic prediction of pre- versus postcapillary pulmonary hypertension. *J. Am. Soc. Echocardiogr.* **2015**, *28*, 108–115. [CrossRef] [PubMed]
186. Sadeghipour, P.; Talasz, A.H.; Rashidi, F.; Sharif-Kashani, B.; Beigmohammadi, M.T.; Farrokhpour, M.; Sezavar, S.H.; Payandemehr, P.; Dabbagh, A.; Moghadam, K.G.; et al. Effect of Intermediate-Dose vs Standard-Dose Prophylactic Anticoagulation on Thrombotic Events, Extracorporeal Membrane Oxygenation Treatment, or Mortality Among Patients With COVID-19 Admitted to the Intensive Care Unit: The INSPIRATION Randomized Clinical Trial. *JAMA* **2021**, *325*, 1620–1630. [CrossRef] [PubMed]
187. Leentjens, J.; van Haaps, T.F.; Wessels, P.F.; Schutgens, R.E.G.; Middeldrop, S. COVID-19-associated coagulopathy and antithrombotic agents-lessons after 1 year. *Lancet Haematol.* **2021**, *8*, 524–533. [CrossRef]
188. Chawla, L.S.; Eggers, P.W.; Star, R.A.; Kimmel, P.L. Acute Kidney Injury and Chronic Kidney Disease as Interconnected Syndromes. *N. Engl. J. Med.* **2014**, *371*, 58–66. [CrossRef]
189. Yende, S.; Parikh, C.R. Long COVID and kidney disease. *Nat. Rev. Nephrol.* **2021**, *17*, 792–793. [CrossRef]
190. He, L.; Wei, Q.; Liu, J.; Yi, M.; Liu, Y.; Liu, H.; Sun, L.; Peng, Y.; Liu, F.; Venkatachalam, M.A.; et al. AKI on CKD: Heightened injury, suppressed repair, and the underlying mechanisms. *Kidney Int.* **2017**, *92*, 1071–1083. [CrossRef]
191. Venkatachalam, M.A.; Griffin, K.A.; Lan, R.; Geng, H.; Saikumar, P.; Bidani, A.K. Acute kidney injury: A springboard for progression in chronic kidney disease. *Am. J. Physiol. Renal. Physiol.* **2010**, *298*, 1078–1094. [CrossRef]
192. Al-Aly, Z.; Xie, Y.; Bowe, B. High-dimensional characterization of post-acute sequelae of COVID-19. *Nature* **2021**, *594*, 259–264. [CrossRef]
193. Maldonado, D.; Ray, J.; Lin, X.B.; Salem, F.; Brown, M.; Bansal, I. COVAN Leading to ESKD Despite Minimal COVID Symptoms. *J. Investig. Med. High Impact. Case Rep.* **2022**, *10*, 1–5. [CrossRef] [PubMed]
194. Delanaye, P.; Huart, J.; Boquegneau, A.; Jouret, F. Long-term effects of COVID-19 on kidney function. *Lancet* **2021**, *397*, 1807. [CrossRef]
195. Delanaye, P.; Jager, K.J.; Bokenkamp, A.; Christensson, A.; Douburg, L.; Eriksen, B.O.; Gaillard, F.; Gambaro, G.; van der Giet, M.; Glassock, R.J.; et al. CKD: A Call for an Age-Adapted Definition. *J. Am. Soc. Nephrol.* **2019**, *30*, 1785–1805. [CrossRef] [PubMed]
196. Bruchfeld, A. The COVID-19 pandemic: Consequences for nephrology. *Nat. Rev. Nephrol.* **2021**, *17*, 81–82. [CrossRef]

MDPI
St. Alban-Anlage 66
4052 Basel
Switzerland
www.mdpi.com

Pharmaceutics Editorial Office
E-mail: pharmaceutics@mdpi.com
www.mdpi.com/journal/pharmaceutics

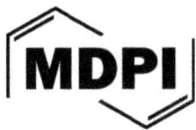

Disclaimer/Publisher's Note: The statements, opinions and data contained in all publications are solely those of the individual author(s) and contributor(s) and not of MDPI and/or the editor(s). MDPI and/or the editor(s) disclaim responsibility for any injury to people or property resulting from any ideas, methods, instructions or products referred to in the content.

www.ingramcontent.com/pod-product-compliance
Lightning Source LLC
LaVergne TN
LVHW070410100526
838202LV00014B/1430